THE COMPLETE NATURAL MEDICINE GUIDE TO THE

50 Most Common Medicinal Herbs

THE COMPLETE NATURAL MEDICINE GUIDE TO THE

50

Most Common Medicinal Herbs

HEATHER BOON, BScPhm, PhD
and
MICHAEL SMITH, BPharm, MRPharmS, ND

Robert
ROSE

We would like to thank the following people for their help in preparing
this second edition of the book: Bob Hilderley (senior editor) for his patience
and guidance through the revision process; Teresa Tsui (student, Canadian College
of Naturopathic Medicine); and Lobna Selim (student, Faculty of Pharmacy,
University of Toronto) without whose hard work and diligence the revision
of our book would never have been possible.

The Complete Natural Medicine Guide to the 50 Most Common Medicinal Herbs
Copyright © The Institute of Naturopathic Education and Research (The Canadian College of Naturopathic
Medicine), 2004.

Disclaimer
The nutritional, medical, and health information presented in this book is based on the research, training,
and professional experience of the authors, and is true and complete to the best of their knowledge.
However, this book is intended only as an informative guide for those wishing to know more about health,
nutrition, and medicine; it is not intended to replace or countermand the advice given by the reader's
personal physician. Because each person and situation is unique, the authors and the publisher urge the
reader to check with a qualified healthcare professional before using any product where there is any question
as to its appropriateness. The authors and the publisher are not responsible for any adverse effects or
consequences resulting from the use of the information in this book. It is the responsibility of the reader
to consult a physician or other qualified healthcare professional regarding his or her personal care.

Canadian Cataloguing in Publication Data
Boon, Heather
The complete natural medicine guide to the 50 most common medicinal herbs /
Heather Boon and Michael Smith. — 2nd ed.

Previously published under title: The botanical pharmacy.
Includes bibliographical references.
ISBN 0-7788-0082-2 (bound).— ISBN 0-7788-0081-4 (pbk.)

1. Herbals. 2. Naturopathy. 3. Herbs — Therapeutic use.
I. Smith, Michael J., 1963– II. Title.

RS164.B66 2003   615'.321   C2003-902879-8

Design and Production: PageWave Graphics Inc.
Editor: Bob Hilderley, Senior Editor, Health
Cover Photography: Mark T. Shapiro
Illustrations: Kveta / Three in a Box

The publisher acknowledges the financial support of the Government of Canada through the Book
Publishing Industry Development Program.

Published by Robert Rose Inc
120 Eglinton Ave. E., Suite 800, Toronto, Ontario Canada M4P 1E2 Tel: (416) 322-6552.

Printed and bound in Canada.
2 3 4 5 6 7 8 9 10 GP 09 08 07 06 05 04

To my parents, Shirley and Glenn Boon,
who encouraged me to pursue my academic dreams
and to my husband, Dr. Albert H.C. Wong,
who challenged me in lively debates regarding
the art and science of healing.
— *Heather Boon*

To my parents, Anne and Jack Smith, for their love,
support and frequent and much needed counsel.
— *Michael Smith*

Contents

Foreword

Everyone involved in the delivery of healthcare is now aware of the increased interest in complementary and alternative medicine (CAM), especially herbal or botanical medicine. According to several recent North American surveys, a growing number of people are using some form of complementary or alternative medicine, 15-25% of the population in Canada, for example,[1,2] which is comparable to a much-quoted *New England Journal of Medicine* report that 34% of American survey respondents had used at least one unconventional therapy in the past year.[3] Significantly, only one-third of these people reported seeing a complementary healthcare provider, indicating a high level of self-medication.

Botanical or herbal medicine is becoming big business for pharmacists. A "Trends Report" in *Pharmacy Post* indicated that three out of every four Canadian community pharmacies now sell herbal and/or homeopathic products and that approximately half of those surveyed intended to increase these sections.[4] Another report suggests that the average "medium sized" community pharmacy in Canada sells at least 35 plant-derived products (including natural source vitamins), marketed by at least 8 phyto-pharmaceutical manufacturers.[5] In addition, *Pharmacy Practice* reported that Canadians spent $175 million on herbal products in 1996, which is an increase from the $150 million spent in 1995.[6] Similar trends prevail in the United States. The popularity of herbal medicine continues to grow day-by-day.

Although some see botanical medicine as a new "niche" for pharmacy,[7] the debate about whether botanical medicine belongs in pharmacies or in health food stores is becoming heated among pharmacists and physicians.[8] The opponents of the sale of botanical products in pharmacies emphasize the fact that most pharmacists have little or no training in this field and perpetuate the notion that herbs have not been 'scientifically' tested for their medicinal action and safety in human studies.

Patients are looking for authoritative information about medicinal herbs — their effectiveness, their safety, and standard dosages — that they can rely on for 'self medication' and that they can can bring to the attention of their physician or pharmacist for their preventative or therapeutic effects. While questions about echinacea and ginseng could once be ignored as a passing trend, now healthcare professionals are expected to be knowledgeable about many common herbs. This book is written for the patient and the healthcare professional looking for current and authoritative scientific information so as to improve understanding of the medical properties of common herbs and to promote communication between patient and doctor.

Initially, this project was planned as a correspondence course with the objective of training pharmacists about botanical medicine. After much deliberation, it was decided that the best approach would be to prepare a series of monographs reviewing the herbal medicines most often seen by pharmacists in clinical practice. A very special team had to be created to make sure this project was a success. As the one of the primary sites of training in CAM in Canada, the Canadian College of Naturopathic Medicine (CCNM) agreed to manage the day-to-day running of the program. In order, to ensure that the information was correct and balanced, an advisory board of experts was established to review all the material. The majority of the monographs were also submitted to the Canadian Council on Continuing Education in Pharmacy (CCCEP) for its approval. The project was completed in the summer of 1998, which culminated in the publication of the reference book *The Botanical Pharmacy* in 1999, addressed specifically to pharmacists and botanical medicine professionals. In 2003, the information was up-dated to include research conducted in the interim, revised to increase the accessibility of the information for the common reader, and published as *The Complete Natural Medicine Guide to the 50 Most Common Medicinal Herbs*.

One of the cornerstones of pharmaceutical and medical care is helping patients and customers to make informed decisions about their healthcare. Likewise, patients owe it to themselves to learn as much as possible about any preventative or therapeutic treatment they may be considering. As patients' options expand to include botanical medicine or medicinal herbs as an acceptable form of healthcare, pharmacists and physicians are being asked to wade through large amounts of (mis)information to help patients make the most informed choices possible. When patients choose to make use of botanical products, it is important for pharmacists and physicians to provide monitoring and report adverse effects as well as herb-drug or herb-herb interactions when necessary. This potential new role requires a pharmacist or physician who has a good working knowledge of botanical medicine and can apply problem-solving skills to "fill in the gaps" of our current knowledge of these products.

The authors hope that this book will provide healthcare professionals with a foundation of knowledge from which they can counsel patients about the use of botanical products with confidence. For patients and consumers, while this book will not answer all your questions about medicinal herbs, we hope that it will be a useful resource for understanding the safe use of these herbs and for posing informed questions to your pharmacist or physician. Your good health is what we all want to ensure.

Introduction

Information Sources

In reading this book, not only is it important to realize what medicinal herbs are but also what they are not. Herbal medicine is a complex subject, both a science and an art. No book could cover all the subtle nuances of this fascinating therapy. We have intentionally concentrated on the published 'scientific' material, but attempted to incorporate empirical information wherever possible. While many conventional practitioners are not familiar with the traditional elements of herbalism, this empirical knowledge plays a pivotal role in the practice of botanical medicine.

In obtaining this information, we conducted an extensive search of MEDLINE and the Complementary Medicine Index (CMI). In addition, a manual search of the journals, periodicals and texts held in the Learning Resource Center at The Canadian College of Naturopathic Medicine was commissioned. Given that much of the information available on the subject is published in a language other than English (notably German), a selection of articles was translated for this project.

Legislation

We also consulted the laws governing the manufacture and the sale of herbal medicines in Canada and the United States of America. Here is a summary of those regulations designed to ensure safety in using medicinal herbs.

Canada

In Canada, all botanical medicines are regulated by the Federal Government. The regulations for Natural Health Products (NHPs) have recently undergone extensive modification, with new regulations taking force in January 2004.

Prior to this date, all herbs legally for sale in Canada were regulated as either foods or drugs (with drug identification numbers or DINs) as stipulated by the Food and Drugs Act. The manufacturer of any herb marketed as a food could not print any medicinal claims on the label of the product. In addition, food labeling regulations did not provide for the inclusion of cautions, adverse effects and other warnings.

As part of a series of provisional measures, some herbal products were classified as drugs in a special category called "Traditional Herbal Medicines." Traditional Herbal Medicines could only be intended for self-medication use; all the active ingredients had to be herbal; and the therapeutic indication had to be supported by herbal reference texts at the dose provided.[1] Manufacturers of Traditional Herbal Medicines were allowed to make approved medicinal claims on product labels; however, the products also had to indicate that they were for use by adults only (some exceptions exist); that they should not be used in pregnancy or lactation; and that the term "natural" could only be used to describe a product sold in its original state (i.e., without processing or refinement).[1]

Labeling standards existed for only a few herbs, including chamomile, echinacea root, ephedra, feverfew leaf, ginkgo, peppermint, St. John's wort and valerian. In addition, while all Traditional Herbal Medicines were required to adhere to Good Manufacturing Practices (GMPs), establishment licenses were not necessarily required.[2] No products for sale in Canada as non-prescription products (i.e., sold directly to the public without consultation with a health care providers) could suggest that they are treatments for conditions listed in Schedule A of the Food and Drugs Act, which includes such conditions as arthritis, asthma and cancer.

In response to public demand, the Federal Minister of Health created a new Federal Office of Natural Health Products (ONHP) in March 1999 as part of Health Canada. The mission of the new Office, now known as the Natural Health Products Directorate (NHPD), was to "ensure that all Canadians have ready access to natural health products [including herbs] that are safe, effective and of high quality, while respecting freedom of choice and philosophical and cultural diversity."[3] On December 22, 2001 the proposed new regulations governing the manufacture, packaging, labeling, storage, importation, distribution and sale of natural health products (including herbs) in Canada were published in *Canada Gazette* Part I,[4] as the first step in the implementation of new statutory regulations. The new regulations are part of the current Food and Drugs Act, but are specific to NHPs, effectively identifying them as a category distinct from foods and drugs. Requirements apply to all persons who sell NHPs, namely manufacturers, distributors, importers, packagers and labelers. A transition period of up to 6 years for certain elements of the regulations was proposed to allow those affected sufficient time to come in to compliance with the new regulations. In June 2003, the new NHP regulations were published Canada *Gazette Part* II[5] and made available on the NHPD website.

> http://www.hc-sc.gc.ca/hpfb-dgpsa/
> nhpd-dpsn/regs_cg2_cp_e.html

The definition of a natural health product has two components: a functional and a substance component. The functional component is related to the intended function of a substance and states that NHPs include those substances that are manufactured, sold or represented for use in:

(i) the diagnosis, treatment, mitigation or prevention of a disease, disorder, or abnormal physical state or its symptoms in humans;

(ii) restoring or correcting organic functions in humans; or

(iii) maintaining or promoting health or otherwise modifying organic functions in humans.[4]

The substance component of the NHP definition provides for an "Inclusion" list that outlines the medical ingredients that can be contained within NHPs, and an "Exclusion" list that specifically identifies those substances that are not considered NHPs.

Regarding herbal medicines, the 'Inclusion' list specifically identifies that the following will be classified as NHPs:

(i) a plant or plant material, alga, fungus or non-human animal material;

(ii) an extract or isolate of this material, the primary molecular structure of which is the same as that which it had prior to its extraction or isolation, as natural health products.[5]

In addition, the NHPD and the Food Directorate provide a list of herbs that are considered NHPs, regardless of their dosage form (this would include bulk form). These specific herbs are not allowed to be sold as foods because of their known physiologic or pharmaceutical properties and lack of food purpose. This list is available on the NHPD website.

Under the new regulations, all NHPs sold in Canada require product licenses. The intent of requiring pre-market approval is to provide a mechanism for assessing and managing the benefits and risks associated with the use of NHPs. The regulations set out the requirements for submitting an application for a product license that includes the quantity of the medical ingredients, the purpose for which the NHP is intended to be sold and supporting safety and efficacy data.

Site licenses are required for all buildings where NHPs are manufactured, packaged or labeled prior to sale. In addition, importers and distributors require a site license for all locations where NHPs are stored and handled prior to sale. One of the key prerequisites for obtaining a site license is the adoption and maintenance of good manufacturing practices (GMPs). A draft guidance document on good manufacturing practices for natural health products, developed in consultation with stakeholders, is available on the NHPD website. This document provides standards for material control, process control, a self-inspection program, a contractor inspection program, recall procedures, quality control, assessment of stability, record keeping, sterility procedures, testing of samples, and recall reporting. In recognition of the diversity in capacity of industry stakeholders, the proposed GMPs are results/outcomes based; they do not dictate the processes utilized to achieve the results.

The new regulations focus on ensuring that NHP labels will "assist consumers in selecting products that meet their particular needs and expectations, and in understanding the merits and limitations of the products they choose."[4] All NHP labels contain such information as brand name, product number (issued with the product license), dosage form, net amount of the NHP, name and address of the product license holder, recommended use and route of administration.

Key information, as designated by the regulations, must be provided in both French and English. Any other language(s) may be used in addition.[4] Manufacturers are allowed to make use claims on the labels of NHPs as long as they are backed up by suitable evidence.

A Standards of Evidence framework is being developed in conjunction with the new regulations. The aim of this framework is to ensure that product claims are supported by appropriate evidence that can include both scientific and traditional evidence depending on the type of claim being made. All claims must be pre-approved by the NHPD before the product is granted a license.

In order to assist consumers, practitioners and members of the NHP Industry, an education program has been developed to complement the new NHP regulations.

The United States of America

Herbal products in the United States are regulated as "dietary supplements" as defined by The Dietary Supplement Health and Education Act of 1994 (DSHEA). This definition also encompasses nutritional supplements such as vitamins, minerals, amino acids and botanical medicines. Companies marketing "dietary supplements" cannot make specific therapeutic claims regarding their products (i.e., about using them to diagnose, prevent, mitigate, treat or cure a specific disease.) However, they may make "statements of nutritional support" or "structure and function claims" (statements explaining how the product may affect the structure of function of the body) and "general health claims" (claims about the effects on "well-being" achieved by consuming the supplement). Under the DSHEA regulations, manufacturing companies may also indicate to customers possible areas of concern such as potential side-effects and contraindications.[6]

Manufacturers are required to ensure that they can substantiate any claim made and that any statements made about their products are truthful and not misleading, but they are not required to seek pre-approval from the FDA. In all cases where the claims have not been approved by the FDA, the following disclaimer must be placed on the label: "This statement has not been evaluated by the Food and Drug Administration. This product is not intended to diagnose, treat, cure or prevent any disease."[7]

Despite the fact that most herbal products are regulated as "dietary supplements," pharmaceutical companies have the option to apply for regulation for herbal products via the same system as applies to conventional non-prescription drugs. However, the lack of patent protection for these products and the time (average of 15 years) and money (average US $500 million) needed to submit a New Drug Application (NDA) make this an unpopular option.[6]

In response to concerns over questions of product quality, US regulatory authorities are exploring ways in which herbal Good Manufacturing Procedures (GMPs) can be implemented.

Botanical Dosage Forms

Herbal medicines are prepared in a variety of forms, including solids, teas, liquids, and standardized extracts.[8-11]

Herbal Teas:
Decoctions and Infusions

A time-honored method of taking herbal medicines is in the form of a tea. There are primarily two kinds: decoctions and infusions. A decoction is normally reserved for fibrous plant material such as stems, bark, roots and rhizomes. It is made by boiling the plant material until it is reduced to a specific volume. Steeping the more delicate plant parts (flowers, leaves) in either hot or cold water makes an infusion. The temperature of the water will influence the constituent(s) extracted.

The use of these dosage forms is often limited by poor palatability and the fact that only water-soluble constituents are extracted.

Liquid Dosage Forms:
Tincture and Fluid (Liquid) Extracts
A tincture is made by macerating/percolating the plant material in a mixture of water and alcohol. The components extracted are determined by the alcohol/water ratio used in the solvent. While the percentage of alcohol can be as high as 90%, it is more commonly in the range of 25% to 60%. The strength of the tincture is usually given as the ratio of solid herbal product used compared to the total volume of the solution. The commonest range is between 1:3 to 1:5 (plant: total solution).

A fluid (liquid) extract is also an hydroalcoholic product; however in these products one unit of the preparation is equivalent to one unit of the original plant product (i.e., they are more concentrated than tinctures). While this increased potency definitely has its advantages, questions have been raised about the way in which some commercial products are manufactured. Many of the commercially available fluid extracts are made by simply evaporating the solvent from a tincture and then reconstituting the residue to the appropriate volume. This method can cause degradation of the more unstable constituents. Unfortunately, in practice, the terms tincture and fluid extract are often used interchangeably. In addition, it is uncommon for liquid dosage forms to indicate either alcohol content or strength on the label.

Tincture and fluid (liquid) extracts are usually ingested in a little water. Using warm water allows the evaporation of most of the alcohol present, reducing its undesirable effects. These dosage forms have advantages of: containing both alcohol and aqueous soluble components; and allowing prescribers to combine herbs. As with herbal teas, poor palatability is often a problem.

A glycerite is a 'tincture-like' product in which glycerin is used as a solvent. They appear particularly useful in the management of pediatric conditions or where alcohol is strictly contraindicated.

Solid Dosage Forms
Herbal medicines are available in a range of solid doses, including capsules, tablets, freeze-dried products and lozenges. While capsules usually simply contain the dried herbs, tablets are often made from concentrates. Concerns have been raised regarding the small quantity of herbs often present in these dosage forms.

Standardized Extract
A standardized extract is a product in which a specific concentration of a particular constituent or group of constituents is guaranteed. While all the original constituents may still be present, they are often not in the proportions found in the original herb. While this approach is attractive to the conventional medical model, it is dependent on the existence, extraction and identification of a discrete single (or group of) active constituent(s). The effect of this approach to the synergy that is reputed by herbalists to exist between components has yet to be clarified.

In order to assure quality, some preparations may be standardized to a 'marker' component guaranteeing that the correct plant was harvested and used. This 'marker' agent need not necessarily be the active constituent.

Dosage Considerations
Botanical medicine is not practiced in a homogenous manner. Different groups follow distinct philosophies that favor specific dosage systems. Suggested dose regimens may come from herbal traditions (Chinese, Ayurvedic), established European pharmacopoeias or as a result of clinical and pharmacological evaluation. This situation presents the practitioner or consumer with a dilemma regarding a standard dosing regimen for any given herb. As a general rule, doses used by practitioners trained in North America are usually lower than those used

by their European counterparts. For this project, the authors have attempted to include a variety of dosage regimens commonly seen in North America.

Safety Issues

A misconception often shared by practitioners and the public alike is that complementary therapies are completely safe. Unfortunately, this is not the case. Adverse effects from a number of complementary therapies, including botanical medicine, have been noted. The dangers of complementary medicine can be classified as falling into one four categories.

Sins of Omission

Sins of Omission are those in which the patient deteriorates because the CAM practitioner does not recognize the seriousness of the patient's condition and does not refer the patient to appropriate medical care.[12] The quality of education and the professional character of the complementary healthcare provider play a role in determining both their safety and competence.[13] While many "professional" associations of Canadian herbal practitioners do exist, none have the authority to regulate the practice. With the exception of the practice of naturopathic medicine in Ontario, Manitoba, Saskatchewan, and British Columbia, no federal or provincial regulations exist regarding the practice of herbal medicine. This results in little uniformity between herbal practitioners. Cases in which a patient self-medicates inappropriately would also fall in this category.

Intrinsic Procedural Risks

Intrinsic procedural risks are those arising as a direct result of the administration of the therapy.[12] Examples of adverse reactions which result directly from the use of a specific herbal product, including allergic responses, have been noted.[14-21] Complications and ill effects have also been noted due to: misidentification of the herbal content,[21-23]

intentional/unintentional adulteration of the product with heavy metals or pharmaceuticals,[21,24-27] and suspected interactions with conventional medication.[28-29]

Situational Amplifications

Situational amplifications occur in cases where CAM therapy aggravates an existing condition.[12] The use of some herbs, especially as part of a 'detoxifying' protocol, may exacerbate a patient's condition at the onset of treatment.[7] Also, critical and objective evidence regarding the use of herbal medicines in certain scenarios such as pregnancy is lacking. Most information in this area comes from anecdotal and historical sources, the importance of which has yet to be investigated.[30]

Worthless Procedures

The final category is the delivery of worthless procedures for financial or other gains on the part of the practitioner.[12] Unfortunately, as the popularity of 'natural' medicine increases, so does the opportunity for misrepresentation of its use. This is especially a concern when effective treatment (either conventional or unconventional) exists for the condition.[31]

Caveat Emptor

One aim of this book is to protect patients from these dangers by providing the most current and accurate information available on the 50 common herbs reviewed, with any false or dubious claims noted, with any adverse effects, cautions or contraindications, and drug interactions prominently recognized. Although herbal medicines have been shown to be effective for preventing and treating health problems, we are not advocating any one herb or herbal procedure, nor are we suggesting that medicinal herbs can replace other conventional drug treatments for serious illness. We strongly recommend you consult with your doctor, medical or naturopathic, and your pharmacist before taking any medicinal herb for any health condition.

Format of Reviews

A challenge we faced was to organize the monographs using a common accessible format despite the fact that the nature and quantity of information varied so much from herb to herb. The reviews of each herb follow a basic outline: Thumbnail Sketch; Introduction (Family, Synonyms, Description, Parts Used, Traditional Use, Current Medicinal Use, Medicinal Forms); and Relevant Research: Preventative and Therapeutic Effects (Constituents, Adverse Effects, Cautions/Contraindications, and Drug Interactions). Given the different types of information available for each herb (scientific, anecdotal, cross-cultural), as well as the quality and quantity of the available information, the Preventative and Therapeutic Effects section may be organized in different ways.

The information also increases in level of complexity, with the Thumbnail Sketch section providing a concise summary of the entire review, the Introduction a presentation of basic botanical information, and the Relevant Research section a summary of published scientific studies and empirical evidence. The research is carefully documented for further reference by the avid reader and the healthcare professional. A list of terms commonly used in herbal medicine that may not be familiar to most members of the public and the conventional healthcare team may be found following this Introduction.

Glossary of Botanical Medicine Terms

Adaptogen
An agent that supports the body's ability to accommodate varying physical and emotional stresses.

Alterative
An agent with the ability to restore normal body function(s) from an initial unhealthy state. This includes a variety of herbal medicine categories, including: anti-microbials, digestive or hepatic tonics.

Astringent
An agent, normally rich in tannins, that can precipitate proteins resulting in a contraction of tissues.

Bitter
An agent that aids and supports the digestive process, promoting salivation and the secretion of stomach acid and digestive enzymes.

Carminative
A primarily digestive agent that supports and soothes the digestive system relieving gas, spasm and distention.

Cathartic or Purgative
An agent with a pronounced laxative effect, resulting in dramatic evacuation or purging of the bowels.

Cholagogue
An agent that promotes secretion of bile by causing contraction of the gall-bladder.

Choleretic
An agent that promotes the production and secretion of bile.

Demulcent
A normally mucilaginous agent that soothes irritated tissues, notably mucous membranes.

Diaphoretic
An agent that promotes detoxification by promotion of perspiration.

Emmenagogue
An agent that stimulates or harmonizes menstrual flow.

Febrifuge
A fever lowering agent.

Galactagogue
An agent that promotes lactation.

Glycoside
Botanical constituent consisting of sugar and non-sugar (aglycone) components.

Hepatic
General term used to describe an agent that supports healthy liver function.

Nervine
An agent that affects the nervous system, either tonifying, sedating or stimulating.

Phytoestrogen
Compounds, usually flavonoids, which have a weak affinity for estrogen receptors.

Stomachic
An agent that supports gastric functions and promotes appetite.

Tonic
A nurturing agent that invigorates either specific organ(s) or the entire individual.

Vulnerary
An agent that supports wound healing.

Medicinal Herbs for Health Conditions

For centuries, herbal doctors in many different cultures worldwide have recommended herbs for treating various health conditions. While these remedies carry with them the authority of folk wisdom, only recently have herbs been tested using conventional scientific methods to assess their efficacy in treating illness and promoting good health. *The Complete Natural Medicine Guide to the 50 Most Common Medicinal Herbs* presents the "Traditional Use" for each herb discussed, which in some cases has been verified in controlled clinical trials, as well as the "Current Medicinal Use" of each herb, which is based on existing scientific research and medical evidence.

When you look at all the evidence, both traditional and scientific, a single herb can have many uses. The following chart should help you find the most appropriate chapter for any specific condition. A more complete listing of herbs and their respective indications can be found in the Index.

The aim of this chart, as with the book in general, is to help you make informed choices about herbal medicines, not to make recommendations or present prescriptions. For example, while ma huang is listed as a possible treatment for asthma, from reading the chapter you will see that this herb has potentially serious side effects requiring caution in its use. Irrespective of the amount of evidence for a particular herbal medicine, many conditions can only be treated safely and effectively after consulting with an appropriately trained healthcare provider.

Acne
- Tea Tree Oil
- Chaste Tree

Allergies & Hay Fever
- Nettle

Cardiovascular Conditions
- Capsicum
- Garlic
- Ginkgo
- Hawthorn

Anxiety/Tension
- Chamomile (German)
- Kava
- Lemon Balm
- Passionflower
- Scullcap
- Valerian

Appetite
- Dandelion

Arthritis
(Osteoarthritis Rheumatoid Arthritis Gout)
- Devil's Claw
- Capsicum
- Evening Primrose
- Ginger
- Juniper
- Meadowsweet
- Nettle
- Turmeric
- Willow

Asthma
- Cat's Claw
- Ma Huang
- Nettle

Back Pain
- Willow
- Devil's Claw

Bites & Stings (Minor)
- Aloe Vera
- Chamomile (German)
- Calendula

Bladder Infections and Cystitis
❖ Cranberry
❖ Uva Ursi
❖ Juniper

Blood Pressure
❖ Garlic
❖ Hawthorn

Boils and Skin Ulcers
❖ Slipper Elm
❖ Elder

Burns (minor)
❖ Aloe Vera
❖ Calendula

Cancer
❖ Astragalus (adjunctive)
❖ Cat's Claw
❖ Garlic (protective)

Canker Sores
❖ Licorice

Childbirth
❖ Red Raspberry

Cholesterol (high)
❖ Alfalfa

Cold Sores
❖ Lemon Balm

Colic
❖ Chamomile (German)
❖ Peppermint

Common Cold
❖ Echinacea
❖ Elder

Constipation
❖ Aloe Vera

Coughs
❖ Elder
❖ Licorice
❖ Lobelia
❖ Thyme

Depression
❖ St. John's Wort

Dermatitis
❖ Elder

Diabetes
❖ Evening Primrose
❖ Ginseng (American/Canadian)

Diarrhea
❖ Chamomile
❖ Red Raspberry
❖ Slippery Elm

Digestive Disorders
❖ Cat's Claw
❖ Calendula
❖ Ginger
❖ Goldenseal
❖ Juniper
❖ Meadowsweet

Dementia
❖ Ginkgo

Dyspepsia
❖ Devil's Claw
❖ Peppermint
❖ Thyme

Eczema
❖ Burdock
❖ Calendula
❖ Elder
❖ Evening Primrose

Fatigue
❖ Ginseng (Asian & American/Canadian)
❖ Ginseng (Siberian)

Flu
❖ Echinacea
❖ Elder
❖ Peppermint

Fungal Infections
❖ Tea Tree Oil
❖ Thyme

Gastritis
❖ Peppermint

Headache
❖ Meadowsweet
❖ Willow

Hemorrhoids
❖ Horse Chestnut
❖ Dandelion

Impotence
❖ Ginkgo

Indigestion
❖ Devil's Claw
❖ Chamomile (German)
❖ Ginger
❖ Meadowsweet

Immune Conditions
❖ Astragalus
❖ Ginseng (Asian & American/Canadian)
❖ Ginseng (Siberian)

Infections (minor)
❖ Goldenseal
❖ Echinacea
❖ Tea Tree Oil
❖ Thyme

Infertility
❖ Chaste Tree

Insomnia
❖ Chamomile
❖ Hops
❖ Lemon Balm
❖ Passionflower
❖ Scullcap
❖ Valerian

Irritable Bowel Syndrome
❖ Hops
❖ Lemon Balm
❖ Peppermint
❖ Wild Yam

Lactation (Breast Feeding)
❖ Chaste Tree

Liver Conditions
❖ Dandelion
❖ Milk Thistle
❖ Turmeric

Memory
❖ Ginkgo

Menopause
❖ Alfalfa
❖ Black Cohosh
❖ Chaste Tree
❖ Dong Quai
❖ Wild Yam

Menstruation
❖ Alfalfa
❖ Black Cohosh
❖ Cat's Claw
❖ Chaste Tree
❖ Dong Quai
❖ Wild Yam

Migraine
❖ Feverfew
❖ Willow

Multiple Sclerosis
❖ Evening Primrose Oil

Muscle Ache, Cramps, Spasms
❖ Valerian
❖ Kava

Nausea & Motion Sickness
❖ Ginger
❖ Peppermint

Neuralgia (Nerve Pain)
❖ Capsicum
❖ St. John's Wort
❖ Valerian

Pain
❖ Meadowsweet
❖ Willow

Peptic Ulcers
- Chamomile (German)
- Licorice
- Meadowsweet
- Slippery Elm

Premenstrual Syndrome
- Black Cohosh
- Chaste Tree
- Evening Primrose
- Wild Yam

Prostate Conditions
- Nettle
- Saw Palmetto

Pregnancy and Morning Sickness
- Ginger
- Red Raspberry

Psoriasis
- Evening Primrose
- Milk Thistle

Respiratory Conditions
- Echinacea
- Elder
- Goldenseal
- Lobelia
- Ma Huang
- Thyme

Rheumatic Conditions
- Burdock
- Cat's Claw
- Meadowsweet

Skin Rashes and Irritations
- Aloe Vera
- Burdock
- Calendula
- Chamomile (German)
- Echinacea
- Licorice

Sore Throats
- Echinacea
- Slippery Elm
- Goldenseal

Stress
- Astragalus
- Ginseng (Asian)
- Ginseng (Siberian)
- Hops
- Lemon Balm
- Licorice
- Valerian

Tinnitus (ringing in the ears)
- Ginkgo

Tobacco Addiction
  Lobelia

Urinary Tract Infections
- Cranberry
- Echinacea
- Goldenseal
- Juniper
- Uva-ursi

Uterine Spasm
- Black Cohosh

Varicose Veins
- Horsechestnut

Vertigo (dizziness)
- Ginkgo

Vomiting
- Ginger
- Peppermint

Weakness and Debility
- Astragalus
- Ginseng (Asian)
- Ginseng (Siberian)

Weight (Obesity)
- Ma Huang

Yeast Infections
- Tea Tree Oil
- Thyme

Water Retention
- Dandelion

Alfalfa

Medicago sativa L.

THUMBNAIL SKETCH

Common Uses
- High Cholesterol (Hypercholesterolemia)
- Menstruation and Menopause Discomfort

Active Constituents
- Saponins
- Triterpenoidal Glycosides

Adverse Effects
- Diarrhea and Stomach Upset (rare)
- Photosensitivity (theoretical)
- Systemic Lupus Erythematosus (SLE) Reactivation

Cautions/Contraindications
- Systemic Lupus Erythematosus (SLE)
- Pregnancy and Lactation (seeds only)

Drug Interactions
- Anti-Coagulants (possible)
- Hormone Replacement Therapy and Birth Control Pills

Doses
- *Dried Herb:* 5-10 g three times daily
- *Liquid Extract* (1:1 in 25% alcohol): 5-10 mL three times daily

Introduction

Family
* Fabaceae (also known as Leguminosae)

Synonyms
* Lucerne
* Buffalo herb
* Chilean clover
* Purple medick[1]

Medicinal Forms
* Dried Herb
* Liquid Extract

Description
Alfalfa is native to Eastern Mediterranean Europe and the Middle East and was first mentioned in literature by Pliny (AD 23-79) as being introduced to Greece by Darius, King of Persia (550-486 BC). Alfalfa can now be found throughout the world.[2,3] Originally cultivated by the Greeks and Romans, alfalfa is currently produced primarily as a fodder crop in North America. This perennial herb, with clover-like, three-lobe leaves and spiraling seed pods, grows to approximately 36 inches or 1 meter. Its flowers range in color from purplish-blue to yellow.

Parts Used
While sprouted seeds are commonly eaten, the aerial parts are used medicinally.

Traditional Use
Although alfalfa has been used medicinally in Traditional Chinese Medicine (to treat digestive disorders) and Ayurvedic Medicine (for digestive conditions, as a diuretic and in the treatment of arthritis), it is not often mentioned in North American textbooks of herbal medicine.[1]

Current Medicinal Use
Modern day herbalists consider alfalfa to be a good general tonic, due largely to its reputation as an excellent source of vitamins, minerals and protein. While more research is needed, alfalfa may be effective in reducing high cholesterol levels. Evidence from traditional use suggests that alfalfa may also be helpful in managing menopause and menstrual discomfort.

Relevant Research

Preventative and Therapeutic Effects

CONSTITUENTS [4-8]
* AMINO ACIDS: canavanine.
* SAPONINS with the aglycone medicagenic acid.
* ISOFLAVONE FLAVONOIDS: genistein, daidzein, formononetin.
* COUMARINS: coumestans, medicagol.
* ALKALOIDS.
* MISCELLANEOUS: carbohydrates, peptides, pigments, acids, vitamins (esp. vitamins A, B1, B6, B12, C, E, K).

EFFECTS ON CHOLESTEROL
Several studies have demonstrated that the addition of alfalfa meal to cholesterol-containing diets prevented hypercholesterolemia in rats;[9,10] and prevented hypercholesterolemia, decreased hypertriglyceridemia and prevented atherosclerosis in rabbits and monkeys.[9,11-16]

In addition, it has been shown that alfalfa decreased cholesterol, decreased plasma phospholipids, normalized plasma lipoproteins and reduced the extent of aortic and coronary atherosclerosis in monkeys when added to their high-cholesterol diet.[17, 18]

Two human trials have been published.[19,20] One clinical trial was an uncontrolled, non-blinded trial with 11 patients diagnosed with type II and 4 patients diagnosed with type IV hyperlipoproteinemia who were given 40 g of heat prepared alfalfa seeds 3 times daily at mealtimes for 8 weeks (remainder of diet unchanged). Of the patients with type II hyperlipoproteinemia, 9 showed significantly lowered total plasma cholesterol, low density lipoprotein (LDL), and apolipoprotein B, while apolipoprotein A-1 did not change. The 4 patients with type IV did not appear to have the same beneficial effects; however, the small number made it difficult to detect statistically significant effects.[20]

Several researchers have suggested that the alfalfa saponins are the active component of the plant. Rat experiments have indicated that saponins from alfalfa decrease the absorption of cholesterol from the intestine.[9,10,21] This is partially supported by the finding that alfalfa increases the excretion of fecal neutral steroids in rabbits and monkeys, which implies that alfalfa interferes with the absorption of cholesterol.[16,22,23] In addition, in vitro experiments showed that alfalfa plant saponins bound significant amounts of cholesterol from both ethanol solution and from micellar suspension. The amount of cholesterol bound was significantly decreased with the removal of saponins from alfalfa; however, the ability to absorb bile acid was unaffected. The hypocholesterolemic action of alfalfa was thought to be a combination of the saponin-cholesterol interaction and an interaction with bile acids.[24]

MISCELLANEOUS EFFECTS
Cardiovascular Effects
Alfalfa has been used in the management of clotting disorders, primarily due to its high vitamin K content; however, the clinical relevance of this indication is questionable. It may be of use in situations arising from vitamin K deficiency.[1]

Women's Health Care
The isoflavones found in alfalfa (genistein, daidzein) have also been extracted from other plants and shown to have phytoestrogenic properties.[1,2] Consequently, alfalfa has been suggested by many complementary practitioners to be useful in the management of menopause and menstrual discomfort.

Immune System Effects
A Chinese study suggests that polysaccharides isolated from alfalfa may have immunopotentiating effects.[25] This has yet to be confirmed.

ADVERSE EFFECTS
Allergic reactions to alfalfa powder have been reported. In addition, diarrhea and stomach upset may occur occasionally.[1] Photosensitivity reactions have been noted in animals and very rarely skin reactions in humans are seen.[26]

Early animal studies found no toxicity associated with alfalfa or alfalfa saponins;[18,27] however, there was some evidence of growth inhibition in studies where alfalfa was ingested without the addition of cholesterol to the diet.[28-30] Ames mutagenicity testing was negative for a variety of extracts from alfalfa.[31]

Alfalfa may have more severe adverse effects, as was noted in a 1981 case study in which a man who ingested 80-160 g of alfalfa seeds daily on eight occasions for up to 6 weeks at a time (as part of a study) developed pancytopenia.[32] This letter was followed by a report of systemic lupus erythematosus (SLE)-like syndrome in monkeys fed alfalfa sprouts,[33] and a letter reporting two cases in which patients with SLE, which was clinically and serologically in remission, had reactivations of their disease in association with the ingestion of alfalfa tablets.[34] L- Canavanine is the component of alfalfa which appears to be responsible for these unwanted effects (not the saponins which are considered to be the active ingredient needed for positive cholesterol-lowering effects).[33,35,36]

Ingestion of a diet consisting 1.0 to 1.2% of alfalfa saponins by monkeys and rabbits is considered to be harmless.[15,18] Humans currently ingest saponins from a variety of sources, including alfalfa sprouts, soybeans, chick peas, spinach, asparagus and sunflower seeds, without any ill effects.[37]

CAUTIONS/CONTRAINDICATIONS
Patients with a history of systemic lupus erythematosus (SLE) should avoid alfalfa.[34] Seeds should be avoided during pregnancy and lactation.[8]

DRUG INTERACTIONS
Given the possible anti-coagulant action of the vitamin K and the coumarins (e.g., medicagol) found in alfalfa, excessive doses may interfere with concomitant anti-coagulant therapy.[8] However, simple coumarins have more toxicity to rodents and dogs than humans. A more significant risk occurs when the plant becomes infected with mold and the coumarin is converted to the more potent anti-coagulant dicoumarol. Thus quality control for mold-free products is a significant issue here.[38]

In addition, the estrogenic nature of the isoflavones present may interfere with hormone replacement therapy and birth control pills if taken in excessive doses.[8]

DOSAGE REGIMENS
❖ DRIED HERB: 5-10 g three times daily.[8]
❖ LIQUID EXTRACT (1:1 in 25% alcohol): 5-10 mL three times daily.[8]

Aloe Vera

A. vera (L.) Burm.f.

Common Uses
- ❖ *Aloe vera gel:* Minor Skin Irritation, Wounds, Burns
- ❖ *Aloes:* Laxative

Active Constituents
- ❖ *Aloe vera gel:* Polysaccharides (including acemannan)
- ❖ *Aloes:* Anthraquinones

Adverse Effects
Aloe vera gel
- ❖ 'Allergic-type' Reactions (rare)

Aloes
- ❖ Abdominal Cramping (severe)
- ❖ Reversible Pigmentation of Colonic Mucosa
- ❖ Urine Discoloration
- ❖ Nephritis, Gastritis, Vomiting, Bloody Diarrhea, Watery Diarrhea

Cautions/Contraindications
Aloe vera gel
- ❖ *External:* known allergy
- ❖ *Internal:* trace anthraquinone glycosides may be of concern in pregnancy and lactation

Aloes
- ❖ contraindicated in pregnancy and menstruation; as well as appendicitis and abdominal pain of unknown origin. Not recommended for treatment of chronic constipation, or in the presence of hemorrhoids

Drug Interactions
- ❖ *Aloe vera gel:* None known.
- ❖ *Aloes:* Interaction with cardiac glycosides (possible)

Doses
Aloe vera gel
- ❖ *Externally:* A minimum of 70% concentration of aloe vera is necessary for wound healing and anti-inflammatory effects. Pure aloe vera gel is also available
- ❖ *Internally:* No standard dosing.
- ❖ *Anti-Viral:* Oral doses of 800-1600 mg of acemannan.

Aloes
- ❖ *Laxative:* 50-200 mg aloe (dried sap) three times daily.
- ❖ *Hypoglycemic Agent:* 2.5 mL (½ tsp) of the dried sap (aloes) daily.

Introduction

Family
- ❖ Aloeaceae (formerly Aloe was included in the Liliaceae family)[1]

Synonyms
- ❖ Curacao aloe
- ❖ *A. barbadensis* P. Miller
- ❖ *A. vulgaris* Lam[1,2]

Medicinal Forms
ALOE VERA:
- ❖ Gel
- ❖ Ointment
- ❖ Lotion

ALOES:
- ❖ Dried Exudate ('latex' or 'juice')

Description

Aloe is a perennial succulent, native to East and South Africa, that grows wild in the tropics and is now cultivated extensively world wide. There are more than 300 species of Aloe plants;[3,4] however, the species used primarily for medicinal purposes is now known as *A. vera* (L.) Burm.f.[1] Previously it was identified as *A. barbadensis* P. Miller or *A. vulgaris* Lam.[2,3,5] The aloe vera plant grows in a rosette from a base which reaches 8 centimeters or 2.5 inches or more in diameter at maturity. The leaves, which protrude from the base, are long and spear-like with thorny ridges. They can reach 0.5 meters or 18 inches in length and 8 to 10 centimeters or 3 to 3.5 inches across at the base, tapering to a point.[6]

Parts Used

The clear mucilaginous gel from the cells in the inner portion of the leaves (parenchyma) is the part of the plant used medicinally for skin abrasions and infections.[2,3] This gel (often referred to simply as aloe gel) is distinct from the bitter, yellow juice found in the rind of the leaves (just beneath the epidermis), which is a potent laxative.[2] Aloe vera has been cultivated since the 1950s for this bitter yellow juice, which was an important source of drug aloes or 'aloin', known for its purgative effects.[7,8] Its use as a laxative has been all but discontinued in North America. However, the plant continues to be cultivated for the gel, which is primarily used externally to treat a variety of skin conditions. Although these two products (aloes and aloe vera gel) are obtained from the leaves of the same plant, their chemistry, pharmacology and uses are very different and thus they will be described separately.

Aloes (or aloe) is the dried exudate ('latex' or 'juice') collected from freshly cut leaves. Aloes is often sold as a reddish-black or dark-brown solid mass, which tastes bitter and has a characteristic unpleasant odor. This concentrated form was originally produced by boiling the 'latex' in a copper kettle until it reached the required consistency and then it was left to harden. Today, the liquid is more often vacuum-dried, which produces a powdered product.[9]

In contrast, the colorless aloe vera gel is collected from the center of the leaf. It is very sensitive to light and heat, and thus is removed from the leaf mechanically and preserved, buffered and stabilized immediately. This process may differ from manufacturer to manufacturer, which means that the quality of aloe vera gel is highly variable.[9]

Traditional Use

Aloe vera gel has been widely used in the treatment of wounds since before 550 BC.[10] For example, the Greek physician Dioscorides claimed that aloe vera gel could be used to heal skin infections, chapping and hemorrhoids.[11,12] There are many legends about the powers of aloe vera, including that it was the secret of Cleopatra's beauty,[6] which may account for its use in a variety of health and beauty aids, and that it was applied to the body of Jesus Christ after his crucifixion. Aloe vera has been widely used in India as a cathartic, stomachic and anthelminthic;[13,14] in China as a common dermatological remedy;[15] and in Mexico to treat minor skin irritations.[6] It is also a common folk remedy in most of America and the West Indies.[16]

Current Medicinal Use

Research has shown that aloe vera gel promotes minor wound healing (lacerations and burns), possibly through its immune system enhancing, anti-bacterial, or anti-inflammatory activity. While more research is needed, topical aloe vera products may be useful in the treatment of such conditions as psoriasis and dental conditions. Even though aloes has been shown to have anti-viral and hypoglycemic properties, the fact that it is a strong purgative (causes evacuation of the bowels) means that it only has limited clinical uses.

Relevant Research

Preventative and Therapeutic Effects

CONSTITUENTS [9-11,17-26]

Aloe Vera Gel

- ❖ POLYSACCHARIDES: celluolose, glucose, mannose, L-rhamnose, aldopentose, acemannan.
- ❖ ENZYMES: oxidase, amylase, catalase, lipase, alkaline phosphatase, glutathione peroxidase, cyclooxygenase.
- ❖ VITAMINS: B1, B2, B6, choline, folic acid, C, alpha-tocopherol, beta-carotene.
- ❖ ESSENTIAL AMINO ACIDS: lysine, threonine, valine, methionine, leucine, isoleucine, phenylalanine.
- ❖ INORGANIC: calcium, sodium, chlorine, manganese, magnesium, zinc, copper, chromium, potassium sorbate.
- ❖ ALOINOSIDES: including barbaloin (aloins A and B) emodin, aloe-emodin (trace amounts only).

Aloes

- ❖ ALOINOSIDES: including barbaloin (aloins A and B), aloe-emodin, emodin, chrysophanol.
- ❖ CHROMONE DERIVATIVES: aloeresin A, B, C.

Aloe Vera Gel

WOUND HEALING

Most of the medicinal use of aloe vera gel centers around claims that it increases wound healing. In North America, where it is a common household plant, many individuals apply the gel obtained by breaking the leaves to minor cuts, abrasions and burns. However, there is some controversy surrounding its effectiveness and mechanism of action. The first case report of the use of aloe vera for wound healing was published in 1935.[27] Fresh aloe vera gel provided rapid relief from the itching and burning of a woman's acute radiodermatitis (caused by a depilatory X-ray dose to her scalp 8 months earlier). Three similar cases have been reported in the literature.[28, 29] Studies of the effects of aloe vera on wound healing since the 1930s abound. For example, researchers using the fresh leaf demonstrated effective treatment of palmar eczema and puritus vulvae.[30] In addition, a controlled, unblinded study (n=12) found that finger abrasions treated with 50% fresh aloe vera gel in petroleum jelly healed faster than those treated with petroleum jelly alone.[31] Most of these early studies were not blinded or controlled and involved only very small numbers of participants.

Early studies also demonstrated that aloe vera gel was an effective treatment of thermal burns.[32,33] This finding is supported by a recent study which found aloe cream to be more effective than fresh aloe vera gel in the treatment of first-degree thermal burns, but that both dosage forms were equally effective in second-degree thermal burns. Assessment of effectiveness in the treatment of third-degree burns was not possible due to high rates of infection.[34]

However, not all the published studies are positive. Some studies have found that aloe vera gel actually hinders the healing process.[35] Several controlled (but unblinded) studies funded by the US army found no difference in experiments comparing the effects of aloe gel and no treatment on rates of wound healing (in rats and rabbits).[36] A similar study in humans (n=6) with second- and third-degree thermal burns also found no improvement with aloe vera treatment.[36] Unfortunately, these researchers did not use the fresh herb and they do not identify the commercial preparations used.

In addition, studies into the effects of aloe vera on the healing of full-thickness wounds have found either insignificant or negative results.[37,38] The most well-known of these involved the treatment of 21 women with wound complications after cesarian delivery or laparotomy for gynecologic surgery. In this non-blinded study, wounds treated with standard management healed significantly faster than those treated with aloe vera.[38] In contrast, a recent controlled study assessing the effect of a commercial preparation of aloe vera on partial-thickness wounds showed a significant increase in healing.[39] It has been suggested that aloe vera should not be used to treat full-thickness wounds because it causes the dermal layer to fuse too quickly, inhibiting the wound from healing properly; however, its use in partial-thickness wounds continues to be supported by many authors.

One open label study of factory assembly-line workers (n=29) with occupationally-related dry, irritated, emollient-dependent hands assessed the effects of a glove that delivers aloe vera gel to the gloved hand.[40] Each participant wore a dry-coated aloe vera glove on one hand only for 8 hours daily for 30 days, followed by 30 days of rest, followed by 10 days of repeated use. Photos of participants' hands at the end of the study were evaluated by blinded research staff. The research team reported that the aloe vera gloves produced a uniformly positive effect on skin integrity, decreased the appearance of fine wrinkling and decreased erythema. There was a statistically significant improvement in the mean global ratings of the gloved hands compared to the non-gloved hands at the end of the study.[40] However, it is not clear how much of this effect was simply due to wearing gloves as compared to the aloe vera that was in the gloves.

Several mechanisms of action for the wound healing properties of aloe vera gel have been suggested. The first is that aloe vera is occlusive and may simply act as a protective barrier.[41,42] Several early non-blinded and/or uncontrolled studies, which found that the application of aloe vera gel increased the healing rate of frostbite injuries, provide some support for this hypothesis (because no vehicle control was used).[43-45] In another example, guinea pig thermal wounds treated with aloe vera healed faster than those treated with silver sulfadiazine, but again, there was no vehicle control.[46] Other researchers have demonstrated increased capillary perfusion after the application of aloe vera topically and suggest that this may provide further insight into the mechanism of action of aloe vera.[47,48]

EFFECTS ON THE IMMUNE SYSTEM

The most recently suggested mechanism of action is that aloe vera gel may directly stimulate the immune system.[49] Most of these studies involve the oral ingestion or intramuscular/

subcutaeneous (im/sc) injection of acemannan, an active ingredient isolated from aloe vera gel. Acemannan has been shown to enhance phagocytosis in a dose-dependent fashion;[50] increase numbers of circulating monocytes and macrophages;[51-52] permit monoctye driven signals to enhance T-cell response to lectin;[49] increase lymphocyte response to alloantigen;[49] enhance the release of cytokines, including interleukin-1, interleukin-6, interferon and tumor necrosis factor in vitro;[52-54] and activate macrophages.[55,56] One study demonstrated that the immune response of chickens to Newcastle disease virus was increased by adding acemannan to a Newcastle vaccine.[57] A study of avian polyomavirus in birds with similar results has also been published.[58] Acemannan has also been shown to have anti-viral activity.[59,60] Although most of these experiments have been *in vitro* studies, the concentrations of acemannan used appear to be achievable *in vivo*.[61]

ANTI-BACTERIAL ACTIVITY

In the early 1950s, it was suggested that aloe vera gel had an anti-biotic action.[62] Early studies found that aloe vera gel inhibited *Myobacterium tuberculosis* and *Bacillus subtilis in vitro*.[63,64] In addition, aloe vera juice was shown to be bacteriostatic to *Staphylococcus aureus*, *Streptococcus pyogenes*, and *Salmonella paratyphi*; however, the juice was also reported to be unstable.[65] More recent studies provide similar results. Different concentrations of aloe vera extracts have been found to be bactericidal to a variety of bacteria including: 1) *Streptococcus agalctiae*, *Enterobacter cloacae*, *Citrobacter species*, *Serratia marcescens*, *Klebsiella pneumoniae*, *Pseudomonas aeruginosa* (at a concentration of 60%); 2) *Staphylococcus aureus* (at a concentration of 70%); 3) *Escherichia coli* (at a concentration of 80%); and 4) *Streptococcus faecali*, a yeast — *Candida albicans* (at a concentration of 90%).[19,66] Other studies have not found any antibacterial activity against *Staphylococcus aureus* or *Escherichia coli*.[67]

ANTI-INFLAMMATORY ACTIVITY

Many studies have demonstrated the anti-inflammatory properties of aloe vera and other Aloe species.[19,26,68-75] For example, researchers have shown that aloe vera gel and hydrocortisone decrease inflammation in an additive, dose-related manner when they are used concurrently.[76] Another study found direct anti-inflammatory activity which could be attributed to known sterols isolated from aloe vera gel (e.g., lupeol, campesterol). In this study, aloe vera gel also appeared to block hydrocortisone's inhibitory effects on wound healing.[74] Another research team demonstrated that constituents of an aqueous gel-extract of aloe vera inhibited the release of reactive oxygen species by human PMNs, reducing the harmful effects of this release at the site of inflammation.[77]

　　Three primary mechanisms of action for the anti-inflammatory effects of aloe vera have been postulated: 1) anti-bradykinin activity has been found in some Aloe species (e.g., A. arborescens, A. saponaria);[26,69] 2) emodin, aloe-emodin and aloin were shown to produce salicylates when metabolized, which appear to inhibit thromboxane production by competitive inhibition through stereochemical means;[19,78] and 3) magnesium lactate, a constituent of aloe vera, is a known inhibitor of histidine decarboxylase and thus may prevent the formation of histamine in mast cells.[3,19] The first hypothesis has been demonstrated in other Aloe species,[26,69,79] but there is little evidence of such action in studies with aloe vera. The second hypothesis has more support in the literature. A clinical case report in which a commercial preparation of aloe vera was applied to a monkey who was accidentally scalded provides some support because the amount of thromboxane A_2 produced by the monkey was decreased.[80] Other studies also provide support for this finding.[19,44,48,78,81] However, one researcher noted that many of the vehicles used in commercial aloe vera preparations (e.g., petrolatum, mineral oil, and aquaphor) are inhibitors of prostaglandin production themselves.[81] This emphasizes the need for well-designed (i.e., vehicle-controlled) studies of aloe vera.

It has been reported that decolorized (anthraquinone-free) aloe vera gel is a more potent inhibitor of inflammation than the colorized form.[82] One study in support of this hypothesis found that high concentrations of anthraquinones increased the production of prostaglandins, while trace amounts appeared to decrease the inflammatory response.[6] However, another study found that an aloe vera gel extract containing anthraquinone was more effective than an anthraquinone-free product.[83] In addition, one researcher demonstrated that anthraquinone is necessary for the absorption of aloe vera given orally.[71]

PROTECTION AGAINST RADIATION

Investigation of the effectiveness of aloe vera gel in the treatment of radiation burns began in the late 1930s when radiation-induced burns or ulcers were a common model to test the ability of aloe vera to increase wound healing. Several early studies demonstrated an increased rate of healing.[33,84-87] One of the best was a study with 20 albino rabbits in which 4 different treatments (fresh aloe vera gel, commercial aloe vera ointment, dry gauze bandage and nothing) were applied to the four quadrants of a wound caused by beta radiation. Visual assessment over a period of 58 days led to the findings that both aloe vera treatments resulted in statistically significant accelerated healing.[86]

A more recent double-blind, placebo-controlled study in 194 women receiving breast or chest wall irradiation found no difference between the 98% pure aloe vera gel and a placebo.[88] This negative finding is supported by another randomized, double-blind study which compared 98% pure aloe vera gel with topical aqueous cream (applied three times daily throughout and for 2 weeks after radiation therapy) by women (n=225) who had undergone lumpectomy or partial mastectomy for breast cancer and then received radiation therapy post-operatively. In this case aloe vera gel did not significantly reduce radiation-induced skin adverse effects such as erythema, pain, itching, and dry or moist desquamation.[89]

DIABETES

Aloe vera has been used in diabetes for its enhancement of wound healing. Researchers have demonstrated in a controlled (unblinded) study of mice that aloe vera increases the rate of healing, provides pain relief, and decreases edema as compared to a saline control in both normal mice and those with streptozotocin-induced diabetes.[90]

MISCELLANEOUS

Anti-Cancer

Acemannan, a compound isolated from aloe vera, has been reported to have anti-tumor activity.[91-93] For example, it has been used to in the treatment of fibrosarcomas in dogs and cats.[94] In addition, Roidex (a formulation of squalene, vitamin A, vitamin E and aloe vera) demonstrated more chemopreventive and curative properties than squalene alone in the prevention and treatment of mouse skin tumors.[95] Aloe juice has also been reported to have antimetastatic activity and to enhance the activity of 6-fluorouracil and cyclophosphamide.[96]

Anti-Viral

Acemannan has also been reported to have anti-viral activity,[59,60,97-98] and it has been suggested that it may play a role as an adjuvant treatment in HIV/AIDS.[51,59,99,100]

Psoriasis

A recent double-blind, placebo-controlled clinical study of 60 patients diagnosed with psoriasis vulgaris found that treatment with 0.5% aloe vera extract (without occlusion) was a significantly better treatment than placebo.[101]

Peptic Ulcer
Aloe vera gel has been taken internally for the treatment of peptic ulcers.[41] One group of authors claim several complete cures among 12 patients diagnosed with duodenal lesions (X-ray confirmation). However, no follow up studies appear to have been performed.[41]

Dental Conditions
Several studies report the effectiveness of aloe vera gel in increasing the rate of healing after dental procedures.[102,103]

Veterinary Use
Effective use of aloe vera in animals has been reported for the treatment of ringworm, allergies, abscesses, fungal infections and different types of inflammation.[104] Although aloe vera as a 'panacea' in veterinary medicine has been questioned,[105] a detailed investigation of 2 cases using the commercial preparation (Dermaide Aloe®) to treat the severe accidental thermal burns of 2 dogs showed that aloe vera accelerated the rate of healing, decreased the production of prostaglandins and inhibited infection by *Pseudomonas aeruginosa*.[78] Its use was also reported to be beneficial in the treatment of a monkey who was accidentally scalded.[80]

Final Notes
Variation in the quality of aloe vera has been documented and may account for some of the negative or inconclusive studies.[6,106,107] In addition, aloe vera has been reported to be biochemically unstable and may deteriorate in a short time period,[6,108] which may also explain some of the conflicting study results. More good-quality, clinical trials are needed to provide conclusive evidence of aloe vera's effectiveness in the management of skin conditions.

Aloes
LAXATIVE
The anthraquinone glycosides are responsible for the well-documented laxative effect of aloes.[9] They induce the intestinal secretion of water and electrolytes and modify intestinal motility. Laxative effects occur approximately 8 hours after the ingestion of aloes, which is metabolized by intestinal bacteria to form the active compound, aloe-emodin-9-anthrone.[109,110] This substance has been shown to inhibit rat colonic $Na+$, $K+$-ATPase *in vitro*, and *in vivo* to increase the paracellular permeability of rat colonic mucosa.[111] Due to its strong purgative effect, aloes is not commonly recommended for use as a routine laxative (see adverse effects).

DIABETES
Aloes' use as a hypoglycemic agent has been demonstrated in 5 non-insulin dependent patients and in an animal model (mice) of diabetes.[112,113] The mechanism of action for this effect has yet to be determined, although it is hypothesized that it may be mediated through stimulation of the synthesis and/or release of insulin from the beta-cells of the Islets of Langerhans.[113]

MISCELLANEOUS
Aloes has been used to flavor products used to discourage nail biting (it has a very bitter taste).[9] Several hydroxyanthracene derivatives have been shown to inhibit a variety of viruses *in vitro*, including herpes simplex (types 1 and 2), varicella-zoster, pseudo-rabies and influenza. It was not active against adenovirus or rhinovirus.[114]

ADVERSE EFFECTS
Aloe Vera Gel
Adverse effects associated with the external application of aloe vera gel have been very rarely reported in the literature. Contact dermatitis, possibly due to an allergic reaction, has been reported in several cases.[81,115-119] There is one report of wide-spread dermatitis after the topical application of aloe vera gel to stasis dermatitis,[120] and one report of an acute bullous allergic reaction.[121] One case of cathartic effects after topical application of aloe vera gel to the mucosal surface has also been reported.[81]

Aloes
Adverse effects are most common with chronic use, which tends to result in tolerance. In addition, chronic use may lead to a reversible pigmentation of the colonic mucosa. After aloes use is discontinued, the pigmentation disappears in 4 to 12 months. Urine may become orange (if pH is acidic) or reddish purple (if pH is alkaline). This is caused by the renal elimination of the hydroxyanthracene derivatives. Severe abdominal cramping is common.[122] Nephritis, gastritis, vomiting, bloody diarrhea with mucous, and watery diarrhea leading to osmotic imbalances have been reported.[9]

CAUTIONS/CONTRAINDICATIONS
Aloe Vera Gel
❖ EXTERNAL: known allergies.
❖ INTERNAL: trace anthraquinone glycosides may be of concern in pregnancy and lactation.[122]

Aloes
Contraindicated in pregnancy, lactation and menstruation; appendicitis and abdominal pain of unknown origin; spasmodic obstipation. Not recommended for treatment of chronic constipation, in the presence of hemorrhoids or chronic renal disease.[9,122]

DRUG INTERACTIONS
Aloe Vera Gel
None known.

Aloes
Although no clinical examples appear to have been published, the anthraquinone glycosides have been known to induce hypokalemia which may interfere with the action of cardiac glycosides.

DOSAGE REGIMENS
Aloe Vera Gel
❖ EXTERNALLY: A minimum of 70% concentration of aloe vera is necessary for wound healing and anti-inflammatory effects.[123] Pure aloe vera gel is also available.
❖ INTERNALLY: No standard dosing.
❖ ANTI-VIRAL: Oral doses of 800-1600 mg of acemannan.[51,124]

Aloes
❖ LAXATIVE: 50-200 mg aloes (dried sap) three times daily.
❖ HYPOGLYCEMIC AGENT: 2.5 mL (1/2 tsp) of the dried sap (aloes) daily.[112]

Astragalus

Astragalus membranaceus Moench

THUMBNAIL SKETCH

Common Uses
- ❖ Resistance to Disease
- ❖ Stress Ailments (including viral infections and fatigue)
- ❖ Adjunctive Therapy to Chemotherapy and Radiation Treatment

Active Constituents
- ❖ Astragalan
- ❖ Astragalosides

Adverse Effects
- ❖ None known

Cautions/Contraindications
- ❖ None known

Drug Interactions
- ❖ None known

Doses
- ❖ *Dried Root* (as tea): adult dose normally 9-15 g daily in divided doses
- ❖ *Tincture* (1:5): 2-6 mL three times daily
- ❖ *Powdered Solid Extract* (2:1): 250-500 mg three times daily
- ❖ *Formulas:* Astragalus is often seen in combination formulas with other similar herbs such as Chinese privet (*Ligustrum lucidum* Ait. Oleaceae), codonopsis (*Codonopsis pilosula* (Franch) Nannf., Campanulaceae) and Asian ginseng (*Panax ginseng* C.A. Meyer., Araliaceae), and is often mixed with Chinese licorice.

Introduction

Family
- ❖ Fabaceae (also known as Leguminosae)

Synonyms
- ❖ Milk-vetch root
- ❖ Membranous vetch
- ❖ Yellow vetch; Huang qi (Chinese)[1,2]

Medicinal Forms
- ❖ Dried Root (as a tea)
- ❖ Tincture
- ❖ Powdered Solid Extract

Description
Astragalus is an herbaceous perennial, with hairy stems and 12-18 pairs of leaflets on each leaf, that grows up to 1 meter or 39 inches in height.[3] It is native to northern China and Tibet, growing both in the grassland and in lightly forested areas that are well drained.[2,7]

Parts Used
The part of the plant used medicinally is the root, which is harvested from 4-7 year-old plants and dried.[7] In the Orient, the seeds of *Astragalus complanatus* R.Br. have also been used medicinally.[4]

Traditional Use
Astragalus has long been a part of Traditional Chinese Medicine. In fact, it was included in the classic *Shen Nong Ben Cao Jing*, which was written 2000 years ago.[2] It is thought to strengthen the body's 'vital energy' or qi and was often used in conditions of physical weakness and during chronic illness. It was believed to both strengthen and invigorate.[2] It is one of the most widely used herbs in Fu-zheng therapy — the use of herbs to augment the host defense mechanisms.[2,5-7] The species of Astragalus which has been used for medicinal purposes, *Astragalus membranaceus* Moench (and its variety mongholicus), has been extensively studied in the Orient. Within Traditional Chinese Medicine, astragalus is considered a sweet and warming tonic used to increase stamina, endurance and resistance to disease.[8] As a classic tonic it is considered superior to Asian ginseng in young adults.[8]

Current Medicinal Use
In many instances, the traditional uses and current medicinal uses are one and the same. For example, astragalus is currently used as an immune stimulant and thought to be helpful for the common cold.[8] Research into its use as an adjunctive therapy for cancer patients, most notably to reduce the side effects of conventional treatments such as chemotherapy, is just beginning.

It is important that cancer patients considering taking astragalus should consult with an appropriately trained healthcare provider first.

Relevant Research

Preventative and Therapeutic Effects

CONSTITUENTS [7-11]
- ❖ TRITERPENE GLYCOSIDES (SAPONINS): astragalosides, acetylastragalosides, isoastragalosides, astramembrannins.
- ❖ POLYSACCHARIDES: astragalans.
- ❖ FLAVONOIDS: kaempferol, quercetin, isorhamnetin, astragalin g-aminobutyric acid.
- ❖ MISCELLANEOUS: free amino acids (including arginine, glutamic acid, canavanine, alanine), trace minerals (including zinc, manganese, magnesium), sterols.

EFFECTS ON THE IMMUNE SYSTEM

The immune effects of astragulus have been investigated in a multitude of *in vitro* and *in vivo* studies. Astragulus has been shown to: significantly increase the spontaneous incorporation of [3H]thymidine in mononuclear cells;[6] increase the proliferation of lymphocytes;[6,12] potentiate IL-2 production and activity;[13-15] activate T cell blastogenesis;[16] increase T cell cytotoxicity;[5,16] enhance the secretion of tumor necrosis factor (TNF);[9] potentiate the phagocytic function of the reticuloendothelial system (RES);[17] increase natural killer (NK) cells' cytoxicity;[16,18] and increase the activity of peritoneal macrophages.[17] Astragalus has also been shown to augment the interferon response of mice who are exposed to viruses.[19]

In addition, many studies have investigated the effects of astragalus when it is given in situations of immunosuppression.[7,12,15,16,20] For example, in a large clinical study, 572 cancer patients were given Fu-zheng therapy (which included astragalus) in combination with standard medical treatment for 2 months. The study results suggested that patients experienced protection of adrenal cortical function during radiation and chemotherapy treatment, and reduced bone marrow depression and gastrointestinal effects.[7] This is supported by a controlled study in which mice were given astragalus concurrently with mitomycin C. In this study, astragalus showed protective effects against immunosuppression in the mice. The authors of the study hypothesized that this resistance to immunosuppression may be correlated with the observed stimulation of the reticuloendothethial system (RES), activation of T cell blastogenesis and increased NK cell cytotoxicity.[16] In addition, a randomized, controlled, clinical trial of 115 patients with leukopenia who were treated with two concentrations of astragalus preparation (15 g twice daily BID vs. 5 g BID) for 8 weeks found that there was an obvious rise in the white blood cell counts (WBC) of both groups, but that the group with the larger dose had a significantly greater increase, suggesting a dose-dependent effect.[12] However not all studies were positive. In another controlled study an extract of astragalus in combination with the herb *Ligustrum lucidum* W.T. Aiton (Oleaceae) did not prevent cyclophosphamide-induced myelosuppression in mice.[20]

CARDIAC EFFECTS

A variety of trials have investigated the effect of astragalus in patients (or animal models) with Coxsackie B virus (CBV) myocarditis. One controlled clinical trial of patients (10 in the treatment group; 8 controls) with CBV myocarditis who were treated with astragalus i.m. (8g/day) for 3-4 months or given conventional treatment only, found that the clinical condition of those treated with astragalus was improved in comparison to the control group.[18] Another study found that astragalus treatment increased the survival rate and decreased the percentage of abnormal action potential in mice infected with coxsackie B-3 virus when compared with controls.[21] In searching for the mechanism of action of these effects, researchers have found that astragalus: significantly enhanced the OKT3, OKT4 and OKT4/OKT8 ratio in patients with viral myocarditis;[22] and appeared to inhibit the replication of coxsackie B-3 virus RNA in the myocardial tissue of mice *in vivo*[23] and *in vitro*,[24] and significantly inhibited the $Ca2+$ influx across the myocardial plasma membrane *in vitro*.[24] Several researchers have suggested that astragalus is a rational treatment choice for patients with viral myocarditis.[24]

In other studies of cardiac effects, components of astragalus have been shown to be effective as positive inotropes, which can improve the condition of patients with congestive heart failure. In one uncontrolled study, 19 patients were given i.v. astragaloside IV (an 'active' component of astragalus) for 2 weeks at which point their symptoms of chest distress, and dyspnea were relieved and their capacity for exercise was increased.[10] In another study, 22 patients with positive ventricular late potentials were treated with a 24 g iv drip of astragalus (control group were given lidocaine) for 2 weeks. The researchers reported that treatment with astragalus successfully shortened the duration of late potentials (significantly more than lidocaine).[25] Astragalus treatment has also been shown to be more effective than nifedipine (a calcium channel antagonist) in the treatment of 92 patients suffering from ischemic heart disease,[26] and also effective in increasing cardiac output in 20 patients with angina pectoris.[27] One team of researchers suggested that the cardiotonic action of astragalus may be partially due to its anti-oxygen free radical action. This was based on their study of 43 patients suffering from their first acute myocardial infarction.[28]

MISCELLANEOUS EFFECTS
Anti-Viral Effects
Several researchers have reported that astragalus has an antiviral effect.[29-32]

Anti-Cancer Effects
An *in vitro* study showed that astragalus increased the secretion of both Tumor Necrosis Factor-a and Tumor Necrosis Factor-b.[9] A clinical study of 54 consecutive cases of small cell lung cancer treated with both standard medical treatment and Traditional Chinese Medicine (including astragalus) reported increased survival when compared to average survival statistics of conventional medical treatment alone.[33] This is supported by a controlled *in vivo* study of mice with renal cell carcinoma. The group receiving 500 mcg each of astragalus and *Ligustrum lucidum* intra-peritoneally daily for 10 days had a significantly higher cure rate than saline controls.[34] It has been hypothesized that the anti-tumor effects of astragalus are the result of an augmentation of phagocyte and LAK cell activities.[34,35]

Prevention of Ototoxicity
A study in guinea pigs found that a mixture of astragalus and *Pyrola rotundifolia* L.(Pyrolaceae) significantly reduced the ototoxicity and nephrotoxicity of gentamicin.[36] The ototoxic effects of aminoglycoside antibiotics are thought to be related to a decrease of cAMP, and astragalus has been shown by other researchers to increase cAMP.

Miscellaneous
One study demonstrated that an aqueous solution of astragalus was able to significantly increase the motility to human sperm *in vitro*. The active constituents responsible for this effect are as yet unknown.[37] Another study reported that a decoction of astragalus root was an effective treatment of senile benign renal arteriolosclerosis. Additional studies are needed to confirm these effects.[38]

ADVERSE EFFECTS
None known.

CAUTIONS/CONTRAINDICATIONS
Since astragalus has been reported to increase tumor necrosis factor, theoretically its use may be of concern in the management of HIV. Clarification of this potential effect is necessary.

DRUG INTERACTIONS
None known.

DOSAGE REGIMENS

❖ DRIED ROOT (AS TEA): adult dose normally 9-15 g daily in divided doses; however, doses from 30-60 g daily are also seen occasionally.[2,3,39]

❖ TINCTURE (1:5): 2-6 mL three times daily.[39]

❖ POWDERED SOLID EXTRACT (2:1): 250-500 mg three times daily.[39]

❖ FORMULAS: Astragalus is often seen in combination formulas with other similar herbs such as Chinese privet (*Ligustrum lucidum* Ait. Oleaceae), codonopsis (*Codonopsis pilosula* (Franch) Nannf., Campanulaceae) and Asian ginseng (*Panax ginseng* C.A. Meyer., Araliaceae).[2] It is also often mixed with Chinese licorice.[40]

Black Cohosh

Cimicifuga racemosa (L.) Nutt.

THUMBNAIL SKETCH

Common Uses
- ❖ Menopause Symptoms (hot flashes, anxiety, depression)
- ❖ Premenstrual Syndrome and Dysmenorrhea
- ❖ Uterine Spasm

Active Constituents
- ❖ Terpenoids
- ❖ Formononetin

Adverse Effects
- ❖ Rare, limited to gastric upset.
- ❖ Historical evidence suggests throbbing headaches, nervous and cardiovascular depression can occur at high doses.

Cautions/Contraindications
- ❖ Pregnancy and Lactation

Drug Interactions
- ❖ None known

Doses
- ❖ *Dried Root:* 40-200 mg taken by decoction or as a solid dose daily
- ❖ *Extract (40-60% alcohol):* equivalent to 40 mg of herb daily
- ❖ *Tincture (1:10 in 60% ethanol):* 0.4-2mL daily

  Note: In the case of menopause treatment, the onset of action of this plant can take up to 2 weeks to occur

Introduction

Description

Black cohosh is an upright perennial, with large compound, tooth-edged leaves. It grows up to 2 meters or 80 inches high, producing numerous small white flowers on a wand-like raceme. Black cohosh is native to the temperate climates of the Northern Hemisphere, including North America, where it is found from Maine to Ontario in the north and from Georgia and Missouri in the south.[4] Even though black cohosh has been cultivated in Europe and is especially popular in Germany for its medicinal properties, all commercial stocks come from the United States and Canada.[4] "Cohosh" is the native Algonquin word for "rough," referring to its gnarled root, which is black in color when harvested, with an acrid taste and strong odor.

Parts Used

The plant grows from a thick fibrous root stock, which is the part used medicinally.[5]

Traditional Use

Black cohosh has long been used for its medicinal properties, especially by peoples of the First Nations. The Cherokee and the Iroquois used a tea made from the root to alleviate rheumatic pains, promote lactation and promote menses. Its use was commonly accepted into the eclectic medical movement in the early to mid 19th century, where it was prized as an anti-spasmodic, analgesic and gynecological agent.[1] It has been called "squawroot" and the "menopause herb." The botanical name for black cohosh, *Cimicifuga racemosa*, comes from the latin *cimex* meaning "bug" and *fuga* meaning "to repel," referring to the fact that it appears to act as an effective insect repellent. Black cohosh is also known as bugbane and bugwort.

Current Medicinal Use

As with its traditional uses, black cohosh products are primarily used in women's health care. Research has shown that substances found in black cohosh have 'hormone-like' properties that influence the endocrine system. A growing amount of research, including clinical trials, show that some black cohosh products may be of help in alleviating the symptoms of menopause (hot flashes, anxiety, mild depression), premenstrual syndrome, dysmenorrhea, and uterine spasm.

Relevant Research

Preventative and Therapeutic Uses

CONSTITUENTS [6-12]

❖ TRITERPENOIDS: a complex mixture including actein, cimigoside, 12-acetylactein, cimifugoside, 27-deoxyacetylacteol.
❖ FLAVONOIDS: formononetin.
❖ ACIDS: isoferulic, salicylic, acetic, butyric, palmitic.
❖ MISCELLANEOUS: phytosterols, hydrolysable tannins, cimicifugin, resinous material referred to as acteina.

ENDOCRINE EFFECTS

It has long been known that *Cimicifuga racemosa* contained agents that possess 'hormone-like' characteristics. Using ovariectomized rats, Jarry et al. demonstrated that the administration of an extract of *Cimifuga racemosa* caused a selective reduction in serum concentrations of luteinizing hormone (LH).[6,7] They also noted that three 'endocrine active' agents could be identified in a methanolic extract of this plant. One of these three constituents was identified as formononetin. While formononetin was seen to bind with estrogen receptors, it failed to reduce LH levels, leading to the conclusion that other agents present in the methanolic extract were responsible for this action.[7] Duker et al. demonstrated similar findings during a placebo controlled trial in humans. A group of menopausal women (n=110, mean age 52) were divided into equal groups, one received a placebo and the other 8mg (4mg twice daily) of a commercially available dried hydroalcoholic extract, Remifemin®. After 8 weeks, a selective and significant decrease was seen in LH levels but not follicle stimulating hormone (FSH) levels. In an attempt to determine the 'active constituents' a lipophilic extract was prepared and subjected to sephadex chromatography.

It was discovered that there were in fact three groups of active components:
GROUP 1: Non-estrogen ligands which decreased LH secretion on chronic administration.
GROUP 2: Estrogen ligands which also suppressed LH release.
GROUP 3: Constituents which showed an affinity for estrogen receptors but failed to decrease LH release.

The authors hypothesized that the agents in group 1 could be exerting their effects on LH release by acting at a central site (similar to clonidine). They also suggested that the agents in group 3 failed to exert an action on LH levels because they may be rapidly metabolized. The authors go on to suggest that since pulsatile LH secretion is associated with the presentation of many of the unpleasant consequences of menopause, this may explain the therapeutic action of *Cimicifuga racemosa*.[13] A recent Danish study conducted on immature rats and ovariectomized rats failed to demonstrate any 'traditional' estrogenic effect.[14]

The vast majority of clinical investigations regarding this plant's medicinal action have been carried out in Europe, notably Germany. A systematic review of the clinical trial evidence regarding the efficacy of black cohosh in the treatment of menopausal symptoms included 4 randomized controlled trials,[15-18] and concluded that "in spite of plausible mechanisms of action of *C. racemosa*, its clinical efficacy has not been convincingly demonstrated through rigorous clinical trials. Additional rigorous RCTs and biochemical and chemical investigations are warranted."[19]

In a randomized study conducted over 6 months with women (n=60, age < 40yrs) who had ovarian insufficiency following hysterectomy but with at least one functioning ovary, investigators compared the effectiveness of a commercial product of *Cimicifuga racemosa* (Remifemin®) and conventional hormone based therapies. At a dose of 2 tablets twice daily,

Remifemin® was shown to decrease menopausal symptoms (measured using Kupperman Menopausal Index) comparable to the three conventional therapy groups (estriol 1 mg daily; conjugated estrogen 1.25 mg; combined estrogen/gestagen therapy).[17] In addition, Warnecke demonstrated that Remifemin® (40 drops twice daily) given over 12 weeks showed estrogen-like stimulation of the vaginal mucosa similar to conjugated estrogens (0.625 mg daily) and an improvement in neurovegatitive symptoms comparable to diazepam 2 mg daily.[15] Another randomized placebo controlled double-blind study conducted over 12 weeks on women (n=80) suffering from the unpleasant consequences of menopause also noted positive results. Remifemin® (2 tabs twice daily) was shown to increase proliferation of vaginal epithelium and decrease physical and mental symptoms (Kuppermann menopausal index and Hamilton Anxiety Index) in a fashion superior to both placebo and conjugated estrogen.[16] Similar results have been noted in other clinical studies of Remifemin®, including: effectiveness in cases where conventional therapy is contraindicated[20], refused[21] and in a protocol removing conventional treatment.[22] It should be noted that the vast majority of the clinical trials described above have been carried out with one specific proprietary product. Remifemin® tablets are standardized to 27- deoxyacetein content (1 mg/unit dose).

A recent randomized placebo controlled trial assessed the use of black cohosh (brand not specified) in the management of hot flashes experienced by 85 women diagnosed with breast cancer who had completed their primary cancer treatment including chemotherapy and radiation.[18] Fifty-nine of the study participants were also taking tamoxifen and they were equally distributed among the treatment and placebo groups. Participants were asked to take either black cohosh (dose not provided) or placebo twice daily with meals for 60 days. Women in both groups (black cohosh and placebo) reported benefits in terms of reduced number and intensity of hot flashes. There were no significant differences in the seven outcome measures reported between the two groups except for sweating, with more improvement reported in the black cohosh group. No differences in FSH or LH were identified between the two groups. The authors conclude that black cohosh was not significantly more efficacious than placebo against most menopausal symptoms, including number and intensity of hot flashes. However, since the dose of black cohosh was not provided, it is difficult to compare these findings with the results of earlier studies.

In a review article, Beuscher comments on a study using a combination product containing both black cohosh and an extract of St John's Wort (*Hypericum perforatum* L., Clusiaceae). In this multi-center trial conducted over 12 weeks with women (n=812) suffering from psycho-vegetative symptoms of menopause (including irritability, poor concentration, fear, insomnia, depression), 90% of patients noted an improvement.[2] It should be noted that standardized extracts of St. John's Wort have now been shown to be effective in the management of mild-moderate depression when given as a single agent.[23]

Another randomized, placebo-controlled trial (n=49) found that a phytoestrogen combination containing 60 mg soy isoflavones, 100 mg dong quai and 50 mg black cohosh significantly decreased the frequency of menstrual migraine attacks as well as significantly decreasing the frequency of all migraines, headache severity, doses of triptans and doses of analgesics compared to the placebo group when ingested for 24 weeks.[24] The clinical contributions of the black cohosh in this product cannot be determined from this study.

Commission E, a German regulatory agency, considers black cohosh useful in the management of PMS, dysmenorrhoea and nervous conditions associated with menopause.[25]

MISCELLANEOUS EFFECTS
Cardiovascular Effects
The administration of the resinous material, acteina, has been shown to exert a hypotensive action in various animal models and cause peripheral vasodilation and increased blood flow

in humans.[26] Triterpene compounds extracted from a plant described as "Japanese Cimicifuga" showed hypocholesterolemic activity *in vivo*.[27]

Anti-Microbial Effects
Extracts of a related species, *Cimicifuga dahurica* (Turcz. Ex Fisch. & C.A. Meyer) Maxim, have been shown to possess antimicrobial activity towards both gram+ and gram– bacteria *in vitro*.[28]

Adverse Effects
Adverse effects appear rare, usually being limited to occasional stomach pains.[25] The consumption of large doses (amounts not specified) were noted by early eclectic physicians to cause: severe 'bursting' frontal headaches, sensory and circulatory depression.[1] Given the lack of long-term toxicity studies, treatment should be limited to 6 months.[25]

CAUTIONS/CONTRAINDICATIONS
Cimicifuga racemosa should be avoided in pregnancy and lactation.[12,29]

DRUG INTERACTIONS
No cases of drug interactions could be found for this plant.[25]

DOSAGE REGIMENS
❖ DRIED ROOT: 40-200 mg taken by decoction or as a solid dose daily.[29]
❖ EXTRACT (40-60% alcohol): equivalent to 40 mg of herb daily.[25]
❖ TINCTURE (1:10 in 60% ethanol): 0.4-2mL daily.[29]
   Note: In the case of menopause treatment, the onset of action of this plant can take up to 2 weeks to occur.

Burdock

Arctium lappa L.

THUMBNAIL SKETCH

Common Uses
- ❖ *Internal:* Skin Conditions and Rheumatic Conditions (resulting from 'toxins')
- ❖ *External:* Eczema and Skin Ulcers

Active Constituents
- ❖ Inulin
- ❖ Polyacetylenes
- ❖ Volatile Oil
- ❖ Arctiopicrin

Adverse Effects
- ❖ Temporary worsening of symptoms

Cautions/Contraindications
- ❖ Pregnancy
- ❖ Diabetes

Drug Interactions
- ❖ Oral Hypoglycemic Agents (possible)

Doses
Internal
- ❖ *Dried Root:* 2-6 g of dried root, or decoction, three times daily
- ❖ *Liquid Extract* (1:1 in 25% alcohol): 2-6 mL three times daily
- ❖ *Tincture* (1:10 in 45% alcohol): 8-12 mL of tincture three times daily
- ❖ *Decoction:* 1 part in 20, 500 mL per day

External
- ❖ An infusion or tincture (1:5, 25% alcohol) of the leaf can be used externally as a poultice

Introduction

Family
❖ Asteraceae (also known as Compositae)

Synonyms
❖ Great burdock
❖ Bardane
❖ Begger's buttons
❖ Thorny burr
❖ Bardana
❖ Gobo
❖ Lappa
❖ Edible burdock[1-3]

Medicinal Forms
❖ Dried Root
❖ Extract
❖ Tincture
❖ Decoction
❖ Infusion

Description
Burdock is a biennial plant, native to both Asia and Europe, but now naturalized across North America.[4] The stems grow to 1.5 meters or 5 feet, with oblong leaves, reddish flower heads, and hooked bracts or burrs. The root is white inside and becomes soft and sweet with chewing, with a mucilage-like texture.

Parts Used
While the root is the primary part used therapeutically, the leaves and seeds are also said to have medicinal properties. The roots are more favored in the Western herbal tradition, but the seeds are often used in traditional Asian medicine.[2]

Traditional Use
Within Western herbalism, burdock is considered an important alterative herb (an agent capable of favorably altering unhealthy conditions of the body and tending to restore normal function). In Western and Chinese herbalism, burdock was used as a detoxifying agent to 'cleanse' the blood, removing toxins from the body. Consequently, it was used, internally and externally, for many conditions of the skin, such as acne, boils, abscesses, and eczema, and for situations of chronic inflammation, such as rheumatism and gout.[2]

Current Medicinal Use
Based on traditional evidence, burdock is primarily used in treating chronic skin diseases (eczema and ulcers), rheumatic ailments and infections.

Relevant Research

Preventative and Therapeutic Uses

CONSTITUENTS

Root [2-7]
❖ CARBOHYDRATES: inulin (up to 50%), mucilage, and pectin.
❖ POLYACETYLENES: notably sulfur containing thiophenes.
❖ VOLATILE ACIDS: including acetic acid, propionic acid, butyric acids, and isovaleric acids.
❖ POLYPHENOLIC ACIDS: caffeic acid, chlorogenic acid.
❖ ALDEHYDES: including acetaldhyde, benzaldehyde, and valeraldehyde.
❖ MISCELLANEOUS: arctiopicrin (sesquiterpene lactone), tannin, 'bitters' (lappatin), quercetin (flavonoid), kaempferol (flavonoid).

Leaves [3,4,7]
❖ TERPENOIDS, including arctiopicrin, sterols and triterpenols.
❖ MISCELLANEOUS: mucilage, essential oil, tannins, inulin.

Seeds [2,3]
❖ FLAVONOIDS, essential oil, fixed oils.

TRADITIONAL USES

Burdock root is reputed to be alterative,[1-3,8] diaphoretic,[3,8,9] diuretic,[1-3,8,9] anti-microbial,[1,3,8] antipyretic,[3] anti-tumor,[3] and a mild laxative.[2] Oral consumption is considered useful in the management of many conditions, including chronic skin diseases,[2,3,8] rheumatic conditions,[1-3,8] and infections.[2,3,8] Externally, it is used in the treatment of skin conditions such as eczema and skin ulcers.[3]

ANTI-BACTERIAL EFFECTS

Extracts of the leaves, flowers and roots have all been shown to possess anti-bacterial activity. The leaves are reported to be active against both gram negative and positive bacteria, while the flowers and roots are active only against gram negative bacteria.[10] In addition, arctiopicrin has been shown to have an anti-microbial action against gram negative bacteria.[6,11] The clinical relevance of this anti-microbial action is questionable since the constituents thought to be responsible for this action are not normally found in the dried commercial herb.[5]

MISCELLANEOUS

Bever et al. demonstrated that extracts of *Arctium lappa* root could produce a "pronounced and long lasting decrease in blood sugar" when administered to rats. It also improved carbohydrate tolerance with negligible toxicity. The constituent(s) responsible for this action is/are unknown.[6]

Dietary fiber extracted from the traditional Japanese food "gobo" (burdock root) and added to the basal diet of rats (5%) was shown to protect against the toxic effects of various food colorings (erthrosine, tartrazine, indigo carmine, new coccine, and brilliant blue).[12]

A desmutagenic factor has been isolated from burdock juice.[13] Other investigators have also noted this antimutagenic potential.[3,5]

ADVERSE EFFECTS

A well-publicized instance of poisoning in a 26-year-old woman has been reported. She consumed 'burdock tea' purchased in local health-food store and presented to the emergency room suffering from symptoms characteristic of atropine poisoning (i.e., blurred vision, inability to void, rapid pulse, dry mouth and 'bizarre' behavior). Since tropane alkaloids (like atropine) are not normally found in burdock root, the product was analyzed and was found to contain an atropine concentration of 300 mg/g. It was assumed that the plant had been adulterated with a member of the Nightshade family, probably deadly nightshade (*Atropa belladonna* L. Solanaceae).[5,14,15] Unfortunately, this appears not to be an isolated example, with other instances of probable atropine adulteration being noted.[16,17] This is often cited as a example of the poor quality control surrounding herbal medicines and the need for stricter guidelines.[3,5]

Three cases of contact irritation (1 adolescent and 2 adults) have been noted following the application of medicinal plasters containing burdock root.[18] There is no clinical evidence to suggest that the preparation made from the leaves will cause a similar problem.[3] However, some sesquiterpene lactones are known to be allergenic and some polyacetylenes and thiophenes are known to be photosensitizers. Thus there is a potential for skin irritation with plant parts containing these compounds, especially in the case of presensitized individuals or with inappropriate use (e.g., too concentrated, too long, too frequent exposure or sun exposure soon after use).[19]

While little information is available, concerns have been raised regarding burdock's pronounced 'detoxifying' action. It has been noted that by treating these 'toxic' states, the symptoms of the conditions being treated may worsen temporarily causing undue distress to the patient.[2]

Burdock root has been shown to possess no carcinogenic potential in mice even when given for a prolonged time at a high dose.[20]

CAUTIONS/CONTRAINDICATIONS

Given the hypoglycemic nature shown in animal studies,[6] caution should be used in cases of diabetes.[5]

An extensive review article suggested that burdock possesses uterine stimulant properties,[21] and thus it should be contraindicated during pregnancy and lactation.[3,5]

DRUG INTERACTIONS

While no instance of a drug interaction could be found, given this plant's influence on blood sugar levels concerns have been raised over concomitant use with oral hypoglycemic agents.[5]

DOSAGE REGIMENS [3,5,7]

Internal

❖ DRIED ROOT: 2-6 g of dried root, or decoction, three times daily.

❖ LIQUID EXTRACT (1:1 in 25% alcohol): 2-6 mL three times daily.

❖ TINCTURE (1:10 in 45% alcohol): 8-12 mL of tincture three times daily.

❖ DECOCTION: 1 part in 20, 500 mL per day.

External

An infusion or tincture (1:5, 25% alcohol) of the leaf can be used externally as a poultice.

Calendula

Calendula officinalis L.

Common Uses
- ❖ *External:* Skin Abrasions, Minor Burns, Wounds
- ❖ *Internal:* Digestive Irritation (minor)

Active Constituents
- ❖ Flavonoids
- ❖ Volatile Oil
- ❖ Terpenoids

Adverse Effects
- ❖ Contact Dermatitis (possibly)

Cautions/Contraindications
- ❖ Pregnancy
- ❖ Allergies to plants in the Asteraceae (Compositae) family

Drug Interactions
- ❖ None noted

Doses

Internal
- ❖ *Dried Florets:* 1-4g three times daily (as an infusion)
- ❖ *Liquid Extract* (1:1 in 40% alcohol): 0.5-1 mL three times daily
- ❖ *Tincture* (1:5; 90% alcohol): 0.3-1.2 mL three times daily

External
- ❖ 1-2 teaspoonfuls of dried florets steeped in 240 mL of boiling water for 10 minutes and allowed to cool can be used as a gargle or used to treat skin conditions.

Formulas: Calendula is often combined with other vulnerary herbs such as *Symphytum officinale* L., *Boraginaceae* (Comfrey), *Matricaria recutita* L., *Asteraceae* (German Chamomile) or *Echinacea spp.*, Asteaceae (Coneflower), and may also be used in combination with phytomedicines with a reported anti-microbial action such as *Hydrastis canadensis* L. and Ranunculaceae (Goldenseal).

Introduction

Family
❖ Asteraceae (also known as Compositae)

Synonyms
❖ Gold-bloom
❖ Marigold
❖ Marybud
❖ Pot marigold
❖ Holigold
❖ Mary bud[1-5]

Medicinal Forms
❖ Dried florets
❖ Tincture
❖ Extract

Calendula is also available, either alone or in combination, as many different dosage forms, including vaginal suppositories, creams, salves, tooth pastes and cosmetics.

Description
Calendula is a common garden annual with hairy stem and leaves which stands 30-60 centimeters or 1 to 2 feet high and is easily recognizable by its brilliant orange single flowers with multiple daisy-like florets.[4,6] While native to Egypt, the Middle East and Mediterranean Europe, it can now be found throughout the world.[1,6] The attractive flowers are highly prized by horticulturists and landscapers and often form the center piece in ornamental gardens.[6] Since the flowers are edible, it is also often found in culinary gardens.[1] It is important to note that this plant is distinct from members of the *Tagetes* genus, which are also commonly referred to as Marigolds.[4]

Parts Used
While the leaves and whole aerial part of the plant can be used medicinally,[1] the whole flowers and petals (actually florets) are most commonly used.[6]

Traditional Use
Calendula is one of the best-known plants in Western herbal medicine and has enjoyed a long medicinal history dating back to the early cultures of the Middle East and Indian sub-continent. Its colorful flowers were thought to lift spirits and encourage cheerfulness.[7] Calendula has been used as a cleansing and detoxifying herb. Creams, salves and plasters were and are still used to treat skin conditions and promote wound healing. The flowers are edible and are often added to salads or made into teas and cordials.[1]

Current Medicinal Use
Animal studies have found that calendula has anti-inflammatory, anti-viral, and anti-bacterial properties. As with traditional uses, calendula products are primarily used externally as creams, gels and even as a mouthwash in managing superficial wounds, minor scalds, skin abrasions, mouth sores and mucosal irritations.

Relevant Research

Preventative and Therapeutic Uses

CONSTITUENTS [2-5,8-10]

❖ TERPENOIDS: lupeol, taraxerol, taraxasterol, faradiol, saponins, volatile oil component, campesterol, stigmasterol.
❖ FLAVONOIDS: rutinoside, rutin, isoquercetin, narcissin, neohesperoside.
❖ POLYSACCHARIDES: rhamnoarabinogalactan, arabinogalactans.
❖ MISCELLANEOUS: bitter prinicple called loiliolide (calendin), carotenoid pigments (beta carotene, lycopene, violaxanthin).

ANTI-INFLAMMATORY EFFECTS

Calendula has been reported to have anti-inflammatory properties.[8,11-14] Following topical application both the triterpene[8,12] and flavonoid[13] fractions have been shown to possess an anti-inflammatory action *in vivo*. The most pronounced effect has been noted with the faridol esters extracted from the essential oil.[12] In addition, it has been suggested that the anti-inflammatory action of the isorhamnetin flavonoid glycosides is due to an inhibition of lipoxygenase activity.[13]

Physiological regeneration and epithelization have been noted following topical application of calendula to surgically induced wounds in an animal study. It is thought to act by increasing the metabolism of various proteins during the regenerative phase.[2]

MISCELLANEOUS EFFECTS

As has been seen in other plants, the high-density polysaccharides are reported to have immunostimulant properties *in vitro*.[15] The clinical relevance of the consumption of high alcohol content calendula products has been questioned, since these constituents are predominately water soluble.[1] In addition, calendula has been reported to have anti-bacterial[1,14,16] and anti-viral activity.[14]

Calendula extracts have a reputation in France of having anti-neoplastic effects. Calendula extracts (made from various parts of *Calendula off.*) have been shown to possess *in vitro* cytotoxicity and *in vivo* anti-tumoral activity. These actions appear not to be parallel since the saponin rich extract which exerted the most pronounced anti-tumor activity showed only weak cytotoxic potential.[14]

A related species, *Calendula arvensis* L., has been shown to have molluscicidal activity,[17,18] and is suggested to be potentially useful in killing the snail vector of schistosomiasis.[17]

EXTERNAL USES

Salves or diluted tinctures are reported to be useful in the management of superficial wounds, minor scalds and skin abrasions.[6,7,19-22] Calendula is also used as a gargle or mouthwash for mouth sores and mucosal irritation.[6,19] Due to its astringent properties calendula has been used to stop bleeding and 'dry' discharges.[6] Calendula has also been suggested in the treatment of fungal vaginal infections.[6,20]

No information could be found regarding attempts at clinical evaluation of these indications. In one case, the addition of a compound herbal product to 0.5% hydrocortisone decreased the healing times of abraded skin when compared to hydrocortisone alone. The clinical relevance of this with regard to calendula in particular is slight since the compound product used contained other phytomedicines with known vulnerary properties.[5]

The product Unguentum lymphaticum®, regarded as being useful in the management of lymphedema, was evaluated for efficacy in rats with induced acute lymphedema. Moderate relief was noted only in edema occurring in the animal's legs.[23] Again since this is a combination herbal product, clinical relevance to the specific action of calendula is unknown.

INTERNAL USES

Calendula has been used in the management of indigestion and in the treatment of gastritis and other situations of digestive irritation.[6,7,20] Calendula is also considered to be an emmenagogue and is used in the treatment of delayed menstruation and dysmenorrhea.[7,20] However, no evidence could be found to support these claims.

ADVERSE EFFECTS

One study documents allergic responses, normally manifested as contact dermatitis, to members of the Asteraceae (or Compositae) family including calendula.[24] The relevance of this to internally ingested supplements is unknown.

CAUTIONS/CONTRAINDICATIONS
While no instances of allergic reactions could be found, it should be noted that other members of the Asteraceae family (e.g., calendula, German chamomile, feverfew) have been shown to have allergic potential.[25] Calendula should be used with caution in pregnancy due to a reputed action on the menstrual cycle.[2]

DRUG INTERACTIONS
None reported; however, calendula has been noted to extend the duration of action of hexobarbitol in rats.[1] The implication to pharmacy practice is unknown.

DOSAGE REGIMENS
Internal
❖ DRIED FLORETS: 1-4 g (infusion) three times daily.[2]
❖ TINCTURE (1:5, 90% alcohol): 0.3-1.2 mL three times daily.[2]
❖ LIQUID EXTRACT (1:1 in 40% alcohol): 0.5-1.0 mL three times daily.[2]

External
1 to 2 teaspoonfuls of dried florets steeped in 240 mL of boiling water for 10 minutes and allowed to cool can be used as a gargle or used to treat skin conditions.[20]

Formulas
Calendula is often combined with other vulnerary herbs such as *Symphytum officinale* L., Boraginaceae (Comfrey), *Matricaria recutita* L., Asteraceae (German Chamomile) or *Echinacea* spp., Asteaceae (Coneflower). It may also be used in combination with phytomedicines with a reported anti-microbial action such as *Hydrastis canadensis* L., Ranunculaceae (Goldenseal).

Capsicum

Capsicum annuum L.

THUMBNAIL SKETCH

Common Uses
- *External:* Diabetic Neuropathy, Post-Herpetic Neuralgia, Other Painful Conditions
- *Internal:* Digestive Tonic, Cardiovascular Tonic

Active Constituents
- Capsaicinoids (especially capsaicin)

Adverse Effects
- Redness and Burning Sensation (at site of topical application)
- Allergy (rare)

Cautions/Contraindications
- *External:* Known allergy
- *Internal:* Severe Hypertension, Acute Gastric Irritation, Pregnancy and Lactation

Drug Interactions
- May influence the hepatic metabolism of some drugs; caution in concomitant use of MAOIs and anti-hypertensives

Doses
Internal
- *Dried Herb:* 30-120 mg three times daily
- *Capsicum Tincture* (BPC 1986): 0.3 to 1 mL daily

External
- *Diabetic Neuropathy:* 0.075% capsaicin cream/ointment applied four times daily
- *Post-Herpetic Neuralgia:* 0.025% capsaicin cream/ointment applied four times daily

Note: Capsicum is found in a variety of commercial external analgesic preparations.

Introduction

Family
* Solanaceae

Synonyms
* Chili pepper
* Red pepper
* Cayenne pepper
* Tobasco pepper
* Hot pepper[1-3]

Medicinal Forms
* Dried Herb (fruit and seeds)
* Tincture
* Cream and Ointment

Description

Recognized world wide for its pungency, capsicum may have been cultivated as early as 7000 BC in Mexico and Peru.[4] This perennial shrub grows to 3 feet or 1 meter in height, with bright red oblong fruit, approximately 10 centimeters or 4 inches long, filled with white seeds. While there are over 50 species of capsicum, the common sweet red, green, yellow, and orange peppers, as well as paprika, and numerous types of chili peppers are all now considered to be varieties of the same species.[5]

Parts Used

The dried fruit and seeds are used medicinally.

Traditional Use

Capsicum is one the oldest and most widely used spices in the world. One author estimates that approximately 25% of the world's population uses capsicum on a daily basis.[6]

The spice itself has enjoyed a long history in many healing disciplines. Historically, it was used as a stimulant to the whole body, and thought to aid digestion, the nervous system and circulation.[7,8] During the early part of the last century, it was a key herbal remedy used by the Thomsonian practitioners of North America. Within this 'heroic' school of medicine, the aim was to stimulate the 'vital energy' and expel pathogenic factors by inducing a 'therapeutic' fever.[7] In addition, capsaicin, the main active ingredient in capsicum, has been used for a variety of medicinal purposes, most often pain relief. 'Red hot peppers' are also have many culinary uses.

Current Medicinal Use

While capsicum is used for a number of conditions, its most common current use is topically for diabetic neuropathy, post-herpetic neuralgia and other painful conditions, such as rheumatoid arthritis and osteoarthritis. There are a number of excellent reviews on capsicum.[9-13]

Relevant Research

Preventative and Therapeutic Effects

CONSTITUENTS [2, 3,14,15]

* CAPSAICINOIDS: capsaicin, dihydrocapsaicin, nordihydrocapsaicin, homocapsaicin, homodihydrocapsaicin.
* CAROTENOIDS: lutein, carotein, capsanthin.
* VITAMINS: A and C.

Notes: The nomenclature associated with capsicum is somewhat confusing. Capsicum is generally defined as the dried, ripe fruit of *Capsicum annuum* L. and a large number of varieties and hybrids of this.[1, 4] In contrast, 'capsaicin' is a compound purified from these species — Chemical

Abstracts (CAS) registry #404-86-4, under the name: N-[(4-hydroxy-3-methoxyphenyl)-methyl]-8-methyl-(E)-6-nonenamide. There are two possible stereoisomers of capsaicin, but only the *trans* isomer exists in nature. The *cis* isomer, civamide, is assigned a separate CAS registry number. To complicate matters even further, a third compound often called "synthetic capsaicin" has been synthesized and is often found as an adulterant in products labelled capsaicin. "Synthetic capsaicin" does not have the same chemical formula as either capsaicin or civamide and should not be used in their place. The official name of this adulterant is nonivamide, but it has also been called pelargonic acid vanillylamide. Nonivamide has never been found in capsicum fruit extracts.[4] Because of wide-spread misrepresentation and adulteration of capsaicin products with nonivamide, efficient analytic systems have now been developed to unambiguously distinguish between the two.[16-22] The active constituents of capsicum are considered to be the capsaicinoids.[14,15] Of these, capsaicin is by far the most important.

ANALGESIC EFFECTS

Diabetic Neuropathy

The use of topical applications of capsaicin for the relief of diabetic neuropathy has been extensively studied.[23-29] The formation of The Capsaicin Study Group has resulted in numerous high-quality clinical trials.[24-26] Most studies have employed topical capsaicin 0.075% in a cream base and have concluded that capsaicin is a safe and effective treatment for painful diabetic neuropathy. For example, one 8-week, double-blind, vehicle-controlled study of 0.075% capsaicin cream (Axsain®) applied four times daily by 54 patients with moderate to severe diabetic neuropathy showed symptom improvement in 90% of capsaicin-treated patients, which was significantly better than the control group.[27] A variety of other trials using the same protocol (0.075% capsaicin cream applied four times daily) have confirmed that capsaicin 0.075% cream was more effective than a vehicle control.[24-26, 28-30] This literature review found only one published negative trial with capsaicin.[31]

Post-Herpetic Neuralgia

A lower strength (0.025%) of capsaicin is used for the treatment of post-herpetic neuralgia than for diabetic neuropathy (0.075%). In an uncontrolled study of 33 patients, 55% of the patients completing the study reported good or excellent pain relief; however, burning sensation after the application of capsaicin was so severe in one-third of the patients that the trial was discontinued prematurely.[32] A large (n=208) open-labelled, uncontrolled trial concluded that topical capsaicin was a promising new treatment for post-herpetic neuralgia. This supports the conclusions of several earlier studies.[33] This supports the conclusions of several earlier studies.[34-37] However, the percentage of patients with substantial pain relief varied from 39% to 75%.[35] This variation may be due to different treatment schedules: Watson et al., used capsaicin 0.025% four times daily, while Bernstein et al. asked patients to apply capsaicin 0.025% five times daily for 1 week, followed by three times daily for an additional 3 weeks. Another study using a 5 times daily treatment regimen, but a 0.001% capsaicin cream reported moderate pain relief in 62% of patients with post-herpetic neuralgia.[38] In addition, a case report suggests the use of topical capsaicin (0.025% — Zostrix ®) in the mouth may be an effective treatment for post-herpetic vesicles in the oral cavity. One episode of xerostomia (dry mouth) forced the discontinuation of therapy for one day only.[39] The signature burning sensation of capsaicin makes it very difficult to maintain a blinded trial; thus to date, these findings have not been confirmed by a randomized, double-blind, controlled trial.

MISCELLANEOUS PAIN INDICATIONS

Capsaicin cream has reportedly been effective in the treatment of Post-mastectomy Pain Syndrome;[40-41] rheumatoid arthritis;[42] osteoarthritis;[42-43] cluster headaches;[44-45] reflex sympathetic dystrophy;[46] relief of local stump pain;[47] idiopathic trigeminal neuralgia;[48] relief of sores of oral mucositis caused by chemotherapy or radiation;[49] pain caused by Guillain-Barre syndrome;[50] and painful psoriasis vulgaris.[51] Capsicum plasters applied topically were found to relieve non-specific low back pain,[52] and, when applied at the Korean hand acupuncture point (K-D2) or the Chinese acupuncture point Pericardium 6 (P6), to reduce postoperative nausea and vomiting after abdominal hysterectomy.[53]

MECHANISM OF ACTION

Capsaicin depletes substance P (SP), a substance that mediates pain transmission from the peripheral nerves to the spinal cord.[1,54] It does this via four stages: (1) SP is immediately released from both central and peripheral terminals; (2) SP fibers are functionally impaired; (3) the axoplasmic transport of SP is inhibited; and (4) SP is depleted (this starts after 1 day and may last for weeks).[55] Although generally believed to be specific for type C nociceptive neurons (i.e., unmyelinated, slow-conducting fibers that transmit cutaneous pain information to the central nervous system),[56,57] other research suggests that capsaicin causes damage to all unmyelinated sensory fibers.[58] Myelinated fibers of the A delta category may also be damaged with high doses of capsaicin.[58] It has been suggested that capsaicin may be a useful neurochemical tool for research into the interaction of sensory neurons with other neuronal systems. Excellent reviews of capsaicin's action on a variety of systems, including the gastro-intestinal, thermoregulatory, cardiovascular, respiratory and nervous systems, have been published.[59-69]

MISCELLANEOUS EFFECTS

Oral administration of capsicum has been shown to inhibit the rise of cholesterol in the liver and increase the fecal excretion of both cholesterol and bile acids in rats.[70] Administration of capsaicin did not effect serum levels of cholesterol; however, it did appear to stimulate lipid mobilization from adipose tissue and it lowered the serum trigylceride concentration in lard-fed rats.[71]

A randomized, placebo-controlled, double-blinded study (n=30) found that ingestion of red pepper powder (obtained by grinding the dried fruit of *Capsicum annuum*) was more effective than placebo in decreasing the intensity of dyspeptic symptoms.[72] Participants in the study were asked to take capsules of study drug 15 minutes before each meal: 1 capsule (500 mg) before breakfast, two capsules before lunch and two capsules before dinner for five weeks. Overall symptom scores, as well as epigastric pain, fullness and nausea scores, of the red pepper group were significantly lower than the scores from the placebo group starting from the third week of treatment.

ADVERSE EFFECTS

Capsicum

TOPICAL ❖ Allergic contact dermatitis has been reported.[73, 74]

INTERNAL ❖ Sweating (generally confined to the head and neck), flushing of the face and upper body, salivation, lacrimation, nasal secretion.[54] In addition, the principle agents in capsicum can be very irritating to the mucosal membranes,[3, 75, 76] and these effects are used in the self-defence protect commonly known as 'pepper' spray.[75] A toxicity study of chronic administration of capsicum extract to hamsters reported decreased vitamin A levels in liver tissue and eye toxicity including: a focal increase in corneal epithelial cells, and hyalinisation and thickening of the substantia propria in the eyeballs.[77] No similar effects have ever been reported in humans. Other effects which have been reported in humans include: increased fibrinolytic activity and hypocoagulability of blood.[78] However, these effects have been reported after ingestion of capsicum in the diet, as opposed to medicinal effects.

Capsaicin

TOPICAL ❖ Erythema; burning and stinging sensations (no vesication) common at both the 0.025%[32] and 0.075% concentrations when applied topically, but the intensity is diminished for most patients with continued use (i.e., after 2 weeks); some dry skin.[24-28,32,34,35,59,79,80] Also, inhalation reactions (coughing, sneezing) occurred occasionally.[24, 27] Capsaicin is generally considered to be safe. No changes in cutaneous sensation of temperature or vibration were noted after administration of 0.075% capsaicin four times daily for up to 32 weeks continuously.[25,81,82]

INTERNAL ❖ Increased gastric acid concentration is possible;[83] however, two other studies found no increase in gastric acid secretion.[84,85] *In vitro* experiments suggest that capsaicin is a potent inhibitor of platelet aggregation.[86] Ingestion of large doses has been associated with necrosis, ulceration and even carcinogenesis; however, small amounts appear to have few deleterious effects.[87]

CAUTIONS/CONTRAINDICATIONS

TOPICAL ❖ Known allergy.

INTERNAL ❖ Contraindicated in cases of severe hypertension,[7] and caution should be used in situations of acute gastric irritation.[3,7] During pregnancy capsicum should not be used at doses exceeding normal dietary levels.[3] Although not used medicinally, the leaves and stems of capsicum have been shown to be uterine stimulants in animal studies.[88] In addition, caution is recommended during lactation (due to the pungency of capsicum).[3]

DRUG INTERACTIONS

No specific drug interactions appear to have been reported in the literature; however, since high doses of capsicum have been shown to increase the activity of two hepatic enzymes in rats (glucose-6-phosphate dehydrogenase and adipose lipoprotein lipase),[71] the hepatic metabolism of some drugs may be affected.[3] In addition, since catecholamine amine secretion is increased, caution is suggested with concommitant use of monoamine oxidase inhibitors (MAOIs) and anti-hypertensives.[3]

DOSAGE REGIMENS

External

❖ DIABETIC NEUROPATHY: 0.075% capsaicin cream/ointment applied four times daily.

❖ POST-HERPETIC NEURALGIA: 0.025% capsaicin cream/ointment applied four times daily.

Internal

❖ DRIED FRUIT: 30-120 mg three times daily.[3]

❖ CAPSICUM TINCTURE (BPC 1986): 0.3-1.0 mL daily.[3]

Note: Capsicum is found in a variety of commercial external analgesic preparations, including Heet lotion, Infra-Rub ointment, Sloan's liniment, Zostrix, Zostrix-HP and Axsain.

Cat's Claw

Uncaria tomentosa (Willd. Ex Roem.& Schult) DC
or *Uncaria guianensis* (Aubl.) J.F. Gmel.

THUMBNAIL SKETCH

Common Uses
❖ Gastrointestinal Disorders
❖ Rheumatism
❖ Inflammatory Conditions

Active Constituents
❖ Oxindole Alkaloids
❖ Glycosides

Adverse Effects
❖ None noted

Cautions/Contraindications
❖ Immuno-compromised Patients
❖ Pregnancy and Lactation
❖ Hemophiliacs (undergoing certain treatments)

Drug Interactions
❖ HIV (AZT) and Cancer Medications
❖ Warfarin
❖ Caution with various hormone or immunoglobulin based therapies

Doses
❖ *Standardized Extract* (4:1): 20-60 mg daily
❖ *Decoction* (20g of root bark/liter): 60 mL diluted with 60 mL of hot water daily

Note: Concerns exist about the quality of some North American standardized extracts. Consumers should be extra cautious when selecting cat's claw products.

Introduction

Description

Members of the genus *Uncaria* are found throughout tropical forests in Asia, Africa, South America and Central America.[6] The common name, cat's claw, comes from the curved thorns or 'hooks' used by the plant to fasten itself onto supporting plants.[2] The species found in South America are woody climbing vines, growing up to 100 feet or 30 meters. While many South American plants are referred to as Una de Gato, the species *Uncaria tomentosa* (Willd. Ex Roem.& Schult) DC or *Uncaria guianensis* (Aubl.) J.F. Gmel. are the ones primarily used medicinally.[7] These species are often considered to have identical therapeutic indications.[1,2] They are also very similar in appearance with only slight differences in the presentation of the leaves and the hooks.[7] To further complicate matters, two different forms or phenotypes of *Uncaria tomentosa* exist, which can lead to confusion over appropriate harvesting of the plant.[8] In addition, some of the active constituents found in one phenotype often have the opposite effects to those found in the other.[8]

Parts Used

While the leaves are used by traditional healers, the parts primarily used in commercially available medicinal products are the dried inner stem bark or the root.[4,5] It takes from 3 to 8 years for plants to reach a suitable size to harvest.

Traditional Uses

Cat's claw has long been used by the indigenous peoples of South America to treat a wide range of ailments and diseases, including asthma, digestive upset, wound healing, menstrual problems, urinary tract infections, arthritis and other inflammatory conditions.[4,5] The herb has recently gained popularity in North America and Europe. Given this increase in demand, ecological concerns have been raised with regard to the sustainability of the crop.[6] The Peruvian government has recently invested in an extensive planting campaign.[2] Some consider that Una de gato may offer an alternative (and more suitable) crop to the illegal cultivation of 'coca'.[1]

Current Medicinal Use

The current medicinal uses are very similar to the traditional uses. While more research needs to be done, results from clinical studies show that cat's claw may be helpful in treating arthritic conditions.

Relevant Research

Preventative and Therapeutic Effects

CONSTITUENTS [3, 4, 8-13]

❖ OXINDOLE ALKALOIDS (PENTACYCLIC AND TETRACYCLIC): including uncarine F, isopteropodine, pteropodine, isorhynchophylline, rhynchophylline and mitraphylline.

❖ QUINOVIC ACID GLYCOSIDES.

❖ TRITERPENES: including oleanolic acid.

❖ POLYPHENOLS: including catechins, rutin, quercetin.

❖ MISCELLANEOUS: tannins.

The alkaloid content of plants seems to vary appreciably from one year to the next.[9] The oxindole alkaloids are the constituents given the most attention, with either pentacyclic or tetracyclic compounds being present depending on which type, or phenotype, of *Uncaria tomentosa* is used.[8]

COMMON USES

Uncaria tomentosa has been used traditionally in the management of many conditions, notably rheumatism, peptic ulcers, intestinal disorders, certain cancers, asthma, inflammatory conditions and menstrual irregularities.[5-7] North American practitioners and patients have reported relief in cases of diverticulitis, diabetes, gastritis, colic and 'leaky bowel syndrome'.[14]

Extracts of cat's claw and constituents found in the plant have been shown to have immunomodulating anti-inflammatory, anti-oxidant, anti-viral and anti-neoplastic properties.[3-5]

EFFECTS ON THE IMMUNE SYSTEM

The pentacyclic oxindole alkaloids have been shown to increase phagaocytosis and affect the amount of lymphocytes.[15] Extracts made from the stem bark stimulate interleukin 1 and interleukin 6 in animal models.[16] As was mentioned above, the action of the pentacyclic oxindole alkaloids appear to be opposed by the tetracyclic oxindole alkaloids found in the other phenotype of *Uncaria tomentosa*.[17]

The immunomodulating action of cat's claw has been the focus of much research done by European natural health product manufacturers. In one small uncontrolled study of 13 HIV positive individuals who had refused conventional care, participants were given 20 mg of *Uncaria tomentosa* extract (containing 12 mg of pentacyclic oxindole alkaloids per gram) for up to 5 months. While lymphocyte count was increased, no change was seen in total leukocyte count or T4/T8 cell ratio.[17] There is also such evidence from small clinical studies that extracts of cat's claw may normalize CD4 counts and decrease the incidence of opportunistic infections such as herpes and fungal infections in people who are HIV positive.[17]

A commercial cat's claw extract, C-Med-100, has been shown to enhance immune functions in men who had received a 23 valent pneumococcal vaccine.[17, 18]

ANTI-INFLAMMATORY ACTIONS

A number of constituents found in cat's claw have been shown to be anti-inflammatory probably by decreasing the production of substances such as prostaglandins and tumor necrotising factor alpha.[19] This has led to a number of clinical trials exploring its use in conditions such as arthritis. Results from one small (n=45) randomized placebo-controlled trial investigating the effectiveness of a extract of cat's claw in patients with osteoarthritis of the knee reached inconclusive results. Patients were given either a freeze-dried extract of cat's claw or a placebo for 4 weeks, with hematological parameters assessed at the beginning and end of the study. While the cat's claw extract decreased knee pain on movement and the amount of inflammatory mediators in the blood, there was no change in pain at rest or decrease in knee circumference.[20]

Cat's claw may also have some benefits in patients with rheumatoid arthritis. In a small randomized, placebo-controlled trial, 40 patients with active rheumatoid arthritis treated with conventional care (sulfasalazine or hydroxychloroquine) were treated with an extract of the pentacyclic chemotype of *Uncaria tomentosa*. This was a two-phase study conducted over 52 weeks, with patients randomized to either a placebo group or a group given the cat's claw extract in the first phase (first 24 weeks), with all patients receiving the cat's claw extract for the final phase (remaining 28 weeks). Results showed a modest improvement in joint pain and swelling when the patients were taking the cat's claw extract.[21]

Results from a number of other studies of commercial European products investigating the use of this herb in various types of arthritis also appear promising.[3]

ANTI-MUTAGENIC AND ANTI-CANCER ACTIONS

Extracts of cat's claw have been shown to have anti-mutagenic properties in a number of animal models and in humans.[3,16] It is thought that this action may be related to the anti-oxidant constituents.

Extracts made from the bark of *Uncaria tomentosa* have been shown *in vitro* to exert a protective antimutagenic effect against photomutagenesis induced by 8-methoxy-psoralen (8-MOP) plus UVA in S. typhimurium TA 102.[16] One *in vivo* study, demonstrated that the "mutagenic activity of the urine" of an adult male smoker was "dramatically" decreased when the volunteer consumed an aqueous decoction made from the bark of *Uncaria tomentosa*. This decrease in mutagenicity was maintained for eight days after the administration of the decoction ended. The authors of this study suggest that agents found in the extract have an antioxidant effect. In addition, an oxindole alkaloid (uncarine F) has been shown to exert an anti-proliferative effect against leukemic cell lines *in vitro*. The authors of the study suggest that this agent may prove useful in the management of certain acute leukemias.[10]

Results from European research suggest that extracts of cat's claw, when given with conventional chemotherapy, may increase remission amongst certain cancers, decrease side effects of chemotherapy and even decrease tumor size. While at first glance this seems promising, it is important to remember that this information comes from unblinded trials and case studies. More evidence is required before specific recommendations can be made.[3, 4]

MISCELLANEOUS EFFECTS

Glycosides extracted from the bark of *Uncaria tomentosa* have also been shown to possess anti-viral properties (against vesicular stomatitis virus) *in vitro*.[11]

ADVERSE EFFECTS

Results from bioassays and clinical trials using cat's claw show that the herb appears to be unlikely to cause problems; however, concerns still exist with regards to safety.[3, 22] One report of acute renal failure in a 35 year old Peruvian woman with systemic lupus erythematosus taking a cat's claw product has been documented.[23] In this case it is important to note that the patient was taking a number of conventional drugs and that no attempt was taken to authenticate the herbal product. A potentially important factor given the difficulty in selecting the correct plant.[24]

Like other herbs with a high tannin content, cat's claw may affect the kidneys and liver or irritate the gastrointestinal tract.[25]

CAUTIONS/CONTRAINDICATIONS

Many of the plants commonly referred to as Una de Gato are considered poisonous. The herb should not be taken for serious conditions such as HIV and cancer unless under the supervision of an appropriately trained healthcare provider.[26]

Cat's claw products should be avoided in transplant patients undergoing immunosuppressive therapy.[4] Until more is known, cat's claw should not be taken during pregnancy and lactation, by women wishing to conceive, and children under 3 years of age.[3, 4] The fact that therapeutic action varies between the various forms of cat's claw, product quality issues and potential adulteration problems are concerns for cat's claw products.[26]

A patent for an Austrian product suggests that hemophiliacs receiving fresh blood plasma or therapy with cryoprecipitates should avoid concurrent use of *Uncaria tomentosa*.[7]

DRUG INTERACTIONS
Cat's claw products have been shown to interact with certain medications taken to manage HIV, such as AZT, and cancer. These interactions may be beneficial as noted above. Cat's claw products should be avoided in patients taking warfarin.[26] Due to its effect on the immune system, patients taking immunosuppressive drugs should avoid cat's claw products.[4]

European manufacturers caution against concurrent use with passive vaccines composed of animal sera, intravenous hyperimmunoglobulin therapy, insulin and "other hormone products." The rational behind these concerns could not be found.[7]

DOSAGE REGIMENS
Recommended doses for cat's claw vary depending on the source and condition being treated. Though no specific dosage regimen could be found, a hydroalcoholic tincture (50% water/alcohol) has been proposed as the most effective dosage form because of the increased alkaloid content.[7] Dosage suggestions include:

❖ STANDARDIZED EXTRACT (4:1): 20-60mg daily.[3]

❖ DECOCTION (20g of root bark/L): 60mL diluted with 60mL hot water daily.[3]

❖ DRIED HERB: 3-6 grams of 'herb' taken daily in divided doses as a tea, increasing to 20 grams in advanced diseases.

Note: Concerns have recently been raised about the quality of 'standardized' cat's claw products on the North American market. This, given the challenges faced in harvesting the correct plant, means that consumers should be extra cautious when selecting cat's claw products.[17]

Chamomile (German)

Matricaria recutita L.

Common Uses
Internal
- ❖ Gastrointestinal Discomfort, Peptic Ulcer, Gastritis, Indigestion, Diarrhea
- ❖ Insomnia and Anxiety (mild)
- ❖ Pediatric Colic and Teething

External
- ❖ Inflammatory Skin Conditions
- ❖ Canker Sores and Irritation of the Gums and Mouth

Active Constituents
- ❖ Volatile Oil (chamazulene, (-)a-bisabolol, spiroethers)
- ❖ Apigenin and other Flavonoids

Adverse Effects
- ❖ Contact Dermatitis
- ❖ Vomiting (in very high doses)

Cautions/Contraindications
- ❖ Individuals with a known allergy to members of the Sunflower (Compositae/Asteraceae) family.

Drug Interactions
- ❖ None known

Doses
Internal
- ❖ *Dried Flowers* (usually as an infusion/tea): 2-4 g three times daily
- ❖ *Liquid Extract* (1:1 in 45% ethanol): 1-4 mL three times daily
- ❖ *Tincture* (1:5 in 45% ethanol): 3-10 mL three times daily

External
- ❖ Topical preparations are usually 3-10% w/w of chamomile

Introduction

Family
- Asteraceae (also known as Compositae)

Synonyms
- *Matricaria chamomilla* L.
- Single chamomile
- Hungarian chamomile
- PinHeads
- Matricaria
- Wild chamomile
- Sweet false chamomile[1-5]

Medicinal Forms
- Infusion
- Extract
- Tincture
- Dried Flower Heads

Description

German chamomile is one of two species of chamomile commonly used medicinally, the other being Roman or English Chamomile (*Chamaemelum nobile* (L.) All.). The primary indications of both are similar, even though the constituents are slightly different. Outside of the United Kingdom, German chamomile is the species that has been both evaluated most extensively and used therapeutically.[6]

German chamomile is a relatively small fragrant annual herb, 60 centimeters or 16 inches tall, with a round hollow stem and sharply cut leaves, native to most of Europe and Western Asia and naturalized throughout North America.[4] As a commercially viable crop, more than 4000 tons of the chamomile are produced annually,[5,7] mainly in Eastern Europe, The Balkans and parts of South America.[4] The bulk of this is German chamomile.[5] Most of the cultivated crop is destined for Europe, especially Germany,[5] rather than North America, where the herb has been relegated by the public to the role of a beverage.[8]

Parts Used

The flowers, preferably picked a few days before opening, are the parts used medicinally.[1]

Traditional Use

The fact that the Germans often refer to German chamomile as *'alles zutraut'*, meaning capable of anything, gives some idea of the high regard in which this plant is held.[9,10] Its panacea-like properties and numerous indications have led many people to refer to it rather confusingly as 'European ginseng'. Chamomile tea has been used as a digestive, hypnotic and antispasmodic, finding particular favor in the treatment of children's ailments.[5] It should not be forgotten that chamomile helped Peter Rabbit get over a particularly over-indulgent trip to Farmer McGregor's vegetable garden.[9] It takes a brave skeptic to argue with evidence like that.

Current Medicinal Use

Components of this herb have been shown to have anti-inflammatory, anti-spasmodic, anti-anxiety, and anti-histaminic properties. While what scientific evidence that does exist is promising, most of the supporting evidence for German chamomile comes from its traditional use. Based upon this, German chamomile is used to manage digestive upset (colic, indigestions, gastritis, diarrhea, and peptic ulcer disease), mouth and skin irritations (insect bites, eczema, diaper rash), insomnia and anxiety.

Relevant Research

Preventative and Therapeutic Uses

CONSTITUENTS [1,3,4,7,11]

Flowers

❖ TERPENOIDS: azulene, chamazulene, a-bisabolol, a-bisabololoxide A, B, C, matricin, farnesol.

❖ FLAVONOIDS: apigenin, apiin, luteolin, quercetin, and rutin.

❖ COUMARINS: umbelliferone, herniarin.

❖ MISCELLANEOUS: capric acid, polysaccharides, spiroethers, and tannins.

> *Note:* The yield of the medicinally important volatile oil fraction, rich in terpenoids and spiroethers, is dependent on both the age and locale of the plant.[7] Matricin is converted to chamazulene in the extraction process.[9] While standardization is not universal, German products are normally authenticated by measuring chamazulene and a- bisabolol content.[7,9]

COMPONENT EFFECTS

The medicinal properties of German chamomile may be attributed to several different components.[5,7] While most attention is paid to the volatile oil fraction, it is now becoming increasingly apparent that other constituents have therapeutically useful properties.

Volatile Oil

The constituents of the volatile oil portion are known to have a variety of medicinal properties including anti-inflammatory [5,7,12] and spasmolytic actions.[5,7,13]

(-)-a-bisabolol

(-)-a-bisabolol is reported to be one of the most powerful anti-inflammatory products present in German chamomile oil.[5,7,11,14] This activity is greater than that exerted by a synthetic racemic mixture, (+)a-bisabolol or various bisabololoxides present.[7,11,14] Results from *in vivo* studies suggest an antiulcerogenic action against various noxious substances and traumatic stimuli including indomethacin, stress and ethanol.[5,7,15] It has also been shown to have anti-bacterial and anti-fungal activity.[5,7] An anti-spasmodic property has been demonstrated, which is greater than that of the total oil and equivalent to that of papaverine.[1]

Azulene Component

Azulene components have been shown to possess both anti-allergenic[5,7] and anti-inflammatory properties.[5,7,13] Following oral administration, matricin was shown to exert a more pronounced anti-inflammatory action in the rat paw carrageenin test than either chamazulene or guaiazulene.[5,16] The anti-inflammatory action of chamazulene, but not its precursor matricin, appears to be partly due to inhibition of leukotriene synthesis.[17] In addition, chamazulene appears to have antioxidant properties.[17,18] The hepatoregenerative action of the volatile oil seen in rats is also attributed to the azulene portion.[7]

Cis-spiroethers

Cis-spiroethers have been shown to possess anti-inflammatory[3,7] and anti-spasmodic properties.[12,19] They were shown to have a prolonged spasmolytic action in the digestive tract of mice following oral absorption; however, they were also absorbed into systemic circulation.[19]

Flavonoids

The flavonoid apigenin was shown to have an anti-inflammatory action *in vitro* superior (10x) to matricin, suggesting that the anti-inflammatory action of the whole plant is not solely dependent on the essential oil content.[13] The flavonoids have been shown to have anti-spasmodic activity with apigenin being more potent than papaverine.[12] In addition, recent animal studies have demonstrated that apigenin present in an aqueous extract of German chamomile flower has an affinity for central benzodiazepine receptors, competitively inhibiting the binding of flunitrazepam.[20] It has also been reported that the flavonoids found in German chamomile have anti-histaminic properties.[21]

Polysaccharides
The high molecular weight polysaccharides appear to have immunostimulant properties.[22,23]

Whole Extracts
While the individual agents responsible are as yet unknown, the volatile oil has been shown to decrease uric acid levels *in vivo*.[24] In addition, results from *in vivo* studies show that the essential oil of the herb increases bile secretion and biliary cholesterol concentration.[25] Ethanolic extracts of the German chamomile have also been shown to inhibit the growth of polio and herpes virus *in vitro*.[26]

COMMON USES
Digestive Effect
The most widely accepted use of chamomile is as a digestive aid and carminative. It is considered useful in the management of many gastrointestinal disorders such as: colic, indigestion, gastritis, diarrhea and peptic ulcer disease. This phytomedicine seems particularly suitable when there is an etiology of stress or tension.[9] A commercial product, Kamillosan®, was shown to exert a spasmolytic effect on the smooth musculature of the intestine in isolated guinea pig ileum.[12]

Mouth and Gum Irritations
The treatment of mouth and gum irritation with chamomile mouthwash is an approved indication according to guidelines established by Commission E, a federal German advisory body.[27] It is thought to be effective in the management of minor mucosal irritations.[5,7] In an uncontrolled trial of patients (n=98), chamomile was found to decrease stomatitis resulting from chemotherapy.[28] Unfortunately, these findings were not supported by a later, more sophisticated, double-blind, placebo-controlled trial (n=164) where chamomile mouthwash was shown to be ineffective in decreasing 5-Fluorouracil (5FU) induced stomatitis.[29]

Skin Irritations
The use of chamomile-based products as a topical treatment of many skin conditions, such as insect bites, eczema and diaper rashes, is common place in Europe, especially Germany.[5,9] External application of chamomile has been shown to be effective in decreasing inflammation[7, 30,31] and promoting cellular regeneration.[5] Kamillosan®, a proprietary product containing chamomile, has been shown to aid in the treatment of dermatitis of the lower legs when added to conventional treatment protocols.[5] It has also been used as adjunctive therapy in the management of more serious conditions such as stasis ulcers. Several studies have demonstrated that topically applied extracts of fresh chamomile have greater anti-inflammatory action than those made from the dried flowers.[13,30] The therapeutic action of chamomile may not be limited to the outer layers of skin since *in vivo* studies have shown that the flavonoids applied topically can penetrate to the deeper layers as well.[32]

Insomnia and Anxiety
Chamomile tea is often used to treat insomnia and nervous tension due to its reputed mild hypnotic effect.[5,7,23] A sedative action has been noted during cardiac catheterisation in

humans following oral administration.[5] While a mechanism of action has yet to be determined, as mentioned above certain flavonoids are known to bind to central benzodiazepine receptors. Apigenin has also been reported to exert a distinct anxiolytic action in mice, with a sedative effect being noted at higher doses.[20] Some authors attribute this hypnotic effect to the possible presence of tryptophan in the flowers, a fact that has yet to be substantiated.[5]

ADVERSE EFFECTS

Cases of allergic reactions to chamomile preparations or the plant itself have been widely documented.[5,7,33-40] The vast majority of these are limited to contact skin irritation,[38,40] most commonly amongst people frequently in contact with the fresh plant (i.e., florists and gardeners).[34,38] Two cases of immediate anaphylactic reactions following oral consumption have been noted.[37,39] Even though allergic sensitivity is quite rare, given the possible outcomes it would be prudent to be cautious.[7,33] The sesquiterpene lactones with exocyclic a-methylene rings are considered the constituents primarily responsible for this allergic potential, which is also shown by other members of this family.[5,7,35,41] Contact irritation appears to be more common with topical use of Roman chamomile than German chamomile.[42]

It is important to note that in most cases of allergic reaction to chamomile, including the incidents of anaphylactic reactions, no attempt was made to authenticate the product itself. This has led many to suggest that the vast majority of allergic reactions may be a result of adulteration with other unidentified plants. For example, German chamomile products containing Stinking Dog Fennel (*Anthemis cotula* L.), which has an established allergenic potential, have been sold erroneously under the name of chamomile.[7,35]

Direct adverse reactions to chamomile appear to be very rare.[7] Consumption of large doses has been noted to cause emesis.[3,7,9]

LD_{50} of oral (-)a-bisabolol in rats is 14.85 g/kg and in mice 11.35g/kg[7]

LD_{50} for orally administered chamazulene in rats is 10 g/kg[7]

LD_{50} of oral German chamomile oil in mice is 2.5 mL/kg[25]

LD_{50} of oral German chamomile oil in rats exceeded 5g/kg[43]

CAUTIONS/CONTRAINDICATIONS

Cross-sensitivity is known to exist between different members of the Asteracee (also known as Compositae) family.[7,33-35] Given this, individuals with a known allergy to other members of the Asteraceae/Compositae family (e.g., ragweed, asters, chrysanthemums) should be cautious in taking products containing German chamomile.[3,5,9] Individuals with existing asthma, urticaria or other allergic conditions should also use chamomile products with caution due to a chance of exacerbation of their symptoms.[3]

German chamomile and the constituent (-)a-bisabolol have been shown to have no teratogenic potential in animal studies.[36] Resorption of fetuses and reduction in birth weight were observed in rats given very high doses of German chamomile.[36] However, no specific contraindications or warnings for use in pregnancy or lactation were found in the literature.[9] In addition, no information was found regarding the potential for sensitization of infants when breast-fed by mothers drinking chamomile tea. However, Newall cautions against applying chamomile products to the gums of teething children.[3] While no reason was given, it is assumed that this warning relates to the potential induction of an allergenic response.

DOSAGE REGIMENS

❖ DRIED FLOWER HEADS: 2-4 g three times daily (as an infusion).[1]

❖ LIQUID EXTRACT (1:1 in45% ethanol): 1-4 mL three times daily.[1]

❖ TINCTURE (1:5 in 45% ethanol): 3-10 mL three times daily.[1]

External

Topical preparations are usually 3-10% w/w of chamomile.[1,9]

Infusion

The most popular dosage form of chamomile is an infusion. Instructions for the preparation of an infusion are given below. Since a large proportion of the medicinally active components are contained in the volatile oil, it is important to cover the container while making the infusion.[44]

Pour hot water (150mL) over a heaped tablespoonful of German chamomile flowers (approx. 3 g), cover, and after 5-10 minutes, pass through a tea strainer. Unless otherwise prescribed for gastrointestinal complaints, a cup of the freshly prepared tea is drunk three or four times a day between meals. For inflammation of the mucous membranes of the mouth and throat, use the freshly prepared tea as a wash or gargle.[27]

Note: Since adulteration is common place, attempts should be made to authenticate the source of the plant contained in any product.[7] While not widely available in North America, European products such as Kamillosan® exist that are standardized and authenticated.[5,35]

Chaste Tree
Vitex agnus-castus L.

Common Uses
❖ Premenstrual Syndrome and Menopause Symptoms
❖ Menstrual Cycle Irregularities
❖ Mastodynia (breast pain)
❖ Insufficient Lactation and Hyperprolactinemia (elevated prolactin levels)
❖ Acne (resulting from a hormonal imbalance)

Active Constituents
❖ The action of *Vitex agnus-castus* appears to be determined by a number of different constituents. The iridoid agnuside is often used as a marker molecule to confirm authenticity.

Adverse Effects
❖ Nausea, Headache (rare)
❖ Menstrual Irregularities, Diarrhea, Dyspepsia, Acne, Pruritus

Cautions/Contraindications
❖ Pregnancy
❖ Children

Drug Interactions
❖ Oral Contraceptives and Hormone Replacement Therapy
❖ Interaction (theoretical) with Dopamine Antagonists (such as haloperidol and metoclopramide)

Doses
❖ *Standardized Extract to fruit content* (9g/100 mL): 40 drops daily
❖ *Dried Fruit:* 0.5-1 g three times daily
❖ *Tincture:* 0.2-0.4 mL (1:2) or 3-10 mL (1:5) daily

Note: Agnus-castus may not have an immediate action. Treatment should be uninterrupted and last for several months for most indications.

Introduction

Family
❖ Verbenaceae

Synonyms
❖ Chasteberry

❖ Agnus-castus

❖ Monk's pepper[1]

Medicinal Forms
❖ Dried Fruit
   (berries)

❖ Standardized
   Extract

❖ Tincture

Description
Chaste tree is a deciduous aromatic shrub native to Mediterranean Europe, central Asia and parts of India, but now widely cultivated in sub-tropical regions. The chaste tree grows to 6-7 meters or 20-25 feet, with palm-shaped leaves. Small lilac-like flowers grow in whorls on long spikes and produce purple peppercorn-shaped berries.

Parts Used
The distinctive purple berries are the parts used medicinally.[2]

Traditional Use
Chaste tree has been used since the time of ancient Greece and Rome, where it played a part in religious ceremonies and medicinal practice. It was reputed to decrease libido in women and was used to 'secure' chastity. Wives of Roman legionnaires spread the aromatic leaves of the chaste tree on their beds while their husbands were at war. It was included in monks' diets (Monk's pepper), planted liberally in the grounds of many Catholic monasteries and worn in the clothing in order to promote celibacy.[2-4] Chaste tree has long been considered of particular importance in women's health care, including symptoms of menopause, menstrual problems, breast-feeding difficulty and infertility.

Current Medicinal Use
While more research is needed, a growing amount of scientific evidence supports the use of this herb in women's health issues. Chaste tree berry is primarily used for the unpleasant consequences of menses and menopause (premenstrual syndrome, mastodynia, dysmenorrhea) due to its amphoteric or balancing quality.[5] It is considered one of the major galactagogues or agents for increasing lactation in nursing mothers.[3,4] Chaste tree berry may also be effective in managing cases of acne caused by hormonal imbalance and in promoting fertility.

Relevant Research
Preventative and Therapeutic Effects
CONSTITUENTS [1,2,6-11]
❖ FLAVONOIDS: isovitexin, orientin, castican, chrysophanol D.

❖ IRIDOIDS: aucubin, agnuside, and eurostide.

❖ VOLATILE OIL: a mixture of monoterpenes and sesquiterpenes including cineol, limonene, and pinene.

❖ ESSENTIAL FATTY ACIDS: linoleic acid.

❖ MISCELLANEOUS: vitamin C, carotenes, castine (a bitter principle).

Note: The whole plant extract (rather than one constituent in particular) is considered medicinally active. The flavonoid agnuside is often used as a reference constituent as a measure of authenticity.[3] Ketosteroids, with a structure similar to sex hormones, have been isolated from the leaves and flowers. The clinical relevance of this is unknown since these plant parts are rarely used medicinally.[4]

WOMEN'S HEALTH CARE

Agnus-castus has been reported to be useful in the management of many 'female' conditions, including premenstrual syndrome, mastodynia, premenstrual acne, unpleasant consequences of menopause, insufficient lactation in nursing mothers, menopause and ailments resulting from corpus luteum insufficiency.

Effects on Premenstrual Syndrome

Several clinical trials have reported that chaste tree may provide symptomatic relief for women suffering from premenstrual syndrome (PMS). One randomized, double blind, placebo controlled study (n=178) found that women ingesting chaste tree (extract Ze 440, 1 tablet daily for three menstrual cycles) had an improved combined score (change from baseline to end point) on their rating of their irritability, mood alteration, anger, headache, and breast fullness compared to those in the placebo group.[12] These findings confirmed those of an earlier multi-center, open-label trial (n=50) of the same chaste tree extract. The open-label study reported a significant reduction in PMS symptoms over the 8 menstrual cycles that the women ingested chaste tree (Extract Ze 440) daily as assessed by the validated Moos' menstrual distress questionnaire.[13]

Similarly, a study (n=36) of women diagnosed with PMS found a generalized improvement in both the physical and psychological symptom picture at a dose of 40 drops of a proprietary brand of agnus-castus tincture (Agnolyt®) daily over three months. Normalization in the luteal phase was also noted.[14] This is supported by an uncontrolled, observational study conducted on women (n=1542, mean age = 34.7 years) diagnosed with PMS in which Agnolyt® was shown to be useful. Results were based on patient and physician assessment. A majority of patients noted either complete relief (33%) or improvement (57%) in their symptoms. These favorable results were supported by the physician assessment (71%=very good; 21% =satisfactory). The dose given was 40 drops daily, with improvement being seen after 25 days.[15]

Other Menstrual Disorders

Loch et al. demonstrated in an uncontrolled observational study of 2447 women presenting with a variety of menstrual disorders (including menorrhagia, hypomenorrhea, hypermenorrhea, metrorrhagia and dysmenorrhea) that a *Vitex agnus-castus* tincture (42 drops daily, mean duration of treatment of 153 days) was therapeutically effective. Both patients and physicians noted an appreciable improvement in symptoms. Instances of multiple diagnoses and concurrent drug use were noted but not controlled for.[16] These favorable findings are supported by a multi-center trial in women (n=1571) presenting with menstrual disorders. At a dose of 40 drops of Agnolyt® daily, with a mean treatment time of 135 days, improvement was noted in 89.1% of cases.[17]

A randomized, double-blind, placebo controlled trial (n=97) using another commercial product, Mastodynon® (30 drops twice daily for three menstrual cycles), suggested that chaste tree may decrease the intensity of pain experienced by women with cyclical mastalgia.[18] A significant difference between the chaste tree and the placebo group was noted after 1 and 2 menstrual cycles, but the results were not quite statistically significant after 3 cycles. In another placebo-controlled trial assessing Mastodynon®, Kubista *et al.* demonstrated a 74.5% improvement (as determined by the use of a 'pain scale') in women (n=55) suffering from severe mastopathy with cyclic mastodynia. There was no statistically significant change in prolactin or progesterone levels.[19]

Many studies have indicated that agnus-castus may prove useful in situations of abnormal menstrual cycle, including normalization of menstrual flow in women suffering from polymenorrhea;[20] decreased bleeding in cases of menorrhagia;[20] pregnancies in cases of both long-standing primary and secondary infertility;[20] increase in progesterone levels in women suffering from compromised corpus luteum function;[21] and secondary amenorrhea.[16]

Lactation
As mentioned above, one of the primary indications of agnus-castus is that of a galactagogue (i.e., increasing production of milk in nursing mothers). Two studies have supported this indication.[1,22] In practice, the onset of action takes several weeks, but the increase in production is marked.[2,3]

Hyperprolactinemia
In a randomized double blind, placebo controlled trial in women (n=52) suffering luteal phase defects due to latent hyperprolactinemia, a commercial brand of agnus-castus (Strotan®) given as 20mg daily, was shown to be beneficial. Latent hyperprolactinemia was evaluated by monitoring prolactin levels 15 minutes and 30 minutes after an IV injection of 200 micrograms of Thyroxin Releasing Hormone (TRH). After three months it was noted in the test group that prolactin levels were decreased, shortened luteal phases normalized and progesterone deficits eliminated when compared to the placebo group. With the exception of a luteal rise in 17 beta-estradiol in the test group, all other hormonal parameters were unchanged.[23]

MECHANISM OF ACTION
It has been suggested that the mechanism of action of agnus-castus is centrally mediated, rather than a direct hormone-like action.[24] Weiss hypothesized that by acting at the level of the pituitary, it promotes LH (luteinizing hormone) and inhibits FSH (follicle stimulating hormone) release.[25] This consequently results in an increase in progesterone levels at the expense of estrogen. Many practitioners have noted that chaste tree appears more progesteronal than estrogenic in nature.[4] However, a study demonstrated that agnus-castus did not influence FSH or LH, either basal levels or when stimulated by addition of luteinizing hormone releasing hormone (LHRH).[26]

Latent hyperprolactinemia has long been known to accompany many of the unpleasant symptoms of premenstrual syndrome, particularly mastodynia.[27-29] It has been hypothesized that the medicinal action of agnus-castus is primarily due to its action on prolactin levels.[24] *In vitro* and *in vivo* experiments have shown that components of agnus-castus inhibit secretion of prolactin, decreasing basal levels and when stimulated by administration of thyroxin releasing hormone (TRH).[30,31] Further, this action is antagonized with administration of a dopamine antagonist (haloperidol) suggesting that constituents present in agnus castus bind directly to central dopamine receptors.[30,31] It has also been noted that agnus castus contains an agent or agents with affinity for both the D1 and D2 receptors.[26,32] It appears that the action of agnus castus on prolactin levels is not due to any cytotoxic effects.[32] While this goes some way to explaining the therapeutic properties of agnus-castus, a complete pharmacology is yet to be elucidated and it is unlikely that its medicinal action is solely due to its influence on the dopaminergic system.[24]

Other studies suggest that whether agnus-castus exerts an antagonistic or agonistic action on prolactin levels may be dependent on both basal levels and drug dose.[33] In a recent trial performed in healthy male subjects (n=20), it was demonstrated that at low doses an antagonistic quality was predominant, the reverse being seen at higher doses. It was also noted that there was a 'smoothing out' effect (decrease in the extent and frequency of prolactin concentration peaks and troughs) independent of the dose given. The authors make the assumption that this specific extract of agnus-castus contained both antagonistic and agonistic constituents acting possibly at different sites. It was also noted that the initial level of prolactin concentration also effected the action of the extract-tested. The unblinded nature of this study and the small number of participants should be noted. Male subjects were selected because they tend to have more stable prolactin levels than women.[33]

MISCELLANEOUS EFFECTS

There were numerous instances of pregnancy reported in the trials discussed above, including in women with established infertility.[21,34-36] One randomized, placebo controlled, double blind clinical trial (n=96) suggested that chaste tree (Mastodynon®, 30 drops twice daily for three months) may be beneficial for women with sterility due to secondary amenorrhea and luteal insufficiency.[37]

A number of uncontrolled studies have suggested that agnus-castus may prove useful in the management of acne vulgaris of a hormonal etiology.[38]

It has been reported that chaste tree, either alone or combined with other herbal medicines, may prove useful in the management of the unpleasant consequences of menopause, notably fluid retention, hot-flushing, anxiety and depression.[2]

ADVERSE EFFECTS

Adverse effects seem to be quite rare with agnus-castus. Situations of dry mouth, disturbed sleep, tachycardia, nausea, allergic skin reaction, vomiting, sensation of epigastric pressure, confusion, giddiness, acne, pruritus, alopecia, erythema and headache have been noted in some studies.[15,16,33] Changes in menses including increased flow and changes in cycle have also been noted.[3] One instance of multiple follicular development was described in a patient undergoing unstimulated *in vitro* fertilization treatment upon introduction of a herbal medicine containing *Vitex agnus-castus*.[39] Although no similar situations are reported in the literature,[40,41] the author of the original article suggests caution in this application.[42]

CAUTIONS/CONTRAINDICATIONS

Vitex agnus-castus should not be used in children or during pregnancy.[4] Although it is reputed to stimulate milk production,[1,22] concerns have been raised regarding its use for this purpose given the lack of conclusive information.[1]

DRUG INTERACTIONS

It is advisable not to use *vitex agnus-castus* with oral contraceptives or hormone replacement therapy.[4] *Vitex agnus-castus* should also be used with caution in individuals taking dopamine antagonists such as haloperidol and metoclopramide.[24]

DOSAGE REGIMENS

❖ DRIED FRUIT: 0.5-1g three times daily.[1]
❖ TINCTURE: 0.2-0.4 mL (1:2) or 3-10 mL (1:5) daily.[4]
❖ STANDARDIZED EXTRACT: Many of the clinical trials mentioned above have been carried out using a commercial brand of alcohol based tincture standardized to fruit content (9 g/100 mL of tincture) called Agnolyt®. The suggested daily dose is 40 drops daily.[4]
   Note: Many authors note that agnus-castus does not have an immediate action. Treatment should be uninterrupted and last for several months when used for most of the above indications. In certain situations, the duration of treatment should be appreciably longer (e.g., 5-7 months for anovulatory cycles and infertility and up to 18 months for secondary amenorrhea of longer than 2 years).[3]

Cranberry

Vaccinium macrocarpon Ait.

Common Uses
- ❖ Urinary Tract Infections (prevention)

Active Constituents
- ❖ Fructose
- ❖ An unidentified large molecular weight compound

Adverse Effects
- ❖ None known

Cautions/Contraindications
- ❖ None known

Drug Interactions
- ❖ None known

Doses
- ❖ *Cranberry Juice:* 150-600 mL daily
- ❖ *Concentrated Cranberry Juice Capsules:* 300-400 mg twice daily

Introduction

Family
* Ericaceae

Synonyms
* *Oxycoccus macrocarpus* (Ait.) Pursh[1]

Medicinal Forms
* Juice
* Juice Capsules

Description
Cranberry is a leathery-leaved evergreen bush with characteristic shiny red berries and pale pink flowers, native to the marshland of Northern Europe, Eastern Canada and the Eastern United States.[2]

Parts Used
The ripe berries are the part of the plant used medicinally.

Traditional Use
Folk wisdom has long held that drinking cranberry juice will prevent urinary tract infections. Early clinical trials generally supported this claim; however, there were some negative findings and much controversy over the hypothesized mechanism of action. A recent large clinical trial aimed at ending the controversy found cranberry juice to be clinically effective in the prevention of urinary tract infections, but has generated controversy of its own.

Current Medicinal Use
Cranberry is used primarily for the prevention of recurrent and uncomplicated urinary tract infections, though not as a treatment for acute infections.

Relevant Research
Preventative and Therapeutic Uses
CONSTITUENTS [1,2]
Berries
* PROANTHOCYANIDINS.
* FRUCTOSE.
* FLAVONOL GLYCOSIDES: leptosine.
* CATECHIN.
* TRITERPENOIDS.
* ORGANIC ACIDS: citric acid, malic acid, benzoic acid, quinic acid.
* MISCELLANEOUS: vitamin C, unidentified large molecular weight molecule.

EFFECTS ON URINARY TRACT INFECTIONS
Many early trials of the effectiveness of cranberry for the prevention and/or treatment or urinary tract infections involved small numbers of participants and were not blinded or controlled.[3-6] Similar criticism may be made of relatively recent clinical trials that have suggested that cranberry juice may be useful for the prevention and/or treatment of urinary tract infections.[7,8] One non-blinded, uncontrolled clinical trial involved 28 elderly patients in a long-term health care facility (a population at high risk for urinary tract infections) who drank 120-180 mL of Ocean Spray Cranberry Juice Cocktail® daily for 7 weeks. Mid-stream clean catch urines (or catheterized urines for 3 patients) were obtained biweekly for 7 weeks. The authors report that 19 of the 28 patients showed no evidence of urinary tract infection during the study period, while in the remaining 9 they found leukocytes and/or nitrates in the

urine and significant presence of gram negative bacilli. The authors conclude that their study provides evidence that drinking cranberry juice product may prevent urinary tract infections.[7]

In a similar study, 21 patients took 12 capsules containing 800 mg cranberry (Pharmacaps®) daily. There was no incidence of urinary tract infections in 20 patients. The same cranberry product was tested in 6 patients with pre-existing urinary tract infections and no cures were reported.[9] Larger, randomized, double-blinded studies were definitely needed.

In an attempt to fill this void, a recent randomized, double-blind, placebo-controlled trial was conducted with 153 elderly women who ingested 300 mL of commercially available cranberry beverage or placebo daily for 6 months. The authors concluded that the frequency of bacteriuria with pyuria was significantly decreased (after 4 to 8 weeks) in the cranberry group in comparison with the placebo group. In addition, there was a decrease in the rate of antibiotics prescribed by physicians to treat urinary tract infections in the cranberry group, suggesting a clinically relevant effect of ingesting cranberry juice.[8] However, this study was criticized in several letters.[10-13] These criticisms, including the difficulties of obtaining "clean-voided specimens,"[12] and that the two groups may not have had the same base-line frequency of urinary tract infections,[10,13] are adequately addressed by the authors.[14] Another small, (n=17) randomized, controlled, cross-over trial[15] and a large (n=150) randomized trial[16] confirm these findings. However, a double-blind, placebo-controlled crossover study of 15 children (aged 2 to 18) diagnosed with neurogenic bladder and receiving clean intermittent catheterization reported that ingestion of 30 mL of cranberry juice concentrate (considered equivalent to 300 mL of cranberry juice) daily for 3 months had no effect on bacteriuria in these patients.[17]

MECHANISM OF ACTION
The original hypothesis was that cranberry juice acted by increasing urine acidity;[5,6,18-20] however other studies have challenged this theory.[8,21-23] The most popular theory currently is that cranberry possesses "anti-adherence" properties, which prevent bacteria from attaching to the lining of the urinary tract.[24-26] For example, two compounds have been found in cranberry that inhibit the adhesion of *Escherichia coli* to urinary tract cells. Fructose, found in all fruit juices, and another as yet unidentified compound (found in cranberry and blueberry juice only) have been shown to inhibit *Escherichia coli* fimbrial adhesions.[27]

ANTI-CANCER ACTIVITY
In vitro screening tests have suggested that the proanthocyanidin fraction of cranberry has potential anti-carcinogenic (anti-cancer) activity.[28]

ADVERSE EFFECTS
None reported.

CAUTIONS/CONTRAINDICATIONS
None reported.

DRUG INTERACTIONS
None reported.

DOSAGE REGIMENS
Prevention of urinary tract infections
❖ JUICE: 150-600 mL cranberry juice daily.[7,24]
❖ CAPSULE: 300-400 mg concentrated cranberry juice capsules twice daily.[29]
   Note: Cranberry juice should not be used as a substitute for antibiotics in acute urinary tract infections.

Dandelion

Taraxacum officinale G.H. Weber ex Wiggers

THUMBNAIL SKETCH

Common Uses
❖ *Root:* Liver (Hepatobiliary) Disorders, Dyspepsia, Loss of Appetite

❖ *Leaves:* Water Retention

Active Constituents
❖ Terpenes/Terpenoids

❖ Bitter Principle

❖ Phytosterols

❖ Inulin

❖ Minerals (potassium)

Adverse Effects
❖ Contact Dermatitis (possible)

Cautions/Contraindications
❖ *Root:* Occlusion of Bile Ducts, Empyema, Paralytic Ileus

❖ *Leaves:* Occlusion of Bile Ducts

Drug Interactions
❖ Leaf may potentiate the action of diuretics

Doses
❖ *Dried Root* (infusion or decoction): 3-5 g three times daily

❖ *Root Tincture* (1:5 in 25% ethanol): 5-10 mL of three times daily

❖ *Dried Leaf* (infusion): 4-10 g three times daily

❖ *Leaf Liquid Extract* (1:1 in 25% alcohol): 4-10 mL of three times daily

Introduction

Description

Dandelion is a perennial herb native to Europe, now found throughout North America, that can grow to a height of 30 centimeters or 12 inches.[4] The oblong leaves grow in a rosette from a milky taproot, which sends up one or more leafless flower stems, each bearing a single yellow, multiple-petal flower. The name 'dandelion' is a corruption of the Latin 'dens leonis or lion's teeth that derives from the appearance of the flower. A 'puffball' tuft or cluster of 'parachute' seeds follows the flower.

Parts Used

The leaf and root of the dandelion are used medicinally. The constituents of this plant, and arguably their medicinal action, change dramatically with the seasons. Generally speaking, the roots are best collected between June and August when they are most bitter.[3] Fresh dandelion leaves are commonly used in salads and sandwiches, the dried root is used as a coffee substitute, and the flowers are used in making dandelion wine and spirits.

Traditional Use

Members of the *Taraxacum* genus have been used by many cultures for their therapeutic properties. Dandelion is considered one of the primary herbs in the British herbal tradition, the roots being used for liver and digestive problems and the leaves for their 'diuretic' properties in cases of edema. This latter action is demonstrated eloquently by the French name, *Pissenlit*.[2,3] Dandelion has also been used in conditions as varied as fevers, boils, diarrhea and hemorrhoids.[5] It has been used in China and the Indian subcontinent for various conditions, including snakebites, abscesses, appendicitis, and for its nutritional value.[3]

Current Medicinal Use

Even though dandelion has a long history of medicinal use, very little scientific research has been conducted on the herb. Dandelion has both a choleretic (promoting production of bile) and a cholagogue (causing contraction of the bile duct initiating the flow of stored bile) activity, and is used in assisting the body in detoxifying. Since it is a digestive bitter, dandelion may help in cases of mild dyspepsia and indigestion. Dandelion leaf has mild diuretic properties.

Relevant Research

Preventative and Therapeutic Effects

CONSTITUENTS [1,2,4,6-8]

- ❖ TERPENOIDS (INCLUDING THE TRITERPENOIDS): taraxerol, taraxacin, lactucin, and taraxasterol.
- ❖ ACIDS: chlorogenic acid, caffeic acid.
- ❖ CARBOHYDRATES: fructose, glucose, inulin, and sucrose. (During the summer the fructose in the root is converted into inulin, to be re-converted back in the winter.)
- ❖ VITAMINS/MINERALS: leaves are rich in potassium (297 mg/100 g), vitamin A (14 000 IU/100 g), vitamin C, B complex, zinc, manganese, copper.
- ❖ PHYTOSTEROLS: sitosterol, stigmasterol, taraxasterol, and campesterol. (The composition of the sterol portion found in the leaves undergoes extensive seasonal fluctuation.)
- ❖ FLAVONOID GLYCOSIDES: luteolin 7-glucoside, luteolin 7-diglucosides.
- ❖ SESQUITERPENE LACTONES AND TARAXACOSIDE: Many references are made to the 'bitter principle' (also called taraxin) found primarily in dandelion root. This portion consists mainly of a mixture of sesquiterpene lactones and taraxacoside.[9]

EFFECT ON LIVER FUNCTION

Dandelion root plays a major part in modern herbal practice where it is considered to be a safe treatment used in the management of many liver related conditions.[2,10] It is considered to be a both a choleretic (promoting production of bile) and a cholagogue (causing contraction of the bile duct initiating the flow of stored bile).[1,3] These properties are firmly part of herbal tradition, and the limited clinical data available tend to support them. For example, studies have shown that administration of dandelion increased bile flow in dogs and rats and aided in the management of a variety of gall-bladder conditions.[3,11] In addition, a product in which dandelion is one of nine ingredients has been used to treat hepatitis.[12]

Given the importance of the liver as an organ of elimination within the herbal tradition, dandelion root is thought to be a useful and protective adjunctive therapy to chemotherapy.[13]

DIURETIC ACTION

Racz-Kotilla et al. demonstrated (in rats and mice) that dandelion possessed diuretic properties when given in high doses. This study noted that an extract made from the leaves had a more pronounced diuretic action than the root. They found the 4% aqueous solution of dandelion leaf (15 mL/kg) had a diuretic effect comparable to furosemide at a dose of 80 mg/kg.[14] This appears to confirm the distinction between leaf and root noted by herbalists.[2] Also noted was that a 4% aqueous leaf extract (8 mL/kg) given for thirty days resulted in a marked weight loss.[14] In a more recent *in vivo* trial, no real diuretic effect was noted when an extract of *Taraxacum officinale* was administered to female wistar rats. Although no specifics were given regarding dose, the dandelion root was used in the preparation of the extract. Even though the diuretic action of dandelion has been shown in animal studies, the exact mechanism is as yet unknown. It appears that there may be numerous constituents playing a role in this function, including sesquiterpene lactones (found in the terpenoid portion), inulin and potassium.[15]

Since dandelion is rich in potassium, herbalists often advocate its use with herbs that have the potential for managing hypokalemia (abnormally low concentration of potassium ions in the circulating blood).[2]

MISCELLANEOUS EFFECTS
Anti-Microbial
Extracts made from dandelion pollen have been shown to exert an anti-microbial action against Proteus, Escherichia and Salmonella *in vitro*.[1]

Digestion
Dandelion root is described as a 'digestive bitter' and is often used in the treatment of dyspepsia and to stimulate the appetite.[2,16,17]

Hypoglycemia
A hypoglycemic action was noted in rabbits following esophageal administration. The fall in blood sugar was pronounced at high doses and it has been suggested that dandelion could be acting in a similar fashion to conventional sulphonylurea hypoglycemics.[18] Other trials have found contradictory results.[9]

Genitourinary
Investigators have hypothesized that the historical role of dandelion in the management of kidney stones could be due to the degradation of potential mucopolysaccharide foci by the saponins present in the plant.[19]

ADVERSE EFFECTS
Contact dermatitis has been noted after frequent exposure to the fresh herb.[20,21] This is unlikely to be clinically important since most herbal products are made from the dried material.[15] Even when given as a large part of the diet (32%) for a prolonged period of time (209 days), dandelion root was not shown to have carcinogenic potential in rats.[22]

CAUTIONS/CONTRAINDICTIONS
LEAF ❖ Dandelion leaf should be used with caution in cases of occlusion of the bile ducts.[23]
ROOT ❖ Dandelion root should be used with caution in cases of: occlusion of the bile ducts and/or gall bladder, empyema and paralytic ileus.[23] Possible cross reactivity has been noted between different members of the Asteraceae/Compositae (Sunflower) family, including dandelion, in sensitive individuals.[24] Historical/anecdotal evidence suggests avoidance of excessive doses in pregnancy or lactation but no evidence has been published to support this claim.[6]

> *Note:* Since Dandelion is most often considered to be a weed by many gardeners, it is very often heavily sprayed with a variety of herbicides and pesticides. Thus, clients should be cautioned against collecting this herb from gardens, by roadsides or from crop fields.[3] It has also been noted that *Taraxacum officinale* growing in urban areas may contain enough heavy metals (lead, zinc and copper) to be potential harmful if taken orally.[25]

DRUG INTERACTIONS
No specific interactions between this plant and any pharmaceutical preparations could be found. Houghton suggests caution in using any herbal diuretic with conventional diuretics.[15]

DOSAGE REGIMENS
❖ DRIED ROOT (INFUSION OR DECOCTION): 3-5 g three times daily.[23]
❖ ROOT TINCTURE (1:5 in 25% ethanol): 5-10 mL of three times daily.[23]
❖ DRIED LEAF (INFUSION): 4-10 g three times daily.[23]
❖ LEAF LIQUID EXTRACT (1:1 in 25% alcohol): 4-10 mL of three times daily.[23]

Devil's Claw

Harpagophytum procumbens DC.

Common Uses
❖ Inflammation of Joints (including osteo-arthritis, rheumatoid arthritis and gout)
❖ Indigestion and Dyspepsia

Active Constituents
❖ Iridoid Glycosides (harpaside, harpagoside)

Adverse Effects
❖ Digestive Upset (mild)

Cautions/Contraindications
❖ Peptic Ulcer (active)

Drug Interactions
❖ None

Doses
For digestive indications
❖ *Dried Tuber in Decoction:* 500 mg three times daily
❖ *Tincture* (1:5 in 25% ethanol): 1 mL three times daily

For other indications
❖ *Dried Tuber in Decoction:* 1.5-2.5 g three times daily
❖ *Liquid Extract* (1:1 in 25% ethanol): 1-2 mL three times daily
❖ *Dried Tuber:* 100-250 mg three times daily

Introduction

Family
* Pedaliaceae

Synonyms
* Harpagophytum
* Grapple plant
* Wood spider[1-3]

Medicinal Forms
* Dried Tuber
* Decoction
* Tincture
* Liquid Extract

Description
Devil's claw is native to southern and eastern Africa, notably the veldt of the Transvaal region. It is a trailing herbaceous perennial, growing to 1.5 meters or 5 feet in length, with lobed leaves, whose brilliant 'devil' red/purple flowers and woody barbed, claw-like fruit are responsible for its descriptive name. The plant produces tubers that are harvested as herbs.[2,3]

Parts Used
The secondary storage root or tuber is the part principally used medicinally when dried.[3]

Traditional Uses
Decoctions of dried roots have long been taken as a tea or tonic by the indigenous peoples of Africa for a variety of digestive and rheumatic conditions.[2] After devil's claw was introduced to European herbal medicine by Mehnert, this herb became so popular that by 1976, it was estimated that 30,000 arthritic patients in the United Kingdom alone were using it.[4]

Current Medicinal Use
Devil's claw is primarily used in the management of inflammatory joint diseases, such as osteo-arthritis, rheumatoid arthritis and gout. Since devil's claw is considered to be a 'bitter tonic', it may be of help in the management of various gastrointestinal complaints, including dyspepsia and digestive upsets.

Relevant Research

Preventative and Therapeutic Effects

CONSTITUENTS [1,3,5-9]
* IRIDOID GLYCOSIDES: harpagide, harpagoside, and procumbide.
* PHENOLIC ACIDS: chlorogenic acid, cinnamic acid.
* FLAVONOIDS: kaempferol, luteolin.
  Note: Harpagoside, which appears to be the constituent of most interest, is primarily found in the secondary tubers.[3] The flowers, stem and ripe fruit appear to be devoid of this agent.[10]

MUSCULOSKELETAL (ANTI-INFLAMMATORY) EFFECTS
Devil's claw has been reputed to have anti-inflammatory and anti-rheumatic properties.[9,11-13] It is commonly used in the management of many inflammatory joint diseases such as osteoarthritis, rheumatoid arthritis and gout.[9,12,13]

Many authors have suggested that devil's claw can exert an anti-inflammatory action. Aqueous extracts of devil's claw were shown to possess anti-inflammatory activity in both rats and mice following intraperitoneal administration.[14,15] The activity appeared greater in chronic rather than acute situations.[16] The anti-inflammatory properties were abolished after oral administration[14] or after an acid treatment.[15] Although harpagoside alone did not have appreciable anti-inflammatory properties, it did appear to exert a peripheral analgesic action.[15]

One study reported that an aqueous extract of devil's claw may possess an anti-inflammatory action comparable to phenylbutazone.[1] However, extracts of devil's claw were shown to possess no appreciable action in reducing rat hind paw edema induced by either carragennan or *Mycobacterium butyricum* when compared to standard NSAID agents.[17,18] Even at doses far higher (100X) than the "standard recommended dose" of devil's claw, no inflammatory action was seen nor any inhibitory action on prostaglandin synthetase action noted.[17]

In an attempt to demonstrate a possible mechanism of anti-inflammatory action, Moussard et al. found that 500 mg of devil's claw (standardized to 3% total glucoiridoids per unit dose) had no influence on eicosanoid production. Human volunteers (aged 20-35 years) were divided into a control group (n=9) and treatment group (n=25). The volunteers took either the placebo or 4 caps of devil's claw daily for 21 days. The influence on both cyclooxygenase and lipoxygenase pathways were determined by using the spontaneously clotting whole human blood model performed on samples taken before and after the investigation. There was no statistically significant difference in blood clotting times between the two groups.[19]

Arthritis

The popularity of devil's claw as an herbal remedy has led to a number of clinical trials being conducted most notably in the treatment of osteoarthritis. In one positive trial, 43 patients suffering from a range of degenerative arthritides were treated with 1.5 g daily of devils claw (Arkocaps®). Symptom improvement was noted after eight days, with marked improvement in pain (89%), range of motion (84%) and time needed for stiffness to wear off (86%).[20] Two studies have compared the effects of devil's claw with a conventional treatment for osteoarthritis, diacerhein and found it to be as effective.[21,22] For example, a randomized, double-blind trial compared 4 weeks of treatment with Haradol® (6 capsules daily each containing 435 mg of powdered devil's claw) or diacerhein (100 mg daily) in the management of osteoarthritis of the knee and hip in 122 patients. Overall, both groups reported a decrease in pain and increase in function with no statistical differences reported between the two groups. At the completion of the study, the devil's claw group reported using significantly fewer NSAIDs and fewer adverse effects than the diacerhein group. However, not all trials of devil's claw have been positive. In an uncontrolled trial conducted in the United Kingdom, 13 volunteers (34-71 years of age) suffering from various arthritic conditions (seropositive arthritis, seronegative rheumatoid arthritis, and psoriatic arthritis) were selected because they had failed to respond to conventional pharmaceutical care. Each was given 410 mg of aqueous devil's claw extract three times daily for 6 weeks. While 4 patients showed some improvement in certain areas (more specific details were not published), there was no significant change in the symptoms of the group as a whole as determined by a variety of objective and subjective measures. It should be noted that the patients continued taking their conventional antirheumatic medications for the duration of this trial.[4]

Low Back Pain

Two trials (one an open label trial with 130 patients;[23] the other a double-blind pilot study with 197 patients[24]) suggest that devil's claw may also be beneficial in the management of the symptoms of low back pain.

However, another randomized, placebo-controlled, double-blind four-week study of 118 patients presenting with low back pain found that devils claw treatment was not significantly better than placebo treatment in two out of three outcome measures. The primary outcome measure was the amount of a specific opiod analgesic (Tramadol®) taken by patients in the last 3 weeks of the study. Secondary outcome measures included relief according to the Arhus low back pain index and the number of patients pain-free at the study's conclusion. While the number of patients pain free at the conclusion of the trial was significantly higher in the treatment group than in the placebo group, there was no significant difference between the groups with respect to the Arhus low back pain index or the amount of analgesic ingested.[25] This study has been criticized because the consumption of analgesic could not be equated with the subjective experience of pain.[26]

Additional research in this area is needed.

DIGESTIVE EFFECTS

Weiss classifies devil's claw as a 'bitter tonic' useful in the management of various gastrointestinal complaints including dyspepsia and digestive upsets due to poor gallbladder and/or pancreatic function.[11] An *in vitro* study has indicated that the iridoid components of devil's claw influence guinea pig ileum. Harpagoside was noted to decrease the contractile response caused by either acetylcholine or barium chloride. The authors infer that this could be a result of an action on the mechanism that controls influx of calcium into the cells.[27] Harpagide was also shown to exert a dose dependent action on the contractile response of guinea pig ileum, augmenting the response at low dose but inhibiting it at a higher one.[27]

MISCELLANEOUS EFFECTS

Cardiovascular

Crude methanolic extracts of *Harpagophytum procumbens* exert a dose dependent protective effect on experimental ventricular arrhythmias induced by various means in both rat and isolated rabbit heart.[28,29] Some authors have suggested that this action is in part due to an inhibition of calcium influx into the myocardial cells since it was shown to be protective against arrhythmias induced by digitalis. This action appears to be the result of a synergistic interplay of constituents rather than solely the harpagoside.[29] Also noted was a positive inotropic effect at low doses and a negative inotropic effect at higher doses.[27,29]

Anti-Microbial

Extracts made from the secondary roots of devil's claw exerted weak anti-fungal action against various fungi.[30]

ADVERSE EFFECTS

A "slight digestive upset" was reported by two patients participating in one study.[20] One individual in another study reported morning frontal throbbing headache, tinnitus, severe anorexia and loss of appetite;[4] however, no attempt appears to have been made to determine whether these effects were due to the devil's claw product being investigated.

CAUTIONS/CONTRAINDICATIONS

Given the action of devil's claw as a classic bitter, theoretically it may increase gastric acid secretion. This fact has led to a caution of its use in cases of active peptic ulcer disease.[9,11] Historically, the use of devil's claw has been contraindicated in pregnancy due to its alleged 'abortifacient' action.[1] Although this situation could be due to a simple mistranslation, until more information is known, it is still a valid point of concern.[31]

DRUG INTERACTIONS

No interactions between this herb and any pharmaceutical preparations could be found. Given the influence in animal studies of *Harpagophytum procumbens* on cardiac muscle (mentioned above), its use in high doses may interact with cardiac and hypo/hypertensive therapy.[1]

DOSAGE REGIMENS

For digestive indications [9]

❖ DRIED TUBER IN DECOCTION: 500 mg three times daily.

❖ TINCTURE (1:5 in 25% ethanol): 1 mL three times daily.

For other indications [9]

❖ DRIED TUBER IN DECOCTION: 1.5-2.5g three times daily.

❖ LIQUID EXTRACT (1:1 in 25% ethanol): 1-2mL three times daily.

❖ DRIED TUBER: 100-250 mg three times daily.

Note: Many of the clinical trials have used a dose range of 400-500 mg of dried herb three times daily. While many products are standardized to harpagoside content, it would be prudent to use whole plant extracts until the importance of this constituent is verified.

Dong Quai

Angelica sinensis (Oliv.) Diels

THUMBNAIL SKETCH

Common Uses
❖ Women's Health Care (including the unpleasant consequences of menopause, dysmenorrhea, amenorrhea)

❖ 'Blood' Tonic (dependent on a suitable Traditional Chinese Medicine diagnosis)

Active Constituents
❖ Components of both the alcohol and aqueous soluble portions have been shown to possess therapeutic properties.

Adverse Effects
❖ Diarrhea and Phototoxic Skin Reaction (rare)

Cautions/Contraindications
❖ Pregnancy, Hypermenorrhea (heavy periods), Hemorrhagic (bleeding) Disease

❖ History of Spontaneous Abortion

Drug Interactions
❖ No examples of drug interactions found, but caution is recommended in cases of concomitant administration with oral anti-coagulants

Doses
❖ *Raw Herb:* 3-10 g (or equivalent) daily

Introduction

Family
- ❖ Apiaceae (also known as Umbelliferae)

Synonyms
- ❖ Chinese angelica
- ❖ Tang kuei
- ❖ Dang gui
- ❖ Female ginseng
- ❖ Female tonic
- ❖ Woman's herb
- ❖ Toki
- ❖ Tangwi
- ❖ *A. polymorpha* Maxim. Var. sinensis Oliv[1-4]

Description

Dong quai is a fragrant perennial plant, growing to 2 meters or 6 feet tall, with large green leaves, hollow stems and clusters of white flowers. It is native to southwestern China and Japan, where it is now cultivated extensively.

Similar plants are often used in place of *Angelica sinensis*, including *Angelica acutiloba* (Siebold & Zucc.); Kitag (Korean or Japanese dong quai); *Ligusticum glaucescens* Franch (wild chin quai); and *Levisticum officinale* Koch (European dong quai). While these plants do possess therapeutically useful qualities, they are considered by most to be inferior to *Angelica sinensis*.[5]

Parts Used

The root, with its distinctive aromatic odor and bitter-sweet/pungent taste, is the part used medicinally. The larger roots are more prized than the smaller ones. As a general rule, the larger the root, the sweeter the taste and the better the quality.

Traditional Use

Dong quai is arguably one of the oldest and most established therapeutic agents used within the Traditional Chinese Medicine healing model.[5] It is considered to be a tonic that can strengthen and invigorate the whole individual or specific organ groups. While dong quai exerts its tonifying action on many sites, it is classically considered to be one of the major 'blood' tonics often used to 'build the blood'. Even though it has numerous applications, it was considered to be of particular importance in the management of 'female' conditions, such as menopause and dysmenorrhea.[6,7] It is in the realm of women's health care that most people will encounter the use of dong quai within the Western world.

Another member of the same genus, *Angelica archangelica* L. (Angelica), shares some of the same constituents and actions as dong quai, but it is used primarily as a digestive tonic, especially in cases of dyspepsia and flatulence.[8] *Angelica archangelica* L. is also used extensively in the liquor industry, where it is used as a flavoring in liqueurs such as benedictine and chartreuse.[2]

Current Medicinal Use

Until more conclusive scientific research has been conducted, it is best to use dong quai as it is intended to be used within a Traditional Chinese Medicine paradigm. In the hands of an appropriately trained practitioner, dong quai may be useful in the management of menstrual and menopause conditions, as well as some cardiovascular conditions.

Medicinal Forms

Dong quai can be ingested in various ways: the fresh root may be either steamed or fried in vinegar, or the dried root can be taken as a soup.[1,7]

Relevant Research
Preventative and Therapeutic Effects
CONSTITUENTS [1,2,5,6,9,10]

❖ VOLATILE OIL: ligustilide, n-butylidene phthalide, n- valerophernone-O-carboxylic acid.

❖ FURANOCOUMARINS: psoralen, bergapten, archangelicin.

❖ ORGANIC ACIDS: ferulic acid, succinic acid,myristic acid.

❖ MISCELLANEOUS: vitamin A, vitamin E, various members of the vitamin B group, polysaccharides, including-AR-4E-2, angelica immunostimulating polysaccharide (AIP).

CARDIOVASCULAR EFFECT
Traditional Use
Within the Traditional Chinese Medicine (TCM) model dong quai is prescribed for conditions of 'blood deficiency', a situation that often presents with symptoms including: pale lips and tongue, dull/pale face with sallow complexion, depression and fatigue, poor memory, oligomenorrhea and amenorrhea.[11] While many of these symptoms may be equated with the Western concepts of anaemia and cardiovascular disease, it is important to realize that conditions diagnosed following a TCM tradition cannot be directly equated with a conventional medical diagnosis.[11]

Cardiac Activity
Several experimental studies suggest that extracts of *Angelica sinensis* exert an inhibitory action on cardiac muscle contraction. Both aqueous and alcoholic extracts of *Angelica sinensis* have been shown to antagonize arrhythmias induced by a number of agents (including epinephrine, strophanthin, digitalis, atropine, datura flower) in both *in vivo* and *in vitro* models.[6,9,12] A quinidine-like action (prolonged atrial refractory period, lowered cardiac excitability) was demonstrated in anesthetized dogs given an ether extract of *Angelica sinensis* root.[9,12] In addition, a 2% fluid extract of *Angelica sinensis* has been shown to markedly increase coronary blood flow and decrease myocardial oxygen consumption in the isolated heart of guinea pigs.[9]

Vascular Action
It has been demonstrated that *Angelica sinensis* exerts a predominately hypotensive effect *in vivo*.[6,9,12,13] This drop in blood pressure appears to be rapid and short lived.[6,12] It was thought that this action was in part due to a decreased cardiac out-put, but this has been shown not to be the case. It is more likely due to a vasodilatory action resulting from muscarinic and histaminic receptor stimulation.[9] Early investigations suggested that the hypotensive action was solely due to the non-volatile components, and the volatile constituents were thought to have a stimulating action. This has since been shown not to be the case.[9,12]

Anti-Thrombotic Action
In vitro experiments have demonstrated that aqueous extracts *of Angelica sinensis* could suppress platelet aggregation induced by ADP and collagen.[9,12] The agent thought to be predominantly responsible for this action is ferulic acid. It has been postulated that the decrease in platelet aggregation could be due to inhibition of cyclo-oxygenase and thromboxane A_2 resulting in a subsequent decrease in the production of bio-active eicosonoids.[12] Osthole, extracted from a related species (*Angelica pubescens* Maxim.) has also shown to decrease platelet aggregation by inhibiting thromboxane B_2.[14] It has also been postulated that the anti-thrombotic action could be due to a decrease in fibrinogen levels and blood viscosity.[12] This influence on the blood coagulating system is far from certain with some suggesting that an effect cannot be demonstrated.[13]

Miscellaneous Actions

Angelica sinensis root when added to the feed (5% w/w) of albino rats and rabbits with experimental hyperlipidemia exerted a demonstrable antilipidemic effect. While the exact mechanism is unknown, it does not appear to be due to an effect on cholesterol absorption.[9]

WOMEN'S HEALTH

Traditional Use

Dong quai is considered to be useful in the management of a variety of conditions including: abnormal/suppressed/difficult menstruation;[2,6,9,10] dysmenorrhea;[1,2,6,9-11] dysfunctional uterine bleeding (see contraindications);[2,6,10] premenstrual syndrome;[6] preparation for conception;[1,10,11] aiding recovery after birthing;[1,11] unpleasant consequences of menopause.[15,16] As mentioned above, many of these conditions are diagnosed and treated using models outside of the conventional medical model.

Menstrual Problems

A common Chinese patent formula containing *Angelica sinensis* root (Xiao Yao Powder) was seen to decrease symptoms of premenstrual syndrome (PMS) in 10 women.[9] A randomized, placebo-controlled trial (n=49) found that a phytoestrogen combination containing 60 mg soy isoflavones, 100 mg dong quai and 50 mg black cohosh significantly decreased the frequency of menstrual migraine attacks as well as significantly decreasing the frequency of all migraines, headache severity, doses of triptans and doses of analgesics compared to the placebo group when ingested for 24 weeks.[17] The clinical contributions of the dong quai in this product cannot be determined from this study.

In addition, dong quai root has been shown to have an action on uterine tissue using various animal models. It appears that this effect is dependent on the extract used.[9,12] The volatile oil fraction causes direct muscular relaxation, completely abolishing contractions in a dose dependent fashion.[6,9,12] The active constituent appears to be ligustilide.[12] The volatile oil antagonizes excitation caused by either histamine or epinephrine, while the non-volatile fractions have an opposite action resulting in strong uterine contractions.[6,9,12] The alcoholic extract has a more pronounced effect than the aqueous one.[9] When administered parenterally there is no difference between the fractions, they all cause excitation.[9]

Intrauterine pressure was shown to influence the action of dong quai on rabbit uterine fistula. When the existing pressure was elevated, contraction became slower and more rhythmic.[9] It has been suggested that this action is responsible for dong quai's effectiveness in the treatment of dysmenorrhea.[6,11]

Menopause

A product containing *Angelica sinensis* (Angelica-Paeonia Powder) was shown to alleviate symptoms commonly seen with menopause in 43 cases (specific details of this trial were not available at the time of preparation of this monograph).[9] In addition, a recent trial of a botanical formula containing *Angelica sinensis* (and *Arctium lappa* L., Asteraceae, *Glycyrrhiza glabra* L., Fabaceae, *Leonurus cardiaca* L., Lamiaceae and *Dioscorea villosa* L., Dioscoreaceae) conducted at the National College of Naturopathic Medicine found that symptoms of menopause where decreased when compared to a placebo group. As was correctly noted by the authors, given the small sample number (n=13) no definite conclusions can be made.[16] No conclusions can be drawn for *Angelica sinensis* in particular from this investigation since the other herbal ingredients in the botanical formula have demonstrable therapeutic actions in their own rights.

The many positive actions of dong quai on the female reproductive system have long been considered to result from 'phytoestrogenic' properties. This assumption is now being questioned because many of the actions of this herb are probably not estrogen dependent.[11,18] Studies in mice have found dong quai to be devoid of estrogenic action.[6,9] Conversely, both aqueous and petroleum ether extracts, when given intraperitoneally and subcutaneously respectively are reported to have an estrogen-like action.[13]

As is demonstrated, the evidence supporting the therapeutic usefulness of *Angelica sinensis* comes predominantly from the Asian medical model with there being a distinct lack of quality clinical information. It should also be noted that what little evidence there is from a western conventional standpoint normally involves products in which dong quai is only one of many ingredients. More research is required before the traditional uses of dong quai can be supported using evidence from a biomedical paradigm.

MISCELLANEOUS EFFECTS
Anti-Microbial
An aqueous decoction of dong quai has been shown to exert a weak anti-microbial action against a variety of bacteria, including: *E coli*, *Salmonella typhi*, *Shigella dysenteriae*.[9]

Metabolic
When added to the feed of rats (5-6% of diet), *Angelica sinensis* was shown to reduce or prevent testicular disease resulting from vitamin E deficiency.[9]

Central Nervous System
Parenteral administration of tang kuei essential oil from Japan has been shown to exert tran-quilizing, hypnotic and anesthetic actions in a variety of animal models.[13]

Analgesic Action
Dong quai is used within TCM for various conditions associated with pain primarily due to a TCM diagnosis of "blood stagnation."[11] This analgesic action appears dependent on the quality and origin of the pain.

ADVERSE EFFECTS
Even though tang kuei extract from Japan accelerated the death of mice that had been given carbon tetrachloride, in practice adverse effects caused by *Angelica sinensis* appear to be very rare.[5,13] The LD_{50} of dong quai administered intravenously to mice was 100.6g/kg.[12]

Diarrhea is possible because of dong quai's relaxant action on the smooth muscle of the digestive tract.[2,19] This appears more likely if the individual has a "weak" digestive system already.[6]

Concerns have been raised regarding the presence of furancoumarins (psoralen and bergapten) in *Angelica sinensis* and the subsequent increased possibility of a photosensitization resulting in a dermatitis like skin reaction.[18,19] Examples of phototoxic reactions have been noted when high doses of psoralens from other plants (e.g., celery) have been administered in conjunction with UV light.[19]

There is one report of a case in which a 35-year-old man in Singapore experienced gynae-comastia after self-medicating with dong quai (dose not available, product labeled 100% dang gui root powder) for 1 month.[20] His hormone levels were reported to be normal and his symptoms resolved completely within 3 months after discontinuing dong quai.

It has been noted that parenteral administration of the volatile oil results in severe pain, nausea, hot flushes and chills. These reactions are usually self-limiting.[9] In addition it has been reported that the intravenous injection of the volatile components of the plant may cause renal failure.[12] A case of anaphylactic shock resulting from the injection of a product containing Angelica has also been noted.[9]

CAUTIONS/CONTRAINDICATIONS

Given its action on uterine smooth muscle, dong quai should not be used during the first trimester of pregnancy or in individuals with a history of spontaneous abortion.[6] Given the lack of information, many suggest that consumption of dong quai should be avoided at any stage of pregnancy except when used by an appropriately trained healthcare provider.[2] There are three unpublished case reports of rashes in infants who were being breast fed by women ingesting dong quai. The rashes reported resolved when dong quai was discontinued. Specific details of these cases are not available.[5]

Practitioners of Traditional Chinese Medicine advise that "tonic" herbs, such as dong quai, should not be used during acute illness (i.e., the flu and colds).[6,7] In addition, dong quai should be avoided in cases of hemorrhagic disease and hypermenorrhea.[6]

DRUG INTERACTIONS

Plant medicines rich in coumarins may interfere with concomitant anticoagulant therapy.[21] There is one case report in the literature that describes a 46-year-old African-American woman diagnosed with atrial fibrillation and stabilized on warfarin who experienced a greater than 2-fold increase in international normalized ratio (INR) after taking dong quai (Nature's Way, one 565 mg tablet once or twice daily) concurrently for 4 weeks. The patient's INR returned to acceptable levels 1 month after discontinuing the dong quai.[22]

DOSAGE REGIMENS

❖ RAW HERB: 3-10 g (or equivalent) daily.[23]

Note: Although dong quai is available in liquid extract and tincture preparations, there is little reliable information available on proper dosages.

Echinacea

E. angustifolia DC., *E. purpurea* (L.) Moench,
E. pallida (Nutt.) Nutt.

Common Uses
- ❖ *Internal:* Colds, Flus (supportive)
- ❖ Upper Respiratory Tract and Lower Urinary Tract Infections
- ❖ *External:* Skin Abrasions and Ulcerations

Active Constituents
- ❖ Polysaccharides
- ❖ Glycoproteins
- ❖ Alkamides
- ❖ Caffeic Acid Derivatives (such as echinacoside, cichoric acid and cynarin)

Adverse Effects
- ❖ Rare allergic reactions manifesting as asthma attacks, anaphylaxis or urticaria.

Cautions/Contraindication
- ❖ *Internal:* Progressive Systemic Diseases (e.g., tuberculosis, multiple sclerosis)
- ❖ Auto-Immune Conditions (e.g., diabetes mellitus, lupus, rheumatoid arthritis)
- ❖ HIV/AIDS (use controversial)
- ❖ *External:* none known

Drug Interactions
- ❖ Opposes Effects of Immunosuppressants (theoretical)

Doses
Internal
- ❖ *Dried Herb:* 1 g three times daily
- ❖ *Hydroalcoholic Tincture* (1:5 in 45% ethanol): 2-5 mL three times daily
- ❖ *Liquid Extract* (1:1 in 45% ethanol): 0.5-1.0 mL three times daily
- ❖ *Expressed Juice (E. purpurea):* 6-9 mL daily in divided doses

External
- ❖ Semi-solid preparations should contain at least 15% expressed juice *(E. purpurea)*

Introduction

Family
❖ Asteraceae (also known as Compositae or Sunflower family)

Synonyms
❖ Purple coneflower
❖ Purple Kansas coneflower
❖ Black simpson
❖ Red sunflower
❖ Comb flower
❖ Cock up hat
❖ Missouri snakeroot
❖ Kansas snakeroot
❖ Indian head[1,2]

Medicinal Forms
ROOT
❖ Dried Root
❖ Tincture
❖ Liquid Extract
AERIAL PARTS
❖ Expressed Juice (liquid or semi-solid)

Description

There are nine Echinacea species indigenous to the North American mid-west from Saskatchewan to Texas,[3] but only three species of this perennial are collected or cultivated as medicinal herbs. *Echinacea angustifolia* is the smallest of these plants, growing to only 0.5 meters or 18 inches. Although commercial cultivation of *Echinacea angustifolia* has been initiated, much of the medicinal supply is still wild-harvested. The tap root of *Echinacea angustifolia* can reach 1 to 1.5 meters or 3 to 5 feet in length. *Echinacea pallida* is larger, growing to approximately 1 meter or 40 inches in height. *Echinacea purpurea*, the most common purple cone flower, can grow from 0.5 to 1.5 meters or 18 inches to 5 feet tall. The entire medicinal supply of this third species is cultivated.[3,4] Each species features several spreading, soft-purple flower rays and a conical disk composed of numerous purple, tubular florets, from which the name "purple cone flower" derives. The genus name may derive from the Greek 'echinos' for sea urchin or hedgehog after its bristly leaves and cone.

Echinacea angustifolia is the favored species in North America and is often the only species listed in North American reference texts. It has been argued that it is largely the favorite simply because of familiarity — it is native to North America and knowledge about this species has been handed down through generations of herbalists and Native healers. However, *E. angustifolia* is largely still harvested from wild sources, which raises concerns about both the sustainability and quality of the supply. Limited efforts are currently underway to cultivate *E. angustifolia* for medicinal purposes.

In contrast, *Echinacea purpurea* is the only species currently commercially cultivated. In addition, the vast majority of both pharmacological and clinical studies have been conducted with *E. purpurea* — primarily with the commercial product Echinacin®, which is the expressed juice of the aerial parts of the plant, with alcohol added as a preservative. Echinacin® was used in the creation of the Commission E monograph in Germany.

Parts Used

Traditionally, the roots are primarily used medicinally; however, there is scientific evidence that the aerial parts of *E. purpurea* also have some medicinal action.[4,5]

Traditional Use

Echinacea species were used extensively as medicinal herbs by native North American tribes,[6] reportedly to treat a variety of ailments, including mouth sores, toothaches, colds, sore throats, burns and snake bites.[1,7-9] Its use for snake bites gave rise to several common names (Missouri and Kansas Snakeroot).

H.F.C. Meyer, a German physician working in Nebraska, is credited with introducing echinacea to the medical profession when he began selling a patent formula containing a root extract of *E. angustifolia* in the 1870s. In 1887 Meyer brought echinacea to the attention of John King, a well-known Eclectic physician, and John Uri Lloyd, a prominent pharmacist and manufacturer, who undertook a number of trials of the product and then began marketing echinacea products as anti-infective agents.[1,2] By 1915, echinacea products were available from many other pharmaceutical companies, including Merck, Wyeth and Parke Davis.[2] Although the Eclectics embraced the use of echinacea, it was widely criticized by the 'regular' medical establishment of the time, who argued that there was no scientific evidence to support its use.[10] However, from 1916 to 1950 *E. angustifolia* and *E. pallida* roots were listed as official drugs in the National Formulary of the United States.

To meet the growing European demand for echinacea, a German company (Madaus AHG) attempted to import *E. angustifolia* seeds from the United States; however, the species imported was subsequently demonstrated to be *E. purpurea*. The majority of European research on echinacea in the last 50 years was conducted using the Madaus product Echinacin®, which is made from the expressed juices of the aerial parts of *E. purpurea* combined with 22% ethanol (as a preservative).[1,11]

Current Medicinal Use

Several hundred articles and three major books have been written about echinacea.[12-14] In addition, Bauer and Wagner provide an excellent review.[9] A large proportion of the literature was originally published in German. Echinacea has been shown to have immunological activity. While the results from clinical trials are sometimes conflicting, there is a growing body of information to show that it may be useful in treating colds, flus and infections of the upper respiratory tract and lower urinary tract when administered internally. This herb also has anti-inflammatory activity, used in managing skin abrasions and ulcerations when administered externally.

Relevant Research

Preventative and Therapeutic Effects

CONSTITUENTS [9,15-22]

Although the three species are often considered interchangeable clinically, their chemical constituents differ. One study found no characteristic chemical differences between the aerial parts of the three species; however, the alkylamides in the roots did differ significantly.[22] *E. angustifolia* may be distinguished from *E. purpurea* because the former contains isobutylamides, echinacoside and cynarin, and the latter contains distinctive polyacetylenes and polyenes.[19] Echinacoside (the chemical to which many echinacea products are standardized) has been found in both *E. angustifolia* and *E. pallida* (but not *E. purpurea*); however, cynarine, a quinic acid derivative has only been detected in *E. angustifolia* and may be useful for discriminating between it and the other two species.[9] In addition, echinacein, the isobutylamide generally thought to cause the 'tingling of the tongue' associated with echinacea products, has only been identified as a constituent of *E. angustifolia*.

E. angustifolia

- ❖ CARBOHYDRATES: sucrose, pentosans, fructose.
- ❖ POLYSACCHARIDES: inulin storage (fructans), hetero-polysaccharides (structural).
- ❖ PHENOLIC COMPOUNDS: caffeic acid derivatives, echinacoside, 3-malonylglucoside cynarin (roots only), chlorogenic, isochlorogenic acid (leaves and stems).
- ❖ FLAVONOIDS: a variety including luteolin, kaempferol and quercetin derivatives, rutoside.
- ❖ FATTY ACIDS: linoleic, oleic, cerotic and palmitic acids.
- ❖ POLYACETYLENES: a variety of polyynes and polyenes.
- ❖ ALKYLAMIDES: echinacein and a variety of others including pyrrolidides, piperidides, isobutylamides (pattern of alkylamides differs from E. purpurea).
- ❖ ALKALOIDS: tussilagine, isotussilagine (pyrrolizidines that do not contain 1,2-unsaturated necine ring system necessary to confer liver toxicity).
- ❖ MISCELLANEOUS: betaine hydrochloride, phytosterols, n-triacontanol, behenic acid ethyl ester.

E. purpurea

- ❖ CARBOHYDRATES: fructose.
- ❖ POLYSACCHARIDES: a variety of hetero-polysaccharides (structural) including arabinogalactan, xyloglucans.
- ❖ PHENOLIC COMPOUNDS: caffeic acid derivatives, chicoric acid, caftaric acid & derivatives (mainly aerial parts).
- ❖ FLAVONOIDS: several, including a variety of kaempferol, quercetin and rutin derivatives, Rutoside.
- ❖ FATTY ACIDS: linoleic, oleic, cerotic and palmitic acids.
- ❖ POLYACETYLENES: a varitey of polyynes and polyenes.
- ❖ ALKYLAMIDES: echinacein and a variety of isobutylamides (pattern of alkylamides differs from E. angustifolia).
- ❖ ALKALOIDS: tussilagine, isotussilagine (pyrrolizidines that do not contain 1, 2-unsaturated necine ring system necessary to confer liver toxicity).
- ❖ MISCELLANEOUS: glycine betaine, cyanidins, glycoproteins.

E. pallida

- ❖ The polyacetylenes of E. pallida are very susceptible to oxidation, thus the chemical composition of the roots depends on storage conditions.[19]
- ❖ CARBOHYDRATES: sucrose, petosans.
- ❖ POLYSACCHARIDES: inulin storage (fructans), hetero-polysaccharides (structural).
- ❖ PHENOLIC COMPOUNDS: caffeic acid derivatives, echinacoside, des-rhamnosyl-verascoside, 6-0-caffcoyl-echinacoside (roots only), caftaric acid & derivatives (mainly aerial parts), chlorogenic, isochlorogenic acid (leaves and stems).
- ❖ FLAVONOIDS: a variety, including luteolin, kaempferol and quercetin derivatives, rutoside
- ❖ FATTY ACIDS: linoleic, oleic, cerotic and palmitic acids.
- ❖ POLYACETYLENES: a variety of polyynes and polyenes; ketoalkynes and ketoalkenes.
- ❖ ALKYLAMIDES: traces.
- ❖ MISCELLANEOUS: betaine hydrochloride, cyanidins.

IMMUNOLOGICAL ACTIVITY

The immunostimulatory action of echinacea appears to depend on the synergistic action of several constituents; although several different compounds have been shown to possess immunological activity, echinacea's effects on the immune system cannot be attributed to any single compound.[9] Most of the scientific research has been conducted with isolated fractions of *E. purpurea* (often a polysaccharide extract) and *E. angustifolia*. Very little research has reported on *E. pallida*.

In vitro and In vivo Studies

Research teams have demonstrated that extracts of *E. purpurea*: increase phagocytosis significantly *in vitro*[23-29] and *in vivo*;[22-24,28,30] increase proliferation of phagocytes in spleen and bone marrow;[24] stimulate migration of granulocytes to the peripheral blood;[24,26] stimulate macrophages to excrete tumor necrosis factor (TNF);[16,17,23,25] stimulate macrophages to secrete interleukin-1 (IL-1)[16-24] and interleukin-6 (IL-6);[24] stimulate monocytes to produce IL-1, IL-6, and tumour necrosis factor;[24] stimulate macrophages to produce interferon-B_2;[16] independently and directly activate macrophages to cytotoxicity;[16,17,30,31]; increase properdin levels;[32] increase the number of PMN and activate the adherence of PMN to the endothelial cells.[25] In addition, studies revealed that *E. purpurea* extracts appear to have no direct action on T lymphocytes,[31] no induction of lymphokine (MAF) production;[31] no significant stimulation of B cell proliferation;[16,31] and no enhancement of specific immune responses (antibody production).[24]

Studies with *E. angustifolia* extracts have demonstrated a statistically significant increase in the phagocytic activity of peritoneal macrophages in mice.[33]

Given that the majority of studies discussed above were completed with defined-composition extracts, it is difficult to extrapolate the results of these studies to consumption of the varied commercially available preparations of Echinacea species in clinical settings.

Human Trials

Roesler et al. demonstrated that many of the effects of *E. purpurea* extracts previously noted *in vitro* or in animal models were also found when an extract was given i.v. to human test subjects.[25] Effects demonstrated in humans include: adherence to endothelial cells;[25] phagocytosis;[23,32,34,35] migration from bone marrow into the peripheral blood;[25] and production of IL-6.[36] However, direct conclusions about the efficacy of marketed echinacea products are not possible from these findings.

A randomized, placebo-controlled study of 42 male triathletes reported that ingestion of 8 mL of the pressed juice of *Echinacea purpurea* (Echinacin EC 31®) daily for 28 days prior to competition appeared to reduce soluble interleukin 2 receptor release and facilitate interleukin-6 release in response to exercise and possibly reduced the incidence of respiratory infections.[37] In contrast to earlier studies, a double-blind, placebo-controlled crossover study (n=20) of the nonspecific immune response after the oral ingestion of the freshly expressed juice of *Echinacea purpurea* (dose not specified, identical in composition to the commercially available German product Esberitox®) for 14 days reported that echinacea did not enhance phagocytic activity of polymorphonuclear leukocytes nor that of monocytes when compared with placebo. In addition, in this study the echinacea dose did not influence the production of tumor necrosis factor alpha, a cause for concern with echinacea products, nor that of interleukin 1 beta.Unexpectedly, the echinacea did decrease serum ferritin concentration.

Clearly the pharmacology of this herb and its many constituents is complex, emphasizing the need for additional research in determining echinacea's mode of action.

Treatment of Upper Respiratory Tract Infections (including the Common Cold)

Melchart et al. have completed a review of 8 controlled trials that assessed the efficacy of preparations of echinacea alone or in combination with other plant extracts in the treatment of the common cold.[38] All 8 trials were randomized and 7 of the 8 were double-blinded. The authors identify that the quality of the reporting of most studies was poor, making it difficult to assess the validity of the results. This review is a good example of the extra effort that needs to be taken in searching for information related to herbal medicine since most of the studies were performed in Germany and none were published in MEDLINE-listed journals. Overall, 6 trials reported that the echinacea preparation was significantly better at relieving symptoms associated with the common cold than a placebo.[39-44] In contrast, 2 trials reported no significant difference between echinacea and the placebo.[39,45] However, in the Braunig trial, only the effects of the low dose were found to be indistinguishable from placebo,[39] and in the Dorn trial the patients in the treatment group had more severe symptoms at baseline.[45] The authors concluded that "preparations containing extracts of echinacea probably can be effective in the prevention and treatment of common colds. Still, the evidence is far from compelling and conclusive for clinical decision making."[38] One of the biggest challenges was identified as the great heterogeneity and unclear compatibility of the echinacea products being investigated in the clinical trials. In addition, the poor quality of the reporting of the studies made the review difficult. The authors also suggest that publication bias may be a concern with respect to studies of echinacea. Relating this information to the herb itself is challenging, since only 2 of the trials included in this review assessed the effect of echinacea as a single agent; the others assessed proprietary combination products. A second review of 9 treatment trials has also concluded that "echinacea may be beneficial for early treatment of acute upper respiratory tract infections."[46]

Three randomized, controlled trials (2 positive and 1 negative) have been published since these reviews. One study compared the efficacy of Echinaforce® (*Echinacea purpurea* preparation from 95% herb and 5% root), *Echinacea purpurea* concentrate (same preparation at 7 times higher concentration) , another brand of *Echinacea purpurea* root preparation or placebo (dose: 2 tablets three times daily). Participants (n=246) started taking the study medication immediately after the onset of the first symptoms of a common cold and continued taking the product until they felt better or for a maximum of 7 days. Those taking Echinaforce® or the Echinacea concentrate experienced a relative reduction in the symptom complaint index compared to the placebo group.[47] A subsequent multi-center, double-blind, placebo-controlled trial of patients (n=263) suffering from the common cold found that those ingesting 3 tablets of a proprietary product (Esberitox®N) containing echinacea and 2 other herbs (Radix baptisiea / *Baptisia tinctoria* and Herba thujae / *Thuja occidentalis*) three times daily for 7 to 9 days had significantly more symptom relief than those ingesting a placebo. The therapeutic benefit as measured by total score of symptoms, bronchitis score, rhinitis score and patients' overall rating of the cold severity appeared greater than placebo on day 2, reached statistical significance on day 4 and continued until the end of treatment.[48] Since both Baptisia and Thuja have historically been used for upper respiratory tract infections, it is difficult to determine how much of these results can be attributed to Echinacea.

The third randomized, double-blind, placebo-controlled trial investigated the efficacy of a dried, encapsulated whole-plant Echinacea (each capsule contained 50% or 123 mg of *E. angustifolia* root, 25% or 62 mg of *E. purpurea* root and 25% or 62 mg of *E. purpurea* ariel parts) as a treatment for the early symptoms of the common cold compared with a placebo (alfalfa). A total of 148 students with common colds of recent onset were given asked to take 4 capsules six times daily (for a total of 6 g daily) for the first day of illness, followed by 4 capsules three times daily (for a total of 3 g daily) for each subsequent day of illness for a maximum of ten days. No statistically significant differences were found between those taking echinacea and those in the placebo group on any of the outcomes measured, which included mean cold duration and severity of cold symptoms. The authors concluded that "compared with placebo, unrefined echinacea provided no detectable benefit or harm in these college students who had the common cold."[49]

Overall, the applicability of most of the clinical studies reviewed to the echinacea products currently available to North American consumers is limited. So although some of these preliminary results appear promising, further research is required to confirm the efficacy of echinacea in the management of acute upper respiratory tract infections or the common cold. Most specifically, it is necessary to determine which specific extracts of echinacea are associated with positive clinical effects in humans.

Prevention of Upper Respiratory Tract Infections (including the common cold)

Melchart et al. recently completed a comprehensive review of placebo-controlled clinical trials that assessed the efficacy of echinacea products for the prevention of upper respiratory tract infections.[38] In total, 5 trials were assessed (3 investigated the effects of echinacea as a single entity and 2 investigated combination products containing echinacea). The authors indicated that 4 of the 5 trials were of acceptable methodological quality and that all were randomized and double-blinded. Of those trials, 1 found a statistically significant lower incidence of infection,[50] while the other trials reported only trends in favor of the treatment group.[51-53] In addition, the study results conflicted with respect to the effect of echinacea on the severity or duration of infections that did occur during the treatment period. Overall, the authors concluded that preparations containing extracts of echinacea probably can be effective in the prevention and treatment of common colds. Still, the evidence is far from compelling and conclusive for clinical decision making."[38]

Two additional studies (both negative) have been published since this review. One used an experimental cold model to evaluate the effectiveness of echinacea (alone) for the prevention of rhinovirus colds. In this randomized, double-blind, placebo-controlled trial participants (n=117) were treated with either echinacea (300 mg three times daily) or placebo for 14 days prior to the virus challenge. They continued taking the study medication for 5 days post virus challenge. Echinacea was found to have no significant effect on either the occurrence of infection of the severity of illness.[54] In the second trial, 109 patients with a history of 3 or more colds in the preceding year were randomly assigned to receive either 4 mL fluid extract of *Echinacea purpurea* or placebo daily and were followed for an 8-week period. Although a trend toward an effect in the echinacea group was noted, no statistically significant differences in the incidence, duration or severity of colds and respiratory infections were noted between those ingesting echinacea and those ingesting the placebo.[55]

Melchart et al. suggest that any prophylactic effect is likely to be moderate in size (15-20% relative risk reduction), and that studies to confirm this would require very large sample sizes and thus would be very costly.[38] Overall, current evidence from clinical trials suggests that prophylactic ingestion of echinacea is unlikely to result in a clinically significant reduction of the incidence, severity or duration of the common cold. Larger (and more costly) clinical trials are necessary to confirm these findings. The expense maybe worthwhile given the popularity of this herb in preventing colds and flus.

OTHER RELATED ACTIVITY

Local Activity in Tissues

Historically, echinacea species were used for the treatment of snake bites and were reported to reduce the spread of venom. Scientific investigation of this phenomenon occurred primarily in the 1950's and centred on the effect of echinacea on hyaluronidase. All these studies were conducted with the German product Echinacin®, which is made from the expressed juices of the aerial parts of *E. purpurea* combined with 22% ethanol (as a preservative).[1,11] Echinacin® has been shown to inhibit hyaluronidase production *in vitro* and *in vivo*.[8,56,57] One study suggested that 0.04 mL of Echinacin® was equivalent to 1 mg of cortisone using a modified spreading test in rats.[58] It has been hypothesized that in addition to a direct effect on hyaluronidase production, Echinacin® may also stimulate changes in fibroblasts resulting in an indirect effect on the hyaluronic acid-hyaluronidase system.[59,60]

Anti-Inflammatory Activity

Investigations of the anti-inflammatory properties of echinacea have primarily been limited to *Echinacea angustifolia*. In 1956, Keller isolated two active fractions from echinacea species and showed that Fraction A had some cortisone-like activity.[61] Later Bonadeo et al. isolated a polysaccharide fraction (which may be identical to Keller's Fraction A) and suggested that its anti-inflammatory mechanism of action may be the formation of a hyaluronic acid-polysaccharide complex which indirectly inhibits hyaluronidase.[62,63] More recently, two research teams have confirmed the anti-inflammatory activity of *Echinacea augustifolia*. A raw extract applied topically inhibited oedema (initiated by croton oil) in the ears of rats in a dose-dependent manner,[64,65] and was found to be more potent than benzidamine (a topical NSAID)[64] and approximately half as potent as topical indomethacin.[65] Given i.v. 1 hour prior to injection with carrageenan, the same extract inhibited oedema in the paws of rats.[65] Most recently, several alkylamides isolated from *Echinacea angustifolia* were shown to inhibit both cyclooxygenase and 5-lipoxygenase *in vitro*.[18] Inhibition of 5-lipoxygenase *in vitro* has also been reported in an alkylamide fraction isolated from *Echinacea purpurea* roots.[66]

In a clinical study, patients with chronic inflammation (9 due to viral infections; 14 due to bacterial infections) were administered Echinacin® (1 ampoule i.m. once daily for 7 days). There was an increase in the total lymphocyte count, with a decreased percentage of T4 cells.[67] Similar results were obtained in another study of patients suffering from contact eczema (n=4), neurodermatitis (n=6), herpes simplex (n=8) and Candida infection (n=10). Echinacin® was applied topically daily for 7 days. After 7 days, the proportion of t-helper cells was decreased, but an overall lymphocytosis was observed.[68]

Anti-Bacterial and Anti-Viral Activity

Echinacea has been shown to have only very weak activity as an anti-viral, anti-bacterial or anti-fungal agent. Several extracts of *E. angustifolia* (echinacoside and an alcoholic extract) have shown limited inhibitory activity against *Staphylococcus aureus*,[69] *Escherichia coli*,[70] *Pseudomonas aeruginosa*,[70] and *Trichomonas vaginalis* [71] *in vitro*. Several compounds isolated from *E. purpurea* were also shown to have weak activity against *Escherichia coli* and *Pseudomonas aeruginosa*.[70] Echinacea does not appear to be clinically useful as an antibiotic.

Several teams of researchers have noted the anti-viral activity of echinacea. The brand Echinacin® (*E. purpurea*) was reported to have some activity (in mice) against encephalomyocarditis virus (EMC virus) and vesicular-stomatitis virus (VSV).[72] In addition, extracts of *E. purpurea* were found to have some activity against influenza, herpes, VSV, and poliovirus *in vitro*.[73,74] Extracts of *E. pallida* have also been reported to exhibit some inhibition of VSV.[75] Given that the anti-viral activity observed requires the presence of 0-2-diethylamino ethyl dextran (DEAE) (*in vivo*)[72] and did not develop in the presence of hyaluronidase (*in vitro*),[73] an "interferon-like" mechanism of action without the induction of interferon has been hypothesized.

MISCELLANEOUS EFFECTS

Anti-Cancer

Echinacin® (*E. purpurea*) 60 mg/m² (i.m. daily days 3-10 and then twice weekly) was given as part of an immunotherapy protocol given to 15 outpatients with metastasizing, far-advanced colorectal cancers that included cyclophosphamide (LDCY) 300 mg/m² every 28 days and thymostimulin 30 mg/m² days 3-10 and then twice weekly. Stimulation of the phagocytic activity of peripheral blood leukocytes was noted 14 days after the low-dose cyclophosphamide and attributed to the effect of the Echinacin®. Mean survival time was 4 months and 2 patients survived more than 8 months.[76] Given the advanced stage of the disease in this patients, comparison of these survival times with others reported in the literature was not possible. A randomized, placebo-controlled trial is needed to assess the effects of this protocol on survival. A second study has suggested that components of echinacea may have the potential to promote anti-cancer activity.[77]

Protection Against Radiation
One study in irradiated rats suggests that *Echinacea purpurea* promoted the effective functioning of the vitamin E redox system by mobilizing the body's stores of liposoluble vitamin A, carotene and vitamin E.[78]

Prevention Against Chemotherapy-Induced Leukopenia
There is one open prospective study with matched historical controls of 15 patients with advanced gastric cancer undergoing palliative chemotherapy who were injected (IV) with 2 mg of the polysaccharide fraction isolated from *Echinacea purpurea* (EPS-EPO VIIa) for 10 days (beginning 3 days prior to chemotherapy). The results of this pilot study suggest that this extract of echinacea (administered IV) might be effective in reducing chemotherapy-induced leukopenia.[79] This evidence is promising and suggests that further research in this area may be warranted.

Prevention and/or Treatment of Skin Photodamage
One study suggests that echinacea species has a dose-dependent protective effect on the free radical-induced degradation of Type III collagen. The authors suggest that echinacea products may be useful in the prevention and/or treatment of photodamage of the skin.[80]

Recurrent Genital Herpes
There is one randomized, double-blind, placebo-controlled crossover trial designed to assess whether an extract of echinacea (*Echinacea purpurea*, Echinaforce® brand) could influence the clinical course of recurrent genital herpes. In total, 50 patients took Echinaforce® (800 mg twice daily) for 6 months; however, no statistically significant benefit could be detected then Echinaforce and placebo were compared (outcomes included frequency and severity of genital herpes recurrences).[81]

COMPARATIVE STUDIES
One study found that the ethanolic root extracts of all three species caused a 20-30% increase in phagocytosis *in vitro* and *in vivo*,[28] with E. *purpurea* appearing slightly (non-significantly) more active than the other two species. Another trial found that *E. purpurea* was significantly more active *in vitro* than the other species;[82] however, Bergner criticizes this trial because the researchers used only 30% alcohol to make the extracts of each of the species and he notes that tinctures of *E. angustifolia* used clinically are usually made with 80% alcohol. The different alcohol concentrations would likely result in the extraction of different compounds from the plant material. He also argues that the sources of the three species were not reported.[83]

ADVERSE EFFECTS
Of all the studies reviewed for this monograph, only one reported any acute toxicity (mild "influenza-like" symptoms after iv administration of 5 mg of polysaccharide extract of *E. purpurea*),[25] and there were no reports of chronic toxicity of echinacea. Many reviews, including the German Commission E, indicate that there are no known toxic effects, although a temperature increase of 0.5-1°C is common with i.v, i.m., or s.c. injections of Echinacin®.[3,8,84] Using the Lorke method on mice, LD_{50} values of >2500 and >5000 mg/kg have been found for a polysaccharide mixture from the aerial parts of E. *purpurea* and from a cell culture of *E. purpurea* respectively.[85] The animals died not from the echinacea, but from the hyperosmolar solution injected in such large amounts.

E. purpurea cell cultures have also been tested for possible gene toxicity in human lymhocyte cultures and found to have no significant toxic effects in short or long term experiments.[86] No hepatotoxic effects have been found (or are expected) with the pyrrolizidine alkaloids in echinacea species because they do not contain the 1,2-unsaturated necine ring system.[87,88] Finally, some concern has been raised given the reported *in vitro* stimulation of the secretion of TNF and the potential role of TNF in cachexia and endotoxic shock;[89] however, Bergner argues that an increase in the secretion of TNF has only been demonstrated by using purified polysaccharides derived from *E. purpurea* cells cultured *in vitro* and that these polysaccharides are not present in most commercial products.[90] Also, as mentioned above, more recent evidence questions whether echinacea effects TNF at all.[37]

In the past, *Echinacea purpurea* roots have been adulterated with *Parthenium integrifolium* L., Asteraceae (Missouri snakeroot), which may have caused other adverse effects.[4] Individuals with allergies to the sunflower family (Asteraceae or Compositae) may experience mild allergic symptoms when ingesting echinacea.[84,91]

One case of echinacea-associated anaphylaxis has been reported in a 37 year old woman who ingested 5 mL (approximately double the manufacturer's recommended amount) of an echinacea tincture (containing *E. angustifolia* whole plant and *E. purpurea* root). The patient experienced an immediate burning of the mouth and throat followed within a few minutes by tightness in the chest, generalized urticaria and diarrhea. Her symptoms resolved completely during two hours of observation in the Emergency Department with no need for further treatment (the patient self-medicated with 75 mg promethazine orally prior to being transported to the hospital).[92] At least 26 cases suggestive of possible immunoglobulin E-mediated hypersensitivity (4 anaphylaxis, 12 acute asthma, 10 urticaria/angioedema) associated with echinacea have been reported to the Australian adverse drug reporting system.[93] In addition, there is a case report of recurrent erythema nodosum that was temporally associated with the use of echinacea.[94] However, as with most herbal adverse event reports, little or no attempt has been made to determine the quality of the echinacea products to rule out potential adulterants that may be the cause the patients' symptoms.

CAUTIONS/CONTRAINDICATIONS
External
None known.[9,84]

Internal
Echinacea should be used with caution by patients with progressive systemic diseases (e.g., tuberculosis, leucoses, multiple sclerosis);[84] or auto-immune conditions (e.g., diabetes mellitus, lupus, rheumatoid arthritis). Use of echinacea is also controversial in HIV/AIDS.

However, Bergner argues that these contraindications are not necessary. He argues that no clinical evidence exists to support these claims and cites historical evidence that echinacea has actually been used to treat tuberculosis,[95,96] and leukemia.[97]

There is currently very little research investigating the safety of echinacea use by women who are pregnant. One prospective controlled cohort study conducted by the Motherisk Program (n=206) concluded that gestational use of echinacea and echinacea products does not appear to be associated with increased risk for major malformation.[98] Additional research in this area is required to confirm these findings.

A recent study reported that echinacea products purchased from retail stores in the United States often do not contain the labeled species and that claims of "standardization" on the labels did not mean that the products were accurately labeled nor that their contents were less variable in concentration than other products.[99] The quality of herbal products such as echinacea can be quite variable depending on the country in which the product is manufactured/sold. This situation makes it difficult to determine efficacy and potential risk for echinacea products.

DRUG INTERACTIONS

None reported by the German Commission E;[84] however, its effects oppose the action of immunosuppressants.

DOSAGE REGIMENS

Echinacea has widely been reported to lose its ability to stimulate the immune system if taken continuously for extended periods of time; however, there appears to be little scientific evidence to clearly support or confirm this claim.[100] Bergner argues that oral doses of echinacea have never been shown to lose their effectiveness, citing recent clinical trials which demonstrated continued effects from echinacea at 8 weeks or more.[100] This opinion is supported by Kerry Bone.[101] However, Hobbs reviews the literature and incorporates his extensive clinical experience to recommend that echinacea products be taken cyclically: 10 to 14 days on with a 3 day rest period.[7] The German Commission E monograph suggests that echinacea should not be taken continuously (internally or externally) for more than 8 weeks.[84]

Internal

❖ DRIED HERB: 1 g three times daily.[102]
❖ HYDROALCOHOLIC TINCTURE (1:5 in 45% ethanol): 2 to 5 mL three times daily.[102]
❖ LIQUID EXTRACT (1:1 in 45% ethanol): 0.5-1.0 mL three times daily.[102]
❖ EXPRESSED JUICE (E. PURPUREA): 6-9 mL daily in divided doses.[84]

External

❖ Semi-solid preparations should contain at least 15% expressed juice *(E. Purpurea)*.[84]
 Note: Many products are standardized to echinacoside content (approximately 4%). This is a method of demonstrating authenticity (for *E. angustifolia*) rather than a measure of therapeutic potency.

Elder

Sambucus nigra L.

Common Uses
- *Internal:* Respiratory Tract Ailments (especially with fever and phlegm colds, flu, sinusitis, hay fever and bronchitis)
- *External:* Eczema, Boils, Dermatitis

Active Constituents
- Flavonoids
- Triterpenes
- Essential Oils
- Sterols
- Phenolic Acids

Adverse Effects
- None noted with berries or flowers of American or European elder.

Cautions/Contraindications
- Pregnancy and Lactation
- Hypokalemic Potential (prolonged use not recommended)
- Limit products made from ripe berries or flowers only

Drug Interactions
- None noted

Doses

Internal
- *Dried Flowers:* 3-5 g three times daily
- *Liquid Extract* (1:1 in 25% ethanol): 3-5 mL three times daily
- *Tincture* (1:5 in 25% ethanol): 10-25 mL three times daily

External
- Elder Flowers can also be used externally in the form of poultices, ointments and salves.

Introduction

Description

Both the *Sambucus nigra* L. (European elder) and *S. nigra* L. ssp. *canadensis* (L.) R. Bolli (American elder) tree are used medicinally. They share similar indications and appearance, except that the European elder is slightly larger, growing up to 10 meters or 33 feet in height as compared to 4 meters or 13 feet for its North American cousin.[1,5] *S. nigra* L. ssp. *canadensis* (L.) R. Bolli is native to the eastern United States and Canada, while *Sambucus nigra* L. is common place throughout the hedgerows of the United Kingdom and Europe.[1,5] Both species can now be found throughout North America. The tree blooms with yellow white flowers in late spring, and the berries turn from through dark red to black.

Parts Used

While the flowers are the part most commonly used medicinally, most parts, notably the leaves and berries, are considered to have therapeutic properties.[1, 3]

Traditional Use

Known as 'Mother Nature's medicine chest', elder has traditionally been used to treat a wide variety of ailments, including coughs, colds, allergies, and arthritis. Elder is also rich in folklore, believed to be a good charm, used to drive away robbers and kill snakes.[6] In rural England, it was considered a grave offence to damage any part of the tree since it was thought to be inhabited by the 'Elder Mother' and intrinsically linked to 'Mother Earth'.[7] Elderberries are also used as food, in making elderberry pie and wine. Another species, Red elderberry (*Sambucus racemosa*), has long been used by the Haida, Saanich and Cowichan peoples of British Columbia in the treatment of many conditions ranging from women's health to those similar to *Sambucus nigra* L. and *S. nigra* L. ssp. *canadensis* (L.) R. Bolli.[8]

Current Medicinal Use

Based on traditional evidence, elder flowers are used in the treatment of many respiratory conditions where there is fever and/or phlegm (colds, flu, hayfever, sinusitis, recurrent ear infections, bronchitis, croup). Ointments, lotions and salves made from elder flowers are used to treat various skin conditions and irritations (eczema, dermatitis, urticaria).

Relevant Research

Preventative and Therapeutic Effects

CONSTITUENTS

Based on investigations of European elder only.

Flowers [1,2,5,9-13]

❖ FLAVONOIDS: quercetin, kaempferol, isoquercetin, rutin, astragalin.
❖ TRITERPENES: ursolic acid, and amyrin, 30 hydroxyursolic acid.
❖ ESSENTIAL OIL: fatty acids and alkanes.
❖ PHENOLIC ACIDS: chlorogenic acid, p-coumaric acid and caffeic acid.
❖ MISCELLANEOUS: mucilage, tannins, potassium, pectin, proteins (plastocynin).

Leaf

❖ Similar to above with cyanogenic glucosides (sambunigrin) also present.[5,9,14]

Berries

❖ Fruit acids, tannins, anthocyanin pigments, pectin, traces of essential oil.[1]

Bark

❖ Phytohemagglutins,[15] lectin, triterpenoids,[2] cyanogenic glucosides.[4]

COMPONENT EFFECTS

Preparations made from various parts of the plant are suggested to be useful in the management of many conditions. Different parts are used for different indications.

Flowers

Elder flowers are used, alone or in combination with other herbal remedies such as peppermint, in the treatment of many respiratory conditions where there is fever and/or phlegm, including: colds,[1,7,9,16,17] flu,[1,7,9,16,17] hayfever,[1,7,16] sinusitis,[1,7,16] recurrent ear infections,[1,7] bronchitis,[1,7] and croup.[1] Gargles made from the flower are used to ease sore and irritated throats.[1] Preparations of elder flower are particularly popular in pediatric cases.[17]

The flowers have also been used for many conditions of the genitourinary tract, such as: cystitis and renal stones.[1] Generally, elder may be indicated in situations where diuresis is required.[7,9,16]

In addition, ointments, lotions and salves made from elder flowers are used to treat various skin conditions, including: eczema, dermatitis, urticaria and generally irritated skin.[1]

Berries

The berries are considered to be useful as an antirheumatic and laxative.[1,7,16] Liquid extracts made from the berries are now commonly used in monodiets, juice fasts and detoxification protocols.

MISCELLANEOUS EFFECTS

Pharmacological findings provide preliminary explanations for some of elder's indications. Extracts of *Sambucus nigra* L. have been shown to exert a diuretic effect in rats, primarily as a result of the flavonoid and potassium content.[9,18] This may explain its use in disorders of the genitourinary tract. As well, a methanolic extract of the branch tips of red elderberry has been shown to exhibit activity against bovine respiratory syncytial virus.[8] Red elderberry has also been shown to have some anti-bacterial[19] and anti-fungal activity.[20] While the extracts of various species of Sambucus have been used as diagnostic tools (e.g., as an indication of immunocompetence), no human clinical trials could be found to substantiate the above indications.[2]

Other miscellaneous actions of elder have also been reported. For example, oral administration of an elder extract has been shown to have mild anti-inflammatory properties in rats,[21] and lectins extracted from European elder have been shown to possess anti-spasmodic properties *in vitro*.[22]

ADVERSE EFFECTS
The flowers and ripe seeds appear to be free from adverse effects and are considered in the USA as being GRAS (generally regarded as safe).[2] Substances found in other parts of the plant, notably the cyanogenic glycosides, have the potential to cause gastrointestinal distress, including nausea, diarrhoea and vomiting.[2] Weiss cautions that the seeds of *Sambucus racemosa* may cause irritation to the mucous membranes.[23] Although the lectins have been shown to have teratogenic potential in pregnant mice, the doses administered were far above those possible in normal practice.[2]

CAUTIONS/CONTRAINDICATIONS
Newall cautions against both use in pregnancy and lactation and against long-term use due to the potential of hypokalemia resulting from prolonged diuresis.[2] No supporting evidence for this concern could be found from empirical sources.

DRUG INTERACTIONS
None recorded.

DOSAGE REGIMENS
Internal
❖ DRIED FLOWERS: 3-5 g of dried flowers taken as a hot infusion three times daily.[9]
❖ LIQUID EXTRACT OF DRIED FLOWER (1:1 in 25% ethanol): 3-5 mL of three times daily.[9]
❖ TINCTURE OF DRIED FLOWER (1:5 in 25% ethanol): 10-25 mL of three times daily.[9]

External
❖ Elder Flowers can also be used externally in the form of poultices, ointments and salves. *Note:* Even though parts from the whole plant have been used historically, medicinal use should be limited to the flowers and ripe berries (which are usually boiled).[2,4] Elder flowers are also taken often in the form of cordials and for nutritious rather than medicinal reasons.[1,23]

Evening Primrose
Oenothera biennis L.

Common Uses
- Atopic Eczema
- Diabetic Neuropathy
- Women's Health Care (including premenstrual syndrome, mastalgia and endometriosis)
- Rheumatoid Arthritis
- Multiple Sclerosis
- Sjögren's Syndrome
- Psychiatric Conditions (schizophrenia, hyperactivity in children, dementia)
- Alcoholism
- Obesity

Active Constituents
- Fixed Oil (containing gamma linolenic acid and linoleic acid)

Cautions/Contraindications
- Mania and Epilepsy

Drug Interactions
- None documented but concerns have been raised regarding use with: phenothiazines, non-steroidal anti-inflammatory drugs, corticosteroids, anticoagulants, and beta-adrenergic antagonists

Doses
- *Adults:* 2-8 grams seed oil daily in divided doses with food
- *Children:* 2-6 grams seed oil daily in divided doses with food

Introduction

Description

Evening primrose is a biennial standing 1 to 3 meters or 3 to 6 feet in height.[3] The stem rises from a fibrous taproot with a flat basal rosette of leaves. The plant blooms in early summer, producing large yellow flowers. The capsular pods that form after the individual blooms die contain brown seeds rich in fixed oil.[4] Evening primrose is actually not a primrose (Family Primulaceae) at all, but a member of the fuchsia (Onagraceae) family. Its name arises from the fact that the flowers open in the evening in order to allow pollination by insects (especially moths). While *Oenothera biennis* L. is native to North America, it is now naturalized throughout Western Europe, brought there accidentally as sea trade increased between the two continents.[4]

Parts Used

While the root and whole plant of evening primrose have been used in the past, the fixed oil from the seeds is now the primary form used therapeutically.[4]

Traditional Use

Evening primrose has been used for both medical and culinary purposes in the past. The root was used as a vegetable because of its pungent flavor,[4] and the whole plant was indicated in the management of many conditions, including: gastrointestinal disorders, asthmatic coughs, neuralgia and whooping cough.[4,5] These numerous indications gave rise to the plant being commonly referred to as 'King's Cureall'.[4]

Evening primrose oil was one the first nutritional/botanical supplements to gain popularity in the renaissance of 'alternative medicine'. The popularity of evening primrose oil supplements is such that in 1993 a survey of complementary medicine use in Australia showed that over 12% of all women supplemented with this product.[6]

Current Medicinal Use

As a source of pre-formed gamma linolenic acid, evening primrose oil may be of use in a number of conditions, especially those with an inflammatory component. Evidence from clinical trails of the efficacy of evening primrose for specific conditions is usually not complete and often conflicting. Despite this, it is commonly used in women's health care for treating premenstrual syndrome, mastalgia endometriosis and atopic eczema. Evening primrose is also used in rheumatoid arthritis, multiple sclerosis, and Sjögren's syndrome, as well as certain psychiatric conditions, such as hyperactivity, dementia and schizophrenia. Irrespective of the reason for taking evening primrose oil, it needs to be taken for a prolonged period of time (over 6 months) for best results.

Relevant Research

Preventative and Therapeutic Effects

CONSTITUENTS [2-4]

Given that the fixed oil of evening primrose oil is the part used medicinally, this analysis of the plant's constituents is limited to the seeds.

Approximately 14% fixed oil, comprising approximately:

❖ Cis-linoleic acid (70%)
❖ Cis-gamma linolenic acid (GLA) (9%)
❖ Oleic acid
❖ Palmitic acid
❖ Stearic acid

ESSENTIAL FATTY ACIDS

In understanding the suggested pharmacology of evening primrose oil, it is necessary to review some basic points regarding essential fatty acid (EFA) biochemistry and nomenclature. By definition, an essential fatty acid is one that the body cannot make. There are two basic types, omega 3 (derived from a-linolenic acid) and omega 6 (derived from linoleic acid). These essential fatty acids are polyunsaturated (containing more than one double bond). The naming of a particular fatty acid is made by determining the position of the first double bond from the methyl end of the carbon-carbon backbone of the molecule. For example, an omega 3 fatty acid contains a double bond between the third and fourth carbon atom. The essential fatty acids have a cis rather than a trans configuration and the omega 3 and omega 6 series are not interchangeable.[7,8]

Both alpha-linolenic and linoleic acid can be modified via desaturation or elongation reactions. While neither alpha-linolenic acid nor linoleic acid have any direct biological effect, their metabolites have pronounced physiological properties. The enzymatic mechanism by which these changes occur is very similar, if not identical, in both the omega 3 and omega 6 series.[8] The physiological action of EFAs occurs in one of two primary ways. EFAs play a role in the physical properties of cell membranes, influencing their flexibility and fluidity and thus they impact membrane based receptors and systems. EFAs also act as precursors of biologically active eicasonoids such as prostaglandins and leukotrienes.[8]

In the omega 6 series, cis-linoleic acid (LA) is converted to gamma-linolenic acid (GLA), which in turn is converted to dihomogamma-linolenic acid (DGLA). The rate-limiting step for this process is the desaturation of LA to GLA by the enzyme delta-6 desaturase. The DGLA can then be metabolized further to form arachadonic acid (AA) by delta-5 desaturase. DGLA can also be acted upon by cyclo-oxygenase to form prostaglandin E_1 (PGE_1). PGE_1 is generally regarded as being beneficial, inhibiting inflammation and platelet aggregation, decreasing blood pressure and regulating the immune system. Conversely, arachidonic acid gives rise to harmful pro-inflammatory mediators.[7,8] While it may be assumed that any increase in GLA would lead to a subsequent increase in both the anti-inflammatory and inflammatory moieties, this appears not to be the case. Administration of large amounts of GLA increases DGLA levels but not AA. It is thought that the beneficial metabolites of DGLA (including PGE_1) play a role in limiting the release of arachidonic acid from its phospholipid stores. Also while the conversion of GLA to DGLA is rapid, the activity of delta-5 desaturase is quite slow.[7,8]

Since the body can manufacture GLA, it should not theoretically be considered an essential fatty acid. In practice this may not be the case due to the inefficiency of the rate limiting enzyme mentioned above, delta-6 desaturase. This enzyme system appears to be compromised in many situations, including aging;[4,8,9] diabetes;[8,10,11] excessive consumption of alcohol;[7,8,12,13] viral infections;[7,8,14,15] and atopic eczema.[7,8] A deficiency in certain nutritional cofactors (e.g.,zinc,[8,16,17] pyridoxine,[4,8,18] and magnesium[4,8]) can also lead to a decreased activity of this enzyme system. The existence of a decreased rate of delta-6 desaturation in atopic individuals is not universally accepted.[19]

The therapeutic rationale for the use of evening primrose oil is that since it is rich in GLA it bypasses the rate limiting delta-6 desaturase stage.[4,8,20]

DERMATOLOGICAL CONDITIONS
Atopic Eczema/Dermatitis
The fact that delta-6 desaturation may be slower in atopic individuals has led to the suggestion that oral administration of evening primrose oil could be beneficial in the management of atopic eczema.[8] A number of clinical studies support this claim, showing that evening primrose oil significantly improved symptoms including itching, inflammation and dryness.[21-29] The evidence is not universally positive with a number of studies showing that evening primrose was not superior to placebo in the management of this condition.[30-34] Consequently, the use of evening primrose oil orally in the management of atopic eczema in North America remains controversial.[35-37] In contrast, evening primrose oil is considered suitable in the management of atopic eczema in many countries, including the United Kingdom, Germany, Australia and New Zealand.[20]

Several explanations for the failure of evening primrose oil in some studies have been suggested. Firstly, omega 3 EFAs (deep-sea fish oil) may be as important as omega 6, implying that combination products containing both may be more beneficial. Also, in some cases of atopy other desaturation steps apart from the delta-6 stage could be involved. Finally, not all cases of atopic eczema are due to disorders of fatty acid metabolism.[8]

Topical application of a cream containing 12.5% evening primrose oil to volunteers (n=20) with dry skin, significantly increased sebum content without changing transepidermal water loss. It should be noted that while the volunteers had an atopic disposition, they did not present with frank atopic dermatitis.[38] Evening primrose oil, when applied topically, did not prevent steroid induced epidermal atrophy caused by the twice daily application of 0.1% betamethasone valerate.[39]

Psoriasis
The supplementation of evening primrose oil and marine oil (i.e., omega 6 and omega 3) have proved unsuccessful in the management of psoriasis.[40]

ASTHMA
Oral administration of evening primrose oil appears not to be effective in the management of various forms of asthma.[19,32,41,42]

DIABETIC NEUROPATHY
As has already been noted, the ratio of linoleic acid and linolenic acid to their respective metabolites has been found to be elevated in diabetes.[8,43,44] In diabetic patients, both delta-6 and delta-5 desaturase enzymes may be impaired.[8,9] This impairment of normal fatty acid metabolism and subsequent production of physiological moieties may play an important role in the development of diabetic neuropathy.[44] By administering pre-formed gamma-linolenic acid (as in evening primrose oil), this imbalance may be corrected. The discovery that evening primrose oil may correct deficient nitric oxide in the nerve ischemia seen in diabetes implies that evening primrose's action may be more complex than was originally proposed.[45,46] Also, recently the role played by cyclo-oxygenase activity in the neuroactivity of evening primrose oil appears to be an important factor to consider.[47,48] A latency period

noted in a recent animal study has led to the suggestion that the action of evening primrose oil may be mediated by metabolically generated compounds rather than one existing in the oil itself.[49]

A beneficial role for the use of evening primrose oil in the correction of the neurovascular disorders seen in diabetics has been demonstrated in a number of animal studies.[8,49-53] Administration of 4 g of evening primrose oil (360 mg gamma-linolenic acid) daily for 6 months to diabetic patients (n=22) suffering from diabetic neuropathy caused an improvement (objective and subjective) when compared to placebo. Glycosylated hemoglobin levels were not influenced by evening primrose oil supplementation.[54] These positive findings were confirmed in a later double-blinded multicenter trial with patients (n=111) suffering from 'mild diabetic neuropathy'. The dose of evening primrose oil was higher than in the previous study (6 grams daily equivalent to 480 mg of gamma-linolenic acid) and the trial was carried out over a year. The response to evening primrose oil appeared more pronounced in those with lower starting glycosylated hemoglobin levels, suggesting satisfactory blood sugar control.[55] It appears that the gamma-linolenic acid content of a supplement does not determine its efficacy in managing diabetic neuropathy. In a recent animal study, evening primrose oil supplementation was shown to out-perform a number of other products rich in GLA (borage oil, blackcurrant oil and 'fungal' oil).[56]

WOMEN'S HEALTH CARE

Premenstrual Syndrome

A number of studies have indicated that evening primrose oil may be of use in the management of premenstrual syndrome.[8,57-61] The benefits are seen only following prolonged administration of 4 to 6 months.[8,20] A proposed mechanism of action is that the PGE1 generated could influence the actions of prolactin which is thought to play a role in the presentation of this syndrome.[8,62] Women with premenstrual syndrome may also have difficulty in converting linoleic acid into gamma-linolenic acid.[63] However, on reviewing the available literature, Budeiri et al. concluded that evening primrose oil offered no benefit. They argued that most of the information comes from easily discounted, open studies and that the well-controlled studies were "small and modest" in design.[64] The above comments regarding the necessity of prolonged administration could play a part in these negative findings.

Mastalgia

Information from both placebo-controlled trials and open trials has shown that evening primrose oil is beneficial in the management of both cyclical and non-cyclical mastalgia.[65-69] However, not all trials have been positive. One randomized, placebo-controlled, double-blind study of 120 women reported that ingestion of 3 g evening primrose oil daily for 6 months did not offer a clear benefit over ingestion of control oils (corn oil and corn oil with wheat germ).[70] The potential advantage of evening primrose oil over other more conventional therapies appears to be the lack of adverse effects.[66,71] While one study suggested it was as effective as bromocriptine,[68] another suggested its effect to be only slightly greater than placebo.[67] The suggested mechanism of action is via prolactin modulation.[8] As with the case of PMS, benefits are only noted after prolonged administration, usually four to six months.[20]

Endometriosis

A combination product containing both gamma-linolenic acid and the omega 3 fatty acid eicosapentaenoic acid (Scotia HGA®) was shown in a placebo-controlled trial to decrease the symptoms of endometriosis in 90% of cases.[8]

Menopause

While evening primrose oil is often used in the management of menopause, it appears to offer no benefit over placebo in treating associated flushing and sweating.[72] One study reported that daily ingestion of Efacal® (a supplement containing 1 g calcium, 4 g evening primrose oil and 440 mg marine fish oil) for 12 months by 42 postmenopausal women was not associated with significant increases in bone mineral density.[73]

INFLAMMATORY AND AUTOIMMUNE CONDITIONS
Rheumatoid Arthritis

Various *in vitro* and *in vivo* trials have demonstrated that PGE_1 has anti-inflammatory properties. Since it has been suggested that evening primrose oil may increase the levels of this moiety, it may be therapeutically useful in the management of this condition.[8,74] In a review of the relevant clinical trials, Joe and Hart conclude that the studies conducted varied in both design and quality and that the evidence supporting its use in the management of this condition is not conclusive. Any benefits noted appeared to be subjective rather than objective.[75] Short-term administration appears to provide no clinical benefits with relief being noted after six months in some studies.[74,76,77] Since two of the clinical trials were of limited duration,[78,79] this has been given as a possible explanation for their lack of positive results.[75]

In a double-blind, placebo-controlled trial of patients (n=38, duration of 9 months) suffering from psoriatic arthritis, a combination product containing evening primrose oil and fish oil (Efamol Marine ®) was seen to offer no therapeutic benefits.[80]

Multiple Sclerosis

An association between multiple sclerosis and levels of linoleic acid has been seen.[74,76,76,81,82] There is some evidence to suggest that evening primrose oil may be beneficial in reducing the severity, duration of relapses of the disease and progression of the disease.[76,83] The patients most likely to respond appear to be those with a recent diagnosis and less severe symptoms.[76,84] The mode of action proposed is that the linoleic acid may be modifying an immune response and that the most benefit may be obtained by combining the therapy with a low animal fat/high polyunsaturated fat diet.[83] The need to use the more expensive evening primrose oil rather than linoleic acid has been questioned.[76]

Sjögren's Syndrome

Abnormalities in fatty acid metabolism have been noted in Sjögren's syndrome.[8] Supplementation with evening primrose oil has been shown to stimulate lachrymation and ease the lethargy often present with this condition.[8,85,86] However, a more recent randomized, double-blind, placebo-controlled trial (n=90) reported that daily ingestion of 800 mg or 1600 mg GLA (extracted from evening primrose oil) for 6 months by patients with primary Sjögren's syndrome had no effect on fatigue compared to placebo.[87]

CARDIOVASCULAR CONDITIONS

Essential fatty acids are known to play an important role in maintaining good cardiovascular health. Problems with essential fatty acid metabolism or inadequate consumption are known to increase cholesterol, increase platelet aggregation and increase blood pressure.[2] Combination products of omega 3 and omega 6 oils may be useful in the management of various cardiovascular conditions.[74,88] Both human and animal studies suggest that evening primrose oil can decrease blood pressure and inhibit platelet aggregation.[8,89]

In a double-blind study, evening primrose oil supplementation was shown to result in symptomatic relief of patients suffering from Raynaud's phenomenon but no change in the objective measures were noted.[90]

PSYCHIATRIC CONDITIONS
Schizophrenia
While the exact pathophysiology of schizophrenia has yet to be determined, it has been suggested that abnormal essential fatty acid metabolism may be implicated. Decreased levels of linoleic acid in plasma phospholipids have been noted in schizophrenics. It has been suggested that they may have difficulty in producing PGE_1,[91] which may play a role in decreasing excessive central dopaminergic function (which is thought to play a role in the pathogenesis of the disease).[8,92] Clinical research to date (placebo-controlled trials, open observational trials and reported case histories) has produced contradictory results.[8,91-93] In a group of psychiatric patients suffering from tardive dyskinesia induced by neuroleptics, evening primrose oil was reported to cause a 'marginally significant' improvement.[92] When four cofactors needed in essential fatty acid metabolism (zinc, pyridoxine, niacin and vitamin C) were added to the protocol, this improvement was increased, and included enhancement of memory and alleviation of schizophrenic symptoms.[8]

Hyperactivity
Abnormalities in essential fatty acid metabolism have been noted in cases of children with hyperactivity disorder, behavioral problems and learning difficulties.[94-97] It is interesting to note that both essential fatty acid requirements and the incidence of hyperactivity are higher in boys than girls.[96] A review of case studies suggests that supplementation with evening primrose oil may prove beneficial in treating hyperactivity.[98] However, in a placebo controlled, double blind study in hyperkinetic children (n=90, age 5 to 15), evening primrose oil supplementation did not improve behavioral patterns or change blood fatty acid composition compared to placebo.[76] It is important to note that the placebo used in this case was safflower oil, a substance rich in essential fatty acids.

Dementia
Supplementation with evening primrose oil may prove beneficial in the management of various kinds of dementia including Alzheimer's disease and that caused by aging.[2,8]

MISCELLANEOUS EFFECTS
Gastrointestinal Disorders
Evening primrose oil has been shown to 'significantly improve stool consistency' when compared to both a fish oil supplement and placebo in ulcerative colitis. No difference in the other symptoms (stool frequency, rectal bleeding, disease relapse, sigmoidoscopic appearance or rectal histology) was seen.[99] In addition, relief was noted in a double-blind, placebo controlled crossover trial in women suffering from irritable bowel syndrome exacerbated premenstrually with supplementation of evening primrose oil.[8]

Post-Viral Fatigue Syndrome
Supplements containing evening primrose have been demonstrated to be effective in the management of 'post-viral syndrome' (a.k.a. chronic fatigue syndrome, myalgic encephalomyelitis) in both placebo controlled trials and in clinical practice.[15,100,101] In a double-blind, placebo-controlled trial of 63 adults with clear cases of 'post-viral syndrome' taking a combination product of evening primrose oil and fish oil (Efamol Marine ®), a pronounced improvement in symptoms (fatigue, myalgia, dizziness, poor concentration and memory) was noted.[15] This study was carried out on volunteers with a clear viral etiology to their condition.[15] However, when a new study team attempted to replicate this 1990 study by Behan et al., their results contrasted sharply with the results from the original study. Although the patients' symptoms generally improved with time, the improvement

was not statistically significant and there were no difference between the treatment and the placebo groups.[102]

Alcoholism

Alcohol is known to have multiple effects on the metabolism of essential fatty acids, causing depletion of linoleic acid stores;[74] inhibiting the conversion of linoleic acid to gamma-linolenic acid;[12,74] and stimulating the conversion of dihomogamma-linolenic acid to arachidonic acid.[74] While alcohol initially increases PGE_1 synthesis, long-term consumption causes a marked drop.[74] Abrupt cessation of alcohol consumption also causes a rapid fall in PGE_1 levels.[74] It has been hypothesized that administration of pre-formed gamma-linolenic acid may play a role in preventing alcohol toxicity and the development of alcohol addiction.[103] Human trials have shown that the administration of evening primrose oil decreases the need for tranquilizer use during the withdrawal phase and promotes the normalization of elevated liver enzymes.[74,76] While long-term administration does not decrease relapse rate, it does appear to appreciably improve recovery of memory and visual-motor coordination.[74] Animal studies have demonstrated that administration of evening primrose oil may decrease the damaging effect on the brain and the teratogenic potential of alcoholism.[74,104]

Renal Disease

Diets enriched with evening primrose oil have been shown to decrease the nephrotoxic effect of cyclosporine in rats.[105,106] Evidence from *in vivo* trials also suggests that evening primrose oil supplementation may prove beneficial in the treatment of urolithiasis.[107-109]

Cancer

In vitro studies have shown that gamma-linolenic acid has anti-neoplastic properties.[74] The clinical relevance of this has yet to be determined. An open-label trial with historical matched controls was conducted to assess the effects of adding 2.8g GLA daily to tamoxifen therapy (20 mg daily) for 6 weeks in 30 patients with endocrine-sensitive breast cancer (20 stage I-II, 14 locally advanced and 4 metastatic). Overall, the addition of GLA seemed to result in a significantly faster clinical response and a greater reduction in estrogen receptor expression.[110] Additional research in this area is recommended.

Obesity

Evening primrose oil has been suggested useful in the management of obesity.[84] Clinical studies on humans have reported mixed results.[84,111-13]

It is important to note that some authors suggest that insufficient vigorous clinical trials exist to justify many of the uses suggested for evening primrose oil.[2,114]

ADVERSE EFFECTS

Evening primrose oil appears to be exceedingly safe.[74,76,115] Adverse effects in humans are very rare and limited to headache, nausea and diarrhea.[4,8] Evening primrose oil has been shown in animal studies to have no carcinogenic properties.[116] At normal therapeutic doses (less than 4 grams daily), it is unlikely that evening primrose oil would be harmful if taken in pregnancy;[117] however, the composition of breast-milk can be manipulated by supplementing the maternal diet with evening primrose oil.[118]

CAUTIONS/CONTRAINDICATIONS

Evening primrose oil should not be used in mania due to a theoretical possibility of exacerbating the symptoms.[84] Evening primrose oil should be used with caution with patients suffering from epilepsy (see drug interactions).[2,76,84]

Historically, evening primrose oil has been used by midwives to hasten cervical ripening in an effort to shorten labor. However, a recent open-label retrospective trial suggestion that oral administration of evening primrose oil from the 37th week of gestation until birth does not shorten gestation or decrease the length of labor and may be associated with an increased incidence of prolonged rupture of membranes, oxytocin augmentation, arrest of descent and vacuum extraction.[119] Additional research is needed before evening primrose oil can be recommended in pregnancy.

DRUG INTERACTIONS

No reports of interactions between evening primrose oil and conventional medication could be found. A possible increase in epileptic attacks has been postulated in schizophrenics on phenothiazines treated with evening primrose oil.[93] The clinical likelihood of this occurring in practice has been questioned.[8,120] A theoretical interaction between gamma-linolenic acid and both non-steroidal anti-inflammatory drugs and corticosteroids has been suggested.[121] Whether this interaction would be synergistic or antagonistic is dependent upon whether the GLA is acting as a precursor of PGE_1 formation or if it modifies membrane composition.[8]

The therapeutic action of a product containing GLA, such as evening primrose oil, may be decreased with patients taking beta-blockers. This is due to the fact that cyclic AMP concentrations is in part mediated by beta adrenergic receptors as well as the action of PGE_1.[8] Evening primrose oil should be used with caution in patients taking conventional anticoagulant therapy.[84] Linoleic acid (in the form of safflower oil) has been shown to decrease neurotoxicity caused by lithium carbonate.[122]

DOSAGE REGIMENS

❖ ADULTS: 2-8 grams seed oil daily.[2,20]

❖ CHILDREN: 2-6 grams seed oil daily in children suffering from atopic eczema.[2,20]

Note: Evening primrose oil is usually taken in divided doses. Most evening primrose oil supplements contain 8% gamma-linolenic acid. Other nutritional supplements exist which may contain more gamma-linolenic acid, such as borage oil (*Borago officinalis* L., Boraginaceae), blackcurrant oil (*Ribes nigrum* L., Grossulariaceae) and algal sources. These sources of GLA are generally considered less biologically active than that from evening primrose oil.[8] The vast majority of clinical evidence exists for evening primrose oil supplements. It is important to remember that both omega 3 and omega 6 essential fatty acids are therapeutically important. Consequently, supplements combining both are becoming increasingly popular in practice.

Feverfew

Tanacetum parthenium (L.) Schultz-Bip.

THUMBNAIL SKETCH

Common Uses
❖ Migraines (prophylactic treatment)
❖ Inflammatory Joint Disease

Active Constituents
❖ Sesquiterpene Lactones (notably parthenolide)

Adverse Effects
❖ Mouth Ulceration and Gastrointestinal Upset
❖ Post-Feverfew Syndrome (including nervousness, tension, fatigue and joint ache)

Cautions/Contraindications
❖ Pregnancy and Lactation
❖ Children (under 2 years of age)

Drug Interactions
❖ Interaction (theoretical) with Anti-Coagulant Therapy (such as warfarin)

Doses
❖ Dried Leaf Preparation (*Tanacetum parthenium* L. Schultz Bip. containing at least 0.2% parthenolide): 125 mg daily
❖ *Dried Aerial Parts:* 50-200 mg daily
❖ *Tincture* (1:5 in 25% ethanol): 5-20 drops daily

Note: For optimal results in the management of recurrent migraines, it is advisable that feverfew be taken continuously for a minimum of 4-6 weeks.

Introduction

Family

❖ Asteraceae (also known as Compositae)

Synonyms

❖ Featherfew

❖ Featherfoil

❖ Motherherb

❖ Flirtwort

❖ Midsummer daisy

❖ Pyrethrum

❖ Febrifuge plant

❖ Altamisa

❖ *Chrysanthemum parthenium* (L.) Bernh.

❖ *Leucanthemum parthenium* (L.) Gren & Godron

❖ *Pyrethrum parthenium* (L.)[1-4]

Medicinal Forms

❖ Dried Aerial Parts

❖ Tincture

❖ Standardized Extracts

Description

Feverfew is an herbaceous perennial native to most of Europe, especially the Balkans, but now naturalized throughout the Americas, Europe and the rest of the world.[5-7] It stands 15 to 60 centimeters or 6 to 24 inches in height with several flowers existing on a common stalk. The flowers may be as large as 2 centimeters or 1 inch with a yellow central disc and a single layer of outer white florets.[5,6] The flowers have a strong odor and the bitter tasting leaves have a 'feather-like' appearance.[5,8] There have been numerous incidents in the past of other members of the Asteraceae family, such as German chamomile and tansy, being sold erroneously as feverfew.[5,6,8] Confusion has also occurred because numerous Latin binomials have been applied to the plant.[5]

Parts Used

The parts used medicinally are the aerial parts, especially the leaves.

Traditional Use

Feverfew has been used medicinally for a variety of indications dating back to Ancient Greece, and it use was been documented in many of the *Materia Medica* written in the Middle Ages. Feverfew was particularly popular in the management of fever (hence its name), headache, migraine, women's health care (threatened miscarriage, labor difficulties, menstrual irregularities), toothache, gastric upset and insect bites.[4,8] The bitter dried powder could be taken orally either mixed with honey or wine, or used topically by adding the herb to baths.[4]

Current Medicinal Use

While not conclusive, results from a number of clinical trials show that feverfew extracts standardized to parthenolide content may be effective in preventing migraines.[9] Claims for its activity in managing arthritis conditions have not been substantiated.

Relevant Research

Preventative and Therapeutic Effects

CONSTITUENTS [3-8,10]

❖ SESQUITERPENE LACTONES: germacranolides (including parthenolide, artemorin and chrysanthemonin), eudesmanolides (including santamarin, reynosin and magnolialide) and guaianolides (including chrysartemin A, partholide and chrysanthemolide).

❖ OTHERS: volatile oils (mainly monoterpene and sesquiterpene derivatives), pyrethrin and various flavonoids.

Note: Qualitative and quantitative differences exist between different chemical races of feverfew. For example, specimens rich in santamarin and reynosin have no parthenolide, and specimens rich in parthenolide have little or no reynosin or santamarin.[11]

PHARMACOLOGICAL ACTIONS

Extracts of feverfew appear to influence production of physiologically active eicasonoids. While feverfew suppresses prostaglandin production,[12,13] it neither inhibits cyclo-oxygenase,[12,13] nor thromboxane A_2 synthesis.[13,14] Unlike classic non-steroidal anti-inflammatory drugs, constituents found in feverfew appear to inhibit cellular phospholipases, hence preventing the release of arachidonic acid and subsequent formation of inflammatory mediators.[15,16] An additional action could be an inhibition of the activating factors of protein kinase C.[17] Compounds present in feverfew may also exert an inhibitory action directly on the prostaglandin synthetase enzyme system preventing the production of prostaglandins from arachidonic acid.[18] It has been suggested that non-sesquiterpene lactones may also play a part in this inhibition of eicasonoid synthesis.[16]

Extracts of feverfew have been shown to exert an antisecretory and anti-aggregatory effect on blood platelets and polymorphonuclear leucocytes.[4,14,15,19] With respect to human platelet activity, there appears little difference between a crude chloroform feverfew extract and parthenolide.[17] Feverfew extract has been shown to decrease deposition of platelets on collagen substrates, leading some to suggest its use as an anti-thrombotic drug.[20] The antisecretory action seems to be dependent on the presence of compounds containing alpha-methylene butyrolactone units (e.g., parthenolide, 3-beta-hydroxyparthenolide, canin and artecanin).[21] This inhibition of secretory and aggregatory activity appears to be due to an action on cellular sulphydryl groups.[22,23] Feverfew extracts have been shown to impede the production of HETE (12-hydroxyeicosateraenoac acid) for which a sulphydryl containing substance (glutathione) is a cofactor.[23] The proposed inhibitory action of phospholipase A_2 activity could also be due to a blockade of important sulphydryl containing components.[4] In addition, feverfew has been reported to inhibit release of serotonin by platelets and vitamin B12 binding protein from polymorphonuclear leucocytes.[19] Feverfew extract has also been shown to protect rabbit aortas against perfusion injury.[24]

Feverfew extracts also appear to inhibit the release of enzymes from polymorphonuclear leucocytes. This action appears more pronounced than that seen with conventional non-steroidal anti-inflammatory drugs such as indomethacin. This action could be responsible for feverfew's reputed effectiveness in the management of various arthritides and certain skin conditions such as psoriasis.[5,6] In addition, an extract of feverfew has been shown to inhibit histamine release from rat peritoneal mast cells stimulated by anti-IgE in a dose dependent manner. The mode of action responsible for this anti-histaminic property is different from that of either quercetin or sodium chromoglycate.[25]

A cytotoxic action for both a crude extract of feverfew and parthenolide has been demonstrated *in vitro*. They were found to inhibit mitogen-induced human mononuclear cell proliferation and interleukin 1 stimulated synovial cells.[26] In addition, sesquiterpene lactones, containing an alpha-methylenebutyrolactone unit, have been shown *in vitro* to exert a cytotoxic activity towards various cell lines. It has been suggested that this action is exerted by influencing DNA replication and synthesis.[21] However, since platelets do not possess DNA and feverfew has been shown to influence their function, it appears that the cytotoxic action may be more generalized.[6]

While numerous mechanisms of action for feverfew and some of its constituents have been identified *in vitro*, the relevance of these mechanisms to the use of feverfew leaf as a migraine prophylactic in humans is not at all clear. While most interest has been focused on the sesquiterpene lactones, notably parthenolide, it is possible that other constituents also exert a biological action. The possibility of a synergy between constituents has also been suggested.[5,6]

EFFECT ON MIGRAINE

Research into this indication was initiated primarily by a group of migraine sufferers in the late 1970s who used feverfew 'successfully' in the treatment of their conditions.[27,28] The public demand led to two documented clinical trials in the 1980s. Following a survey of migraine sufferers in which it appeared that feverfew may be beneficial,[29] a placebo controlled trial was performed. Volunteers (n=17) who had consumed fresh feverfew leaves daily (average of 2.44 leaves) for at least three months and had a history of migraines (common or classic) for two years with no more than 8 attacks per month were selected. One group (n=8) received 'freeze-dried' feverfew (50mg daily) and a second group (n=9) received placebo. Assessment was made by using diary cards scoring the visual symptoms, nausea, headache (including times of onset and relief and of any additional treatment taken) according to a predetermined scale. The group given the feverfew product reported no change in condition, while the group given the placebo noted both an increased frequency of attacks (3.43 attacks/month as compared to 1.22/month before) and increased severity of headache, nausea and vomiting over 6 periods of 4 months. The abrupt withdrawal of feverfew in two of the patients led to the recurrence of some symptoms.[30] The observations and conclusions drawn from this study have been questioned because of the poor methodology.[31]

The efficacy of feverfew in the prophylactic management of migraines was evaluated in a randomized, double-blind, placebo-controlled, crossover trial in 1988. Volunteers (n=76) who had suffered from migraines (classic or common) for 2 years or more (at least 1 attack per month) were selected. Following a one-month single-blind placebo run-in, the volunteers were given either 1 capsule of feverfew daily (mean weight 82mg equivalent to 2.19 mmol parthenolide) or placebo. The treatment was continued for 4 months and patients were then transferred to the other option. Conventional migraine medications were stopped at the beginning of the trial. A symptom diary was used to record number and duration of individual attacks, severity of headache and any associated symptoms. In addition, the overall impression of the patients was assessed by use of a visual analogue scale and the selection of a predefined 'descriptive' in order to describe the change in headache (much worse, worse, same, better, much better). Patients were assessed every 2 months during the double-blind portion of the study. Following treatment with feverfew, an improvement was noted in the number and severity of attacks, degree of vomiting and general improvement (visual analogue scale). There was no alteration in the duration of individual attacks.[32]

Another recent well-designed randomized, double-blind, placebo-controlled, crossover trial of feverfew did not find such promising results.[33] Patients (n=50) were selected who had suffered from migraines since their youth and continued to suffer from at least one migraine, classic or common, at least once per month and had never taken feverfew in the past. The patients involved suffered serious migraines that were not receptive to conventional medication. While all migraine-related medications were stopped at the start of the trial, volunteers were permitted to treat any attacks acutely using conventional symptomatic drugs. After a one-month placebo phase, patients were treated with either a dried alcoholic extract of feverfew leaves containing 0.5 mg of parthenolide or placebo. After four months the patients were crossed over to the opposing group. The severity of the migraine attacks was recorded according to a predetermined scale and the number of headaches during the period month 2 to 4 recorded. There was no significant difference in the number of migraines experienced between the groups. Of the group of 44 volunteers that completed the study, 7 in the feverfew group reported "using considerably fewer anti-migraine preparations." This study has been criticized on a number of points. The investigators noted that unlike the previous studies, the individuals selected had never used feverfew before. Also, the feverfew product used an alcoholic extract rather than dried feverfew leaves. While extracts used were standardized to parthenolide, other necessary active moities could be absent.[33] Concerns about the use of acute migraine drugs during the trial, and their effect on the assessment of the severity of the attacks, have also been raised.[34] In addition, the appropriateness of the criteria used by the investigators to measure changes in symptoms (the International Headache Society's scale) has been questioned.[34]

One final study sought to investigate a dose-response of a new feverfew extract (MIG-99).[35] In a randomized, double-blind, controlled trial, 3 doses of feverfew (2.08 mg, 6.25 mg and 18.75 mg) given three times daily were compared with placebo in 147 patients suffering from migraines with and without aura over a 4 week period. In this study feverfew extract MIG-99 failed to show a significant migraine prophylatic effect in general and a dose-response relationship was not observed. Only in those patients with at least 4 attacks during the 28-day baseline period (n=49) was feverfew shown to be effective and in these patients, the 6.25 mg dose (three times daily) was found to be the most effective.

More recently, two systematic reviews have concluded that although the available studies indicate that feverfew may be more effective than placebo in preventing migraines, the efficacy of feverfew for migraine prevention has not been established beyond a reasonable doubt and future rigorous studies are needed.[36,37]

While the vast majority of feverfew users take feverfew prophylactically for the management of migraines, incidents of it proving useful in the symptomatic treatment of acute migraines have been documented.[4]

EFFECT ON ARTHRITIS
While feverfew has been used in the management of various arthritic conditions, this claim is not supported by clinical research.[27] In a double-blind, placebo controlled study of female patients (n=41) suffering from rheumatoid arthritis, dried feverfew (70–86 mg equivalent to 2–3 μ of parthenolide) taken once a day for 6 weeks was shown to offer no benefits over placebo. Patients were permitted to continue their conventional non-steroidal treatment throughout the study. Concerns were noted that the dose used might have been too low. The authors suggested that these findings did not exclude a benefit in the management of osteoarthritis or soft tissue damage.[38]

MISCELLANEOUS EFFECTS
Parthenolide has been shown to possess anti-microbial properties against a variety of Gram positive bacteria, fungi and dermatophytes.[3,4,39,40] A weaker action has been noted against some Gram negative pathogens.[39] The clinical relevance of this is unknown.

ADVERSE EFFECTS
Adverse effects are considered to be generally rare, primarily presenting as mouth ulceration and gastrointestinal upset.[6,30] Mouth ulceration presented in 12% and swelling of the lips in 7% of patients in one British clinical trial.[41] Mouth ulceration is due to a systemic rather than a direct irritant action, thus encapsulation does not decrease its presentation.[30] Feverfew products may also cause inflammation of the mucous membranes of the buccal cavity resulting in inflammation of the lips/tongue and a loss of taste, which is likely to be reduced when the feverfew is taken as a tablet or capsule.[6] These adverse effects present usually within the first week, but may occur anytime in the first two months of treatment.[3,6] One study described a group of symptoms including nervousness, tension, fatigue and joint aches, which was associated with withdrawal of feverfew products. The phrase 'Post Feverfew Syndrome' was coined to describe this finding.[30] No other reference to this syndrome could be found.

Allergic reactions to feverfew have also been reported.[42] Numerous examples of contact dermatitis have been noted in individuals handling the fresh feverfew plant. The sesquiterpene lactone portion appears to be the component responsible. An appreciable cross sensitivity between feverfew and other plants containing these constituents has also been seen.[43-47]

In a comparative study between a group of migraine sufferers (n=30) who had been taking a variety of feverfew products (leaves, capsules or tablets of feverfew for at least 11 months) and a non-user control group, no significant chromosomal aberrations, sister chromatid exchanges or mutagenicity of urine (Ames test) were noted.[48]

CAUTIONS/CONTRAINDICATIONS

Feverfew is considered an emmenagogue and abortifacient and consequently its use is contraindicated in pregnancy.[49,50] Feverfew should not be administered to children under 2 years of age.[9] Also, feverfew products should not be taken for more than 4 months without consulting a physician. This caution is due to the lack of long-term information regarding toxicity.[9]

Feverfew should not be taken by people with known hypersensitivity to other members of the daisy (Asteraceae) family due to the potential allergenicity of the sesquiterpene lactones present.[47]

DRUG INTERACTIONS

No documented instances of drug interactions occurring with feverfew were found for this review.[6] However, it has been suggested that the effect of feverfew may be reduced when it is taken concurrently with non-steroidal anti-inflammatory drugs or corticosteroids.[38] Theoretically, feverfew may potentiate the action of anti-coagulants such as warfarin.

COMPARISON OF DOSAGE FORMS

In a very detailed review article, D. Awang discusses many concerns related to the practical use of feverfew preparations.[9] Many of the statements made by manufacturers regarding the superiority of a particular product (freeze-dried or certain extracts) cannot be substantiated.[9] The quality, with regard to parthenolide content, of commercial feverfew products has also been questioned. Investigation of commercially available feverfew products found that many did not contain the parthenolide content considered necessary for therapeutic efficacy.[41,50-53] In addition, the parthenolide content of the dried feverfew leaf has been shown to decrease appreciably over time. This led to questions regarding effective shelf life and the need for more specific storage conditions.[4,51,54] Many factors, such as the season in which the feverfew is harvested and the growing conditions, can effect the sesquiterpene lactone content.[4] To further complicate matters, the bioactivity (ability to inhibit the release of serotonin from bovine blood platelets) appears to vary within and between samples. This variance can be independent of the geographical source of the sample of T. parthenium.[55]

The Health Protection Branch of the Canadian Federal government granted a DIN (Drug Identification Number) to a British feverfew product allowing it to make the claim that the product was effective in the prevention of migraine headaches.[7,9] They stipulated that the original harvested plant should have undergone independent 'botanical certification' and that the feverfew leaf product should contain at least 0.2% pathenolide.[9] Medicinal claims can only be made legitimately in Canada for dried feverfew leaf products.[9] Awang also made note that "there is no scientific evidence supporting either the superiority of the wild traditional feverfew or ineffectiveness of non-traditional or cultivated variants."[9] In comparing capsule versus tablet formulations, Awang comments, "while there is no fundamental reason to reject tablets *per se*, it should be noted that their effectiveness would be dependent upon satisfactory disintegration/dissolution characteristics."[9]

Products marketed in France require that feverfew extracts be standardized to 0.1% parthenolide, extracted from both the leaves and stem.[7]

DOSAGE REGIMENS

❖ DRIED LEAF PREPARATION (*Tanacetum parthenium* L. Schultz Bip. containing at least 0.2% parthenolide): 125 mg daily. This dose in this form is considered useful in the prophylactic treatment of migraines by the Canadian Health Protection Branch .[9]
Although it has been argued that administration should be limited to standardized extracts,[32] other dosage forms seen in clinical practice include:

❖ DRIED AERIAL PARTS: 50-200 mg daily.[56]

❖ TINCTURE (1:5, 25% ethanol): 5-20 drops daily.[56]
Note: For optimal results in the management of recurrent migraines, it is advisable to that feverfew be taken continuously for a minimum of 4-6 weeks.[27]

Garlic

Allium sativum L.

Common Uses
- ❖ Cardiovascular (protective effects, including decreased cholesterol levels, decreased blood pressure, decreased platelet aggregation)
- ❖ Anti-Microbial
- ❖ Cancer (protection against cancer, especially stomach and colon cancer)

Active Constituents
- ❖ Sulfur-containing Products (including alliin, allicin, diallyl disulfide and ajoene)

Adverse Effects
- ❖ Heartburn, Flatulence, and Gastro-intestinal Upset (usually only at doses greater than 4 cloves daily)
- ❖ Contact Dermatitis (if the skin is exposed to raw garlic for an extensive period of time)
- ❖ Post-Operative Bleeding

Cautions/Contraindications
- ❖ Pregnancy and Lactation
- ❖ Surgery (discontinue prior to surgery)
- ❖ Organ Transplants (caution should be exercised after organ transplants)
- ❖ Pemphigus

Drug Interactions
- ❖ Anti-Coagulants
- ❖ Anti-Diabetic Therapy (possibly)
- ❖ Highly Active Anti-Retroviral Therapy (HAART) used in treating HIV and AIDs, most notably ritonavir (possibly)

Doses
- ❖ *Fresh Garlic:* 3-30 g (1-8 cloves) daily
- ❖ *Dried Cloves:* 2-5 g of fresh air-dried daily
- ❖ *Dried Powder:* 400-1200 mg of fully dried powder daily
- ❖ *Garlic Oil:* 2-5 mg daily
- ❖ *Allicin:* 2-5 mg daily

Introduction

Family
❖ Liliaceae

Synonyms
❖ Russian penicillin (Allicin)[1]

Description

Garlic is a perennial growing from 30 centimeters to 1 meter or 1 to 3 feet tall, with pale pink or green-white flowers and a bulb composed of a cluster of 'cloves'. Native to central Asia, garlic is now cultivated widely for culinary and medicinal purposes.

Parts Used

The garlic bulb is the part of the plant used medicinally. When intact it is odorless; however, crushing the cells brings the enzyme alliinase into contact with the sulfur-containing compound alliin, converting it to allicin, which produces the characteristic garlic odor. Allicin is relatively unstable and is converted to a variety of other active sulfur-containing compounds.

Traditional Use

Garlic has been used medicinally since approximately 3000 BC. The Latin name *Allium* is derived from the Celtic word for pungent, hot and burning, properties common to all the *Allium* species.[1-3] The species name, *sativum*, means cultivated or planted, referring to the fact that garlic is no longer found in the wild. It was one of the earliest cultivated crops and continues to be extensively grown for both medicinal and culinary purposes.[2,3]

Garlic has been described as an aphrodisiac, as well as a treatment for a large variety of other conditions, including colds, coughs, high blood pressure, hypertension, diarrhea, rheumatism, and snakebites.[2] In addition, garlic oil has been used to 'expel' round worms and was generally considered to be a good antiseptic. Traditionally, garlic was used to treat diabetes in Norway and Central Europe, and it was considered to be a heart remedy in traditional Ayurvedic medicine.[1] In Traditional Chinese Medicine (TCM), garlic was used in controlling dysentery, as an anti-parasitic, anti-febrile and stomachic.[2]

More than 1300 papers have reported on the chemical constituents, mechanisms of action and clinical applications of garlic over the last 100 years,[3] making it one of the most extensively researched medicinal plants. Fenwick and Hanley (1985) provide an excellent review of many of these.[4-6]

Current Medicinal Use

A growing amount of evidence now shows that the sulphur-containing constituents have medicinal properties, including anti-microbial, cardioprotective and potentially anti-cancer actions. Garlic is primarily used to decrease high cholesterol, but does not appear to be effective in decreasing blood pressure. When taken as either a supplement or part of the diet, garlic has been associated with a decrease in some types of cancer, such as colorecectal cancer.

Medicinal Forms

Fresh cloves, oil, powder. When crushed or chopped, it has been estimated that one gram of fresh garlic will release 3.7 mg of allicin, which appears to be the precursor for many of the major active constituents of garlic.[7] Dried garlic contains no allicin but does contain both alliin and alliinase, and thus theoretically should be able to produce allicin. Allinase is inactivated by acids and thus the conversion to allicin does not occur in the stomach. It has been suggested that dried garlic is most effective if it is ingested as an enteric coated formulation so that it is released in the alkaline medium of the intestine. In the intestine the conversion to allicin occurs rapidly, and allicin is quickly combined with cysteine to produce 5-allylmercaptocysteine, which prevents the distinctly odored allicin from being absorbed into the blood stream. Thus this form of garlic is relatively odorless and most likely still effective.[8] Odorless garlic products may be also prepared by coarsely chopping, peeling and rapidly freeze-drying the cloves before powdering so that there is little opportunity for enzymatic conversion of the odorless alliin to the odoriferous allicin and related breakdown products. Some people argue that the potency of a garlic product can be determined by its ability to produce allicin, which in turn yields many of the other active components. Some commercial products are now standardized to their allicin yield.[8]

Oil-based products are less likely to be efficacious because allicin is unstable in an oil base. Similarly, in aqueous products, allicin suffers substantial degradation.[8] A 1992 German study investigating the allicin content of 18 German garlic products found that only 5 had an allicin yield equivalent to the 4 grams of fresh garlic (or more) that the German Commission E considers necessary for therapeutic activity.[7]

Relevant Research

Preventative and Therapeutic Effects

CONSTITUENTS [1-3, 9-11]

❖ ENZYMES: alliinase, peroxidase, myrosinase.

❖ SULFUR-CONTAINING COMPOUNDS: alliin (S-allyl cysteine sulfoxide); allicin (diallyl thiosulfinate) which is formed when the enzyme alliinase acts on alliin when the garlic clove is crushed; allyl methanethiosulfinate; diallyl disulfide (breakdown product of allicin); diallyl trisulfide; allyl methyl trisulfide; S-allyl-mercaptocysteine; ajoene ($C_9H_{14}S_3O$) (formed by combining allicin and diallyl disulfide) which is considered to be unstable and may rearrange to a variety of polysulfides; 2-vinyl-4H-1,3-dithiin; 2-vinyl-4H-1,2-dithiin; S-allylcysteine; allixin.

❖ MISCELLANEOUS: neutral lipids (predominant), phospholipids, glycolipids; essential amino acids (of particular importance are those containing sulfur, for example, cysteine and methionine, as well as arginine; anthocyanins; quercetin and its flavone aglycone analogues; kaempferol glycosides; scordinins (biologically active thioglycosides); tellurium compounds.

Note: The biological action of garlic is generally thought to be due to its organosulfur compounds, specifically those containing the allyl CH2=CH-CH2- group.[1] It has been estimated that one gram of fresh garlic will release 3.7 mg of allicin when crushed or chopped.[11]

CARDIOVASCULAR EFFECTS
Protective Effects
A systematic review including 45 randomized controlled trials and 73 additional studies reporting adverse effects concluded that the trials "suggest possible small short-term benefits of garlic on some lipid and antiplatelet factors, insignificant effects on blood pressure, and no effect on glucose levels. Conclusions regarding clinical significance are limited by the marginal quality and short duration of many trials and by the unpredictable release and inadequate definition of active constituents in study preparations."[12] The ability of garlic to decrease cholesterol, triglycerides and low-density lipoprotein in the blood has been documented by numerous studies.[13-32] However, studies reporting no lipid or cholesterol lowering effect have also been published.[33-40]

Studies over the past 25 years have reported that the ingestion of garlic can decrease serum cholesterol, sometimes as much as 20%; however, the study designs, doses, forms (raw or powder), study populations and blinding mechanisms (the smell of garlic makes it very difficult to conducted blinded studies) vary widely making it difficult to reach firm conclusions regarding the efficacy of garlic for this indication.[6,16,41-43] For example, Kleijnen *et al.*(1989) severely criticized both the quality of commercial garlic products and the methodological quality of the 13 controlled trials they reviewed.[15,16,33,44-53] They concluded that while experiments with fresh garlic are consistent in showing that garlic lowers cholesterol levels, the doses required to achieve this effect are extremely high (a minimum of 7 cloves daily). In addition, it appeared that the effects of garlic ingestion lasted only a few hours. In response to this finding, several manufacturers began producing dehydrated garlic preparations (water accounts for up to 60% of the bulk of garlic), which are standardized to alliin content.

Other reviews of double-blind controlled studies have concluded that ingestion of garlic significantly decreases lipid and cholesterol levels.[54,55] A meta-analysis of five placebo-controlled, randomized trials,[18-20,56,57] which assessed the effect of garlic on total serum cholesterol in individuals with cholesterol levels greater than 5.17 mmol/L (200 mg/dL), concluded that the oral ingestion of the equivalent of ½ to 1 clove of raw garlic daily significantly decreased serum cholesterol levels by approximately 9%.[55] The study suggests that these effects are possible with relatively low doses of garlic. However, problems with the low quality of the trials included in the analysis continues to be of concern. Another meta-analysis of 16 trials (952 subjects combined) found an overall 12% reduction in total serum cholesterol in those taking garlic compared to those taking placebo. This effect was apparent after approximately one month and persisted approximately six months after the therapy was discontinued. Garlic powders were also reported to reduce triglyceride levels by an average of 13%. However, the authors cautioned that more than half the trials reviewed were of poor quality.[58] The most recent meta-analysis of 13 randomized, placebo-controlled studies concluded that although garlic appears to be superior to placebo in reducing total cholesterol levels, the size of the effect is modest and the clinical use of garlic in the management of hypercholesterolemia remains debatable.[59]

A double-blind, placebo-controlled, randomized crossover clinical trial (n=28) of individuals with mild to moderate hypercholesterolemia (5.5 to 8.05 mmol/L) taking 300 mg of garlic powder tablets (Kwai®) or placebo three times daily for 12 weeks found no significant difference between the group taking the garlic and the group taking the placebo on outcome measures of: plasma cholesterol, LDL cholesterol, HDL cholesterol, plasma triglycerides, lipoprotein(a) or blood pressure.[60] Another double-blind, randomized study of 42 healthy adults with total serum cholesterol levels greater than 220 mg/dL who received the same product (300 mg three times daily) reported a significant decrease in total serum cholesterol and low-density lipoprotein cholesterol (LDL) in the garlic group when compared with the placebo group; however, there was no significant change in high density lipoprotein cholesterol (HDL), triglycerides, serum glucose or blood pressure.[61] A third double-blind crossover study comparing 7.2 g aged garlic daily with placebo (for 4-6 months) in 41 men (total serum cholesterol 220-290 mg/dL) reported statistically significant decreases in total serum cholesterol and LDL cholesterol in individuals treated with garlic.[27] Finally, a double-blind, randomized, placebo-controlled study of 46 patients diagnosed with mild to moderate hypercholesterolemia reported that 12 weeks of garlic supplementation (four tablets daily that each contained 220 mg garlic powder, equivalent to approximately 2.6 g fresh garlic and standardized to produce 2.4 mg allciin), in conjunction with a low fat diet, resulted in a significant reduction in total cholesterol and LDL cholesterol compared with the placebo group.[32]

In contrast, a double-blind, placebo-controlled randomized trial found that steam-distilled garlic oil (5 mg twice daily) had no influence on serum lipoproteins, cholesterol absorption or cholesterol synthesis in 25 patients with moderate hypercholeterolemia.[35] Similarly, a randomized, double-blind, placebo-controlled trial found garlic powder (900mg daily) for 12 weeks to be ineffective in lowering cholesterol levels in patients (n=28) with hypercholestrolemia.[37] These findings are supported by a third randomized, double-blind, placebo-controlled study (n=51) that concluded that ingestion of garlic (either 500 mg or 1000 mg daily) for 12 weeks did not significantly effect plasma lipid levels.[38] In addition, a randomized, double-blind, placebo-controlled study of 50 patients diagnosed with moderate hypercholesterolemia concluded that garlic therapy (Kwai® 300 mg three times daily) for 12 weeks had no effect on majr lasma lipoproteins.[39] Another randomized, double-blind, placebo-controlled clinical trial concluded that 8 weeks of garlic (Kwai®, 300 mg three times daily) had no significant effect on cardiovascular risk factors in pediatric patients (n=30) aged 8 to 18 years with familial hyperlipidemia.[36]

In one of the few studies comparing garlic to standard lipid-lowering products, garlic was compared in a double-blind clinical trial with bezafibrate in 98 patients. There was no significant difference in the outcome measures between the two groups — both groups had significant reductions in triglyceride, total cholesterol, and LDL levels, as well as increased HDL levels.[62]

One randomized, double-blind, placebo-controlled trial (n=152) reported that garlic (900 mg powder daily) significantly reduced the increase in ateriosclerotic plaque volume by 5 to 18% (or even effected a slight regression in the volume) compared with the placebo over an observational period of 48 months.[63] Additional research in this area appears warranted.

MECHANISM OF ACTION

Several mechanisms of action have been postulated, including increased bile acid excretion;[64] reduced 3-hydroxy-3-methyl-glutaryl coenzyme A reductase activity;[65-67] and inhibition of squalene epoxidase, the final enzyme in the synthetic pathway of cholesterol by tellurium compounds found in garlic bulbs.[10] All these mechanisms decrease the hepatic production of cholesterol. It appears that components of garlic (e.g., allicin, diallyl disulfide, allyl mercaptan and the vinyl-dithiins) may all play a role in the interference of cholesterol biosynthesis although via a variety of different mechanisms.[68]

In addition, it is suggested that components of garlic may decrease the activity of lipogenic enzymes (e.g., glucose-6-phosphate dehydrogenase and malic dehydrogenase),[64,65] which leads to a decrease in fatty acid synthesis. Another hypothesis is that components of garlic may exert cardioprotective effects by decreasing the levels of glycosaminoglycans (GAGs). The amount of GAGs has been shown to be proportional to the susceptibility of different species to cholesterol induced athersclerosis. GAGs are able to bind to plasma lipoproteins and thus have been implicated in lipid accumulation in developing lesions.[26] One study presents findings that suggest the hypothesis that garlic decreases the susceptibility of isolated LDL to oxidation may not be correct.[69]

Of interest is the finding in several studies of an initial rise in cholesterol, triglycerides and LDL/VLDL blood levels during the first few months of garlic ingestion.[15,57] Researchers have postulated that this initial increase could be due to the garlic causing tissue lipids to move into circulation.[3]

Platelet Aggregation Inhibitory Ability

The anti-thrombotic effects of garlic have been extensively studied.[17,23,24,70-81] Garlic has been shown to inhibit platelet aggregation induced by epinephrine,[75] adenosine diphosphate (ADP),[75,82] and collagen.[82] An excellent review of the inhibition of platelet aggregation by a variety of components of garlic is available in Agarwal 1996.[3]

Clinical Studies

A review of 13 trials, most rated as poor in quality, concluded that although fresh garlic reliably decreases platelet aggregation, it does so only at very high doses (greater than 7 cloves per day) and the effects appear to last for only a few hours.[43] Other studies have found decreased platelet aggregation at significantly lower doses. For example, one double-blind, placebo-controlled, crossover study of 10 individuals randomized to receive either 900 mg (1.3% alliin) daily or placebo found no significant effects at 6 hours; however, at 7 and 14 days those taking the garlic had decreased platelet aggregation caused by ADP and decreased platelet aggregability in response to collagen.[82] In contrast, another clinical study of daily consumption of 600 mg garlic powder in tablet form (equal to 1.7 g of cloves) for 4 weeks found no inhibitory effects of platelet aggregation.[17] Another randomized, double-blind placebo controlled study of healthy volunteers (n=34) taking between 2.4 and 7.2 g of aged garlic extract daily reported that only at the highest supplementation level (7.2 g daily) did garlic show a slight increase in the threshold of ADP-induced aggregation and reduced adhesion to von Willebrand factor. Platelet adhesion to collagen was inhibited only at higher levels of supplementation, but adherence to fibrinogen was potently inhibited at all levels of supplementation.[81] These findings are similar to those of an earlier study.[80]

It has been suggested that garlic causes a slow build up of active constituents , making higher single doses necessary to achieve inhibition of platelet aggregation , but lower doses of garlic may have anti-coagulant effects in long-term administration.[79]

MECHANISM OF ACTION

Both alliin and allicin have been shown to inhibit collagen-induced platelet aggregation; however, allicin is approximately fifteen times more active.[3] In vitro studies indicate that platelet cAMP, cyclooxygenase and thromboxane synthetase activity are not affected by either of these constituents of garlic.[73] It should be noted that the anti-thrombotic effects of allicin are destroyed above 56°C and at a pH greater than 8.5.[73] Several studies have noted decreased or complete lack of the anti-thrombotic action of garlic after it has been exposed to heat.[83,84] The exact antithrombotic mechanism of action is unknown; however, raw garlic has been shown to irreversibly inhibit cyclooxygenase activity in a dose-dependent manner,[83] and decrease thromboxane B_2 levels.[30, 84] Thus, other constituents of garlic must play a role in this effect.

Although allicin is considered to be one of the most potent anti-aggregation constituents in garlic, it is not found in the blood stream after oral ingestion of garlic. Shortly after it is absorbed into the blood stream it is converted to allyl mercaptan.[3] Allicin may also be converted to ajoene, which has been identified as an active anti-thrombotic agent;[85,86] however, ajoene is often not present in commercial garlic pills, or powders of steamed garlic distillates. Ajoene has been shown to inhibit platelet aggregation traditionally induced by a variety of stimulatory agents, including: collagen, ADP, epinephrine, arachidonic acid, platelet-activating factor, and thrombin.[87-90] This activity is increased by prostcyclin (PGI$_2$), forskolin, indomethacin, and dipyridamole.[87,89] Several mechanisms have been postulated for the anti-thrombotic activity of ajoene. It is thought to inhibit the exposure of fibrinogen receptors on platelet membranes.[90,91] Other researchers have suggested that it may interact with a purified hemoprotein, which in turn may play an important role in the activation of platelets.[92]

Other components of garlic have also been implicated as anti-thrombotic agents (e.g., diallyl disulfide and methyl allyl trisulfide); however, studies regarding their anti-thrombotic activity have been conflicting.[2] For example, in one study, methyl allyl trisulfide was shown to be the agent responsible for the complete blockage of platelet aggregation in response to serotonin one hour post oral ingestion of fresh garlic (100-150 mg/kg). It should be noted that no inhibition was seen at 30 minutes or 2 hours post ingestion.[93] In addition, components of garlic may activate calcium-dependent nitric oxide synthase, producing increased amount of nitric acid by which the therapeutic actions of garlic may be exerted. This activation does not appear to be dependent upon the alliin-derived products or arginine.[75,94]

Effect on Blood Pressure

Although several trials have demonstrated garlic's ability to decrease blood pressure,[17,19,20,23,24,27] others have not been able to show such an effect.[3,22,61,95] For example, a double-blind, placebo-controlled study of 42 patients getting 300 mg TID of standardized garlic powder in tablet form found no effects on blood pressure.[61] In contrast, a double-blind, placebo-controlled crossover study of 41 men (total serum cholesterol 220-290 mg/dL) taking 7.2 g of aged garlic or placebo daily for 4 to 6 months reported a 5.5% decrease in systolic blood pressure and a slight reduction in diastolic blood pressure in the group taking garlic.[27] In addition, a study of 47 patients with mild hypertension (mean diastolic blood pressure 102 mmHg) who took 600 mg dried garlic powder (Kwai®) daily (or placebo) for 12 weeks, reported that the supine diastolic blood pressure in the group taking the garlic was significantly lower at 8 weeks and 12 weeks than those in the control group.[19]

A meta-analysis which reviewed 8 randomized controlled trials of a least 4 weeks in duration (all of which used Kwai® garlic powder) concluded that there is currently insufficient evidence to routinely recommend garlic use in patients with hypertension.[19,20,61,62,96-99] Of the eight studies reviewed, only three were conducted in hypertensive subjects and only seven compared garlic to a placebo. Overall, three showed a significant reduction in systolic blood pressure and four showed a significant decrease in diastolic blood pressure.[100]

MECHANISM OF ACTION

The ability of garlic to decrease blood pressure may be due to its ability to inhibit adenosine deaminase, the enzyme which degrades adenosine to inosine, enhancing the physiological effects of adenosine.[101,102]

ANTI-MICROBIAL EFFECT

Garlic has been used as an anti-microbial for hundreds of years in a variety of cultures.[103] Allicin is considered to be the primary anti-bacterial constituent of garlic.[3,104] Garlic has been shown to inhibit the growth of *Staphylococcus aureus*, *Streptococcus* (alpha- and beta-hemolytic), *Escherichia coli*, *Proteus vulgaris*, *Salmonella eneritidis*, *Citrobacter* sp., *Klebsiella pneumoniae*, *Mycobacteria*, and *Helicobacter pylori*.[103,105-107] However, other researchers have been unable to demonstrate any inhibition of *Staphylococcus aureus*.[107]

In addition, garlic has been shown to have a significant anti-fungal effect, especially against fungal skin infections. Studies have demonstrated its effectiveness against *Microsporum, Epidermophyton, Trichophyton* and *Candida albicans*.[103,108] In Asia, garlic preparations are used (alone or in combination with amphotericin B) to treat systemic fungal infections and cryptococcal meningitis. *In vitro* evidence supports garlic's fungistatic and fungicidal activity against *Cryptococcus neoforans*.[109]

CANCER PREVENTIVE EFFECT

Garlic has long had a reputation for providing protection from cancer. Much of the evidence that garlic may reduce cancer deaths comes from epidemiological studies.[110-13] Several good reviews of the evidence (or lack thereof) for this indication for garlic have been published over the last 10 years.[111,114-117] The most recent of these (Ernst 1997) reviews nine epidemiological studies of the association between garlic consumption and cancer.[118-126] Of these studies, 4 reported that garlic had a protective effect against cancer (thyroid nodular disease, stomach cancer, cancer of the larynx, colon cancer); two found positive, but non-significant trends (gastric cardia, cancers of the nasal cavity and sinuses) and 3 found no protective effect for garlic (gastric cancer — 2 studies, stomach cancer). The authors conclude that "the hypothesis that regular consumption of *Allium* vegetables (including garlic, onions and leeks) reduces the risk of cancer is compelling and would seem to deserve testing in intervention trials." [117]

Two specific studies have garnered attention due to their more rigorous designs. The Iowa Women's Health Study followed 41,837 women aged 55 to 69 years for 5 years and found that garlic consumption was inversely associated with risk of colon cancer. The protective association with garlic was stronger than with any other nutrient analyzed in the study.[125] The second notable study followed 58,279 men and 62,573 women aged 55 to 69 for just over 3 years. This study found no protective effect against cancers of the stomach or breast from garlic.[116,127]

An ongoing randomized, multi-intervention trial (N=3599) to investigate the ability of daily long term use of 500 mg vitamin C, 200 IU vitamin E, 75 mcg selenium, 800 mg garlic and 4 mg garlic oil to inhibit the progression of precancerous gastric lesions recently reported that the supplements were well-tolerated and that high compliance rates were achieved to date.[128] Clinical outcomes from this study will be reported in the future.

Animal studies have shown garlic to be effective at inhibiting chemically-induced stomach and colon cancer;[129-131] suppressing the growth of human colon tumor cell xenografts in mice;[132] protecting against the clastogenic effects of known genotoxicants,[133,134] both alone and in combination with selenium;[130,135-137] inhibiting induced mammary carcinogenesis; and inhibiting gamma-radiation-induced chromosomal damage.[138] In addition, diallyl disulfide has been shown to inhibit the proliferation of human tumour cells *in vitro*.[139] Lau (1990) and Dausch (1990) provide excellent reviews of the both *in vivo* and *in vitro* studies in this area.[111,115]

It has been hypothesized that components of garlic may exert their anti-neoplastic effects by modulating gluthione S-transferase dependent detoxification enzymes.[138,140-142] Other researchers have suggested that the sulfur components of garlic may inactivate endogenously formed nitrosamines.[143] In addition, the antibacterial effect of garlic (esp. against *Helicobacter pylori* which is a major risk factor for stomach cancer), may add to the protective effects.[107,144] For example, it may limit the formation of potentially carcinogenic nitrosamines by bacterial conversion in the stomach.[125] One author identified ajoene as a primary antimutagenic compound based on his investigation using the Ames test.[145]

ANTI-DIABETIC EFFECTS

Animal studies have demonstrated the hypoglycemic action of garlic.[146] Allicin has been shown to have a significant hypoglycemic action because it appears to compete with insulin for insulin-inactivating sites in the liver. This results in an increase in free insulin in the bloodstream.[147]

MISCELLANEOUS EFFECTS

HIV and AIDS

One small German study of 10 patients with advanced AIDS and severely low natural killer cell activity (all had opportunistic infections), involved the ingestion of 5 g of garlic (Kyolic® brand) daily for six weeks, followed by 10 g daily for another six weeks. Three patients died before the trial was completed. All seven patients who completed the trial were reported to have normal natural killer cell activity by the completion of the trial. Symptoms from their opportunistic infections were also reported to have improved, including chronic diarrhea and genital herpes.[148]

Anti-Aging Properties

Garlic has a reputation for an ability to prolong longevity and youthful appearance. However, few studies support these claims. Researchers report that ingestion of garlic was able to increase the survival of senscence-accelerated-prone mice (genetically bred to have shorter survival times), but did not affect the survival of another strain of mice bred to have longer survival times. Garlic appears to have improved the performance of mice in several models designed to test learning deficits, memory acquisition and memory deficits.[149,150] The applicability of these findings to human physiological aging and age-related memory deficits is unknown.

Earaches

Garlic oil is a popular folk remedy for the relief of earaches.[151] Traditionally, raw garlic is inserted into the ear. Garlic's usefulness for this indication is thought to be related to the antibacterial action of allicin.

Ischemia

Aged garlic extracts have been shown to provide a protective action in a rat model of brain ischemia.[152,153] The mechanism of action is hypothesized to be either an anti-oxidant action,[152,154] or an inhibitory action on arachidonic acid metabolism.[153]

Anti-Oxidant Effects

Several *in vitro* studies have demonstrated the anti-oxidant activity of garlic.[154-156] This activity is thought to be related to the mechanisms of action of many of its clinical effects, including decreasing blood cholesterol levels and providing protection in ischemic attacks.

Protection from Acetaminophen-Induced Hepatotoxicity

Two animal studies report that pre-treatment with garlic provides protection from acetaminophen-induced hepatoxicity in a time- and dose-dependent manner.[157,158]

Tick Repellent

A brief report of a crossover study of 100 Swedish military service personnel suggested that daily consumption of garlic (1200mg) for 8 weeks may decrease tick bites.[159] This finding has been questioned.[160] Additional studies are required.

ADVERSE EFFECTS

Heartburn, flatulence, and gastro-intestinal upset have been noted, usually at doses equivalent to 5 or more cloves daily.[7,43] In addition, the odoor of garlic is noticeable in the milk of lactating women. Contact dermatitis (caused by direct skin contact with raw garlic) is also possible, although most case reports occur in individuals (often young children) where crushed garlic pastes are applied to the skin for extended periods of time.[43,161-168]

Several cases of allergic reactions to garlic have been reported in the literature. In one case, a cook developed eczematous eruptions on his hands and was found to have a positive type IV patch test for diallyl disulfide, one of the compounds in garlic.[169] In addition, a single case of IgE-mediated urticaria caused by the ingestion of garlic has been reported.[170] Finally, one case of exercise-induced anaphylaxis possibly stimulated by garlic has been described.[171]

Several cases of post-operative bleeding associated with the ingestion of garlic have been reported.[172,174] A 72-year-old man who had been taking garlic for "many years" experienced unusual bleeding following a transurethral resection (TURP); laboratory tests confirmed a decrease in platelet coagulation in the presence of collagen.[172] Another case involved a 32-year-old women undergoing elective cosmetic surgery who also experienced increased bleeding post-operatively. Her heavy dietary garlic intake prior to surgery is suspected to have caused her increased blood clotting time.[173]

Several cases of occupational asthma stimulated by garlic have also been reported in the literature.[175-177]

In animal studies, rats fed high concentrations of garlic for a prolonged period of time suffered from anemia, weight loss and failure to grow.[178] Rats administered 500 mg/kg (equivalent to 10 cloves per day in humans) intraperitoneally once daily were reported to have extensive damage to the lungs (thickening of the alveolar walls) and liver (vacuolation especially near the organ surface). The same dose administered orally cause less damage and those fed low doses of garlic orally (50 mg/kg which is equivalent to 1 clove or 3-4 g in humans) daily had no significant lung or liver damage.[179]

CAUTIONS/CONTRAINDICATIONS

Garlic supplements should be used with caution by pregnant and lactating women.[180] In addition, they should be avoided before undergoing surgical procedures due to possible post-surgical bleeding.[174] One author also recommends caution after organ transplants because it has been reported that garlic enhances the activity of natural killer (NK) cells, which are largely responsible for tissue rejection.[148]

Attacks of pemphigus, a relatively rare autoimmune disorder resulting in lesions of the mucous membranes and skin, may be induced by drugs which contain active thiol groups. This sulfur-containing group is found in garlic; thus, it is suggested that patients with this condition avoid garlic.[181]

DRUG INTERACTIONS

A possible interaction with warfarin has been reported.[182] In addition, it has been suggested that it may potentiate the anti-thrombotic effects of ASA,[183] and may interfere with existing diabetic therapy.[180]

There are two case reports of HIV-infected persons taking garlic who developed severe gastrointestinal toxicity after initiating ritonavir-containing antiretroviral therapy.[184] However, a study evaluating the effect of acute dosing of garlic supplements on the single dose pharmacokinetics of ritonavir did not find any significant changes in the pharmacokinetics of ritonavir in healthy volunteers. The authors caution that their results should not be extrapolated to steady-state conditions, where the possibility of an interaction still needs to be evaluated.[185]

DOSAGE REGIMENS

❖ FRESH GARLIC: 3-30 g (1-8 cloves) daily.[12,186,187] The German Commission E considers a daily dose equivalent to 4 g of fresh garlic to be therapeutically effective.[12,186]

The British Herbal Compendium recommends:

❖ ALLICIN: 2-5 mg daily.

❖ GARLIC OIL: 2-5 mg daily.

❖ DRIED: 2-5 g of fresh air-dried daily.

❖ DRIED POWDER: 400-1200 mg of fully dried powder daily.[188,189]

Ginger

Zingiber officinale Roscoe

Common Uses
- ❖ Digestive Aid (dyspepsia and gastrointestinal upset)
- ❖ Motion Sickness
- ❖ Nausea (following anaesthesia)
- ❖ Nausea and Vomiting due to Pregnancy (see Cautions/Contraindications)
- ❖ Inflammatory Conditions (such as osteoarthritis, rheumatoid arthritis and myalgias)

Active Constituents
- ❖ Components of the Oleoresin Portion (notably the gingerols and shogaols)

Adverse Effects
- ❖ Heartburn and Digestive Upset (rare)

Cautions/Contraindications
- ❖ Gallstones (use only under medical supervision)
- ❖ Pregnancy (doses greater than 1 g daily should only be used in pregnancy when the patient is under medical supervision)

Drug Interactions
- ❖ None noted when ginger is taken at the suggested therapeutic doses

Doses
General Use
- ❖ *Dried Rhizome:* 0.25-1.0 g taken orally as a capsule, tablet, powder or decoction three times daily
- ❖ *Weak Ginger Tincture BP (1:5 in 90% ethanol):* 1.5-3.0 mL three times daily
- ❖ *Strong Ginger Tincture BP (1:2 in 90% ethanol):* 0.25-0.5 mL

General Anti-Emetic
- ❖ *Powdered Rhizome:* 1-2 g single dose

Motion Sickness
- ❖ *Powdered Rhizome:* 2-4 g daily

Introduction

Family
❖ Zingiberaceae

Synonyms
❖ Zingiber
❖ Gan-jiang[1, 2]

Medicinal Forms
❖ Fresh Rhizome
❖ Dried Rhizome
❖ Tincture

Description
While native to southern Asia, ginger is one of the most widely used spices in the world and is now cultivated throughout India, Australia, the Caribbean (notably Jamaica) and parts of West Africa. The plant is an erect perennial, growing up to 1 meter or 40 inches in height, with knife-shaped leaves, white or yellow flowers, and a characteristic 'gnarled', aromatic rhizome.[4,5]

Parts Used
The rhizome (underground stem), which is often referred to as the 'root', is the part used medicinally.[5] Once the rhizomes are harvested, they can be used as fresh ginger (green ginger); syruped ginger (candied ginger); dried ginger (as a spice); or an extract (e.g., volatile oil).[4]

Traditional Use
Very few herbs have more of a medicinal history than ginger.[3] Its use originated in the healing models of the Orient and quickly spread to the ancient cultures of Europe and the Middle East. It was introduced to North America during the exploration of the "New World" in the 16th century.[4] Historically, it has been used for numerous conditions, ranging from dyspepsia and vomiting to cholera and malaria.[2] Ginger has also been used extensively as a culinary spice.

Current Medicinal Use
A growing amount of evidence, including clinical trials, supports the use of ginger in the treatment of a number of forms of nausea, including motion sickness, nausea from pregnancy and potentially even after anaesthesia. Ginger may also prove useful as a digestive aid in treating dyspepsia as well as acting as an anti-inflammatory in the treatment of certain types of arthritis and muscle aches or myalgias.

Relevant Research
Preventative and Therapeutic Effects
CONSTITUENTS [1,4-6]

❖ OLEORESIN: pungent principles notably gingerols, shogaols and zingerone. (Proportion of shogaols increases upon drying; these compounds are largely absent in the fresh plant.)
❖ VOLATILE OILS: complex mixture of various hydrocarbons including: beta-bisabolene, zin giberene, zingiberol, various alcohols and aldehydes.
❖ LIPIDS: free fatty acids, triglycerides, phosphatidic acids and lecithins.
❖ CARBOHYDRATES: up to 50% starch.
❖ MISCELLANEOUS: various amino acids, proteins and vitamins.

DIGESTIVE ACTIONS

Ginger has long been praised in the management of digestive conditions. It is classically described as a 'stimulating carminative', both aiding digestive function as well as tonifing the gastrointestinal system.[7] Like many other spices, it has traditionally been used to enhance digestion by those who believed it increased salivary flow and gastric acid secretion.[8]

GASTROPROTECTIVE ACTION

Historical wisdom suggests that spices promote and/or irritate gastric ulcers.[9] However, several animal studies have demonstrated that ginger has potential gastroprotective properties.[10-12] In these studies, extracts of ginger were administered orally to rats in doses ranging from 500 to 1000 mg/kg resulting in significant decreases in the incidence of stress-induced gastric ulcers initiated by various experimental protocols (including HCl/ethanol, and NSAID). Acetone extracts of ginger compared favorably to cimetidine and misoprostol in one animal study.[12] While an exact mechanism of action has yet to be ascertained, it is suggested that certain components (esp. zingiberene and 6-gingerol) may be influencing the activation of a cellular protective action.[10]

In addition, several studies have demonstrated that extracts of ginger increased gastric pH and decreased gastric secretions.[9,13] In one study with rabbits, the effect of an aqueous extract of ginger (dose 169 mg/kg) on gastric secretion 3 hours after oral administration was comparable to an oral dose of 50 mg/kg of cimetidine.[13] Another study found that the increase in gastric pH due to the ginger extract was very slight when compared to cimetidine.[9] These actions may play a role in the gastroprotective action noted above.

Digestive Aid

Animal studies have shown that dried ginger added to the diet results in increased digestive enzyme action, especially lipase activity.[8] Other studies have reported that an acetone extract of ginger caused an increase in bile secretion.[14] These studies support the historical use of ginger to aid in the digestion of fatty meals.

HAEMATOLOGY EFFECTS

Inhibition of Platelet Aggregation

Several studies have found that ginger inhibits platelet aggregation induced by various means, including adenosine diphosphate (ADP) and epinephrine.[15,16] In one randomized study, volunteers (n =20) ingested 10 g of dried ginger or placebo in addition to 100 g of butter daily for 7 days. Although serum lipids remained unchanged in both groups, platelet aggregation was significantly decreased in the group ingesting ginger.[15] An *in vitro* study of an aqueous extract of fresh ginger found a dose-dependent inhibition of platelet aggregation. However, a recent randomized, double-blind trial (n=8) in the United Kingdom suggests that this effect may be limited to doses greater than 2 g of dried ginger daily or doses of fresh ginger.[17] As with the anti-inflammatory mechanism described below, the anti-aggregation activity of ginger may be due to its influence on prostaglandin and thromboxane synthesis.

Anti-Hypercholestermic

It has been suggested that ginger may be useful in the management of patients with elevated cholesterol levels. In 1978, a study of cholesterol fed rats concluded that oral administration of ginger oleoresin (1.5 mg/kg) resulted in significantly lowered serum and hepatic cholesterol levels as well as increased fecal cholesterol excretion.[18] These findings have been only partially supported by more recent studies. A 1984 study found that oral ingestion of 1 g of fresh ginger by rats offered no immediate protection against a cholesterol rich diet. While ginger, was shown to have an anti-hypercholesterolemic effect, their results suggested that it must be ingested for several days before this action is manifested.[19] A recent report of the isolation and identification of a specific compound (ZT) from ginger, which is assumed to be an HMG-CoA reductase inhibitor, found that ZT exerted an inhibitory effect on cholesterol biosynthesis.[20]

MUSCULOSKELETAL EFFECTS

Ginger has historically been used for its anti-inflammatory properties in many Asian healing models, notably in the Ayurvedic (Indian subcontinent) and Kampo (Japanese) systems of medicine.[21] Attempts have been made to investigate this action in both animal models and human subjects.[22-24] In two reviews of case studies (n=7 and n=56), patients suffering from a variety of arthritic conditions and mylagias were investigated.[22,23] When ginger was ingested, an appreciable decrease in pain and swelling was noted in the majority of cases. The daily doses ingested by these patients ranged from 3-7 g of powdered ginger, with one individual ingesting 50 g of raw ginger daily. No adverse reactions were reported in any of these patients who had taken ginger from periods ranging for 3 months to 2.5 years. Relief was normally noted within 1-3 months and remained for as long as the ingestion of ginger continued. Symptoms returned when the therapy was discontinued, usually within two weeks. It should be noted that these reports were not clinical trials but case studies and no attempt was made to standardize the therapeutic protocols. However, a recent experiment using a rat model of inflammation found that ginger oil (33 mg/kg) given orally for 26 days caused a significant suppression of both paw and joint swelling.[24]

A recent randomized, double-blind, placebo-controlled 6-week study of 261 patients diagnosed with osteoarthritis of the knee and in moderate to severe pain assessed the efficacy of a concentrated extract of 2 ginger species (*Zingiber officinale* and *Alpinia galanga* (EV.EXT 77)) for this indication.[25] Participants ingested ginger or placebo twice daily and were allowed to use acetaminophen if needed. Overall, significantly more participants in the ginger group experienced a reduction in knee pain on standing compared with the placebo group. Reduction of knee pain on walking and reduction in the Western Ontario and McMaster Universities osteoarthritis composite index were also noted. Another randomized, controlled double-blind, double-dummy, crossover study (with a 1-week washout period) compared the effectiveness of ginger (170 mg of EV.ext-33 extract), ibuprofen (400 mg) and placebo in 56 patients with osteoarthritis of the hip or knee.[26] Overall, ibuprofen was found to be better than ginger which was found to be better than placebo. A significant difference was noted between ginger and the placebo only in the first arm of the crossover study, but not in the study as a whole. Additional research in this area is warranted.

While no exact mechanism of action is known, the anti-inflammatory action of ginger could be due in part to its influence on eicasonoid production and other inflammatory mediators.[23,27] Constituents of the oleoresin portion (especially the gingerols) are thought to decrease levels of inflammatory mediators produced from lipid membranes. It has been suggested that by inhibiting cyclooxygenase and 5-lipoxygense respectively, the production of both inflammatory prostaglandins and leukotrienes could be prevented. In addition, aromatic components of ginger may inhibit the inflammatory action initiated by pyrogens such as interleukin 1.[28]

ANTI-NAUSEA EFFECTS

Motion Sickness

Of all its modern-day applications, ginger is perhaps best known for its suggested use in the management of motion sickness. While many clinical trials have been conducted, their results have often been conflicting. In 1982, Mowrey and Clayson reported that 940 mg powdered ginger was superior to 100 mg dimenhydrinate in preventing symptoms of motion sickness in blindfolded subjects (n=36) placed in a tilted, rotating chair.[29] This study has been criticized because all subjects were selected because of their self-reported high susceptibility to motion sickness and because the main outcome measure was the patients' self-assessment of gastrointestinal discomfort.[30]

Another double-blind, randomized, placebo-controlled trial found that 1 g of powdered ginger ingested every hour for 4 hours reduced the tendency to vomiting and cold sweating significantly better than placebo in seasickness. The authors also noted that fewer symptoms of nausea and vertigo were reported after ginger ingestion, but that this difference was not statistically significant.[31] This study has also been criticized because the difference between the effect of ginger and the placebo did not reach statistical significance until the fourth hour of the trial;[30] however, it is also important to note that this is currently the only study carried out in field conditions.

In 1988, a second trial using a rotating chair model of motion sickness found that 1000 mg of fresh ginger, 500 mg and 1000 mg of dried ginger given 2 hours before the test were all no more effective than the placebo.[32] The design of this study differed from the study conducted by Mowrey and Clayson because: 1) a Latin square design allowed each participant to serve as his/her own control; 2) participants were not blind folded; 3) the ginger was ingested 2 hours prior to the test (rather than 20-25 minutes as in the previous trial); and 4) standardized N.A.S.A. outcome measures were used. Finally, a third trial of the efficacy of ginger for the prevention of the symptoms of motion sickness in a revolving chair model was conducted in 1991. In this study, participants were blindfolded and ingested the ginger (500 mg or 1000 mg of powdered or 1000 mg of fresh) one hour prior to the test. The authors concluded that ginger does not possess anti-motion sickness activity.[30]

The most recent randomized, double-blind, placebo-controlled, crossover trial (n=18) of the effects of ginger on motion sickness reported pre-treatment with ginger (1000mg and 200 mg) 1 hour prior to induction of nausea by spinning participants reduced nausea, prolonged the onset of nausea and shortened the recovery time after nausea induced by the spinning.[33]

It is interesting to note that the majority of the negative trials have been conducted in North America leading some to suggest that the quality of ginger and ginger preparations locally available may be influencing the outcome.[34,35] Also of interest is the fact that irrespective of the negative trials, the Commission E, a German government advisory body, has approved the use of ginger in the management of motion sickness. Their suggested dosage of 2-4 g daily is higher than those used in the majority of the studies.[34] In addition, many practitioners suggest that for the prevention of motion sickness, ginger must be ingested for a prolonged period of time starting several days before the journey commences.[35] In conclusion, while ginger is a long established treatment for motion sickness in complementary health-care circles, its efficacy has yet to be conclusively confirmed by clinical trials.

Nausea Associated with Anaesthesia

Many anti-emetics commonly used to control nausea and vomiting following surgery have side effects, which has led to a search for a less toxic agent. Studies of the use of ginger for the prevention of nausea and vomiting post-operatively have been conflicting. One study of 60 women who had major gynaecological surgery found that 500 mg of powdered ginger given 1.5 hours prior to surgery was superior to placebo and comparable to metoclopramide in decreasing the number of incidences of nausea post-operatively.[36] This study was supported by a study of 120 women following laparoscopic gynaecological surgery which found that 1 g of powdered ginger given 1 hour prior to induction of anaesthesia reduced the incidence of nausea and vomiting comparably to metoclopramide and significantly more than a placebo.[37] However, a more recent Australian study of 108 women undergoing laparoscopic gynaecological surgery found that the ingestion of 500 mg or 1000 mg of powdered ginger one hour prior to surgery slightly, but not significantly increased the incidence of nausea and vomiting post-operatively.[38] In addition, two other randomized, placebo-controlled studies of women (n=184 and n=120) undergoing gynecologic laparoscopic surgery reported that treatment with ginger (total of 600 mg given pre and post-operatively or 2 g pre-operatively) did not decrease the incidence of post-operative nausea and vomiting.[39,40]

Nausea Associated with Pregnancy

The use of ginger as an anti-emetic during pregnancy is controversial. To date, three studies provide direct evidence on this issue. In a double-blind, randomized, crossover, placebo-controlled trial of women diagnosed with hyperemesis gravidarum (n=30), 250 mg of powdered ginger ingested four times daily was found to be significantly more effective in relieving symptoms than a placebo. No side effects were observed.[41] It should be noted that it is difficult to generalize the results of this study to those which may be expected if ginger is ingested for the relief of routine morning sickness due to the severity of the symptoms associated with hyperemesis gravidarum.

The second double-blind, placebo-controlled study investigated the effects of ginger (1 g daily) for 4 days in 70 women who were experiencing nausea before 17 weeks gestation.[42] The severity of nausea and the number of vomiting episodes decreased significantly compared to baseline in the ginger group compared to the placebo group. No adverse effect of ginger on pregnancy outcome was identified.

The third randomized, double-blind, placebo-controlled trial investigated the ability of ginger syrup mixed with water to relieve the nausea and vomiting of women (n=26) in their first trimester of pregnancy.[43] Each participant ingested the equivalent of 250 mg of ginger four times per day for 14 days. The women in the ginger group appeared to experience more relief from their symptoms than the women in the placebo group; however, statistical analyses were not performed because of the small numbers of women in each group.

Drug-Induced Nausea

A single animal study found that an acetone extract of ginger (150 mg/kg) ingested orally by rats was comparable to metoclopramide (25 mg/kg) when administered 60 minutes prior to cyclophosphamide (300 mg/kg s.c.). Both provided complete protection from vomiting episodes. The authors suggest that this warrants further investigation.[44]

Mechanism of Action

The exact mechanism responsible for the anti-emetic effects of ginger is unknown. It appears that this is primarily due to a gastrointestinal action, rather than one mediated through the central nervous system.[45] However, several studies have concluded that ingestion of ginger does not affect the gastric emptying rate, as has been hypothesized by many investigators.[30,37] More recently it has been suggested that ginger exerts a more generalized action on the entire gastroinestinal tract. In addition, the lack of centrally-mediated action is being questioned.[46,47] For example, ginger has been reported to antagonize 5-HT$_3$ receptors, which are found in both the wall of the gastrointestinal tract and the brain. Antagonism of these receptors produces anti-emetic effects.[48] A recent study suggests that ginger may have an novel anti-nausea action by decreasing tachygastric activity and preventing the elevation of plasma vasopressin induced by circular vection.[33]

MISCELLANEOUS EFFECTS

Cardiotonic

Ginger has long been praised within many healing models as an effective circulatory stimulant.[49] While clinical evidence confirming its influence on the cardiovascular system is limited, it has been shown that the gingerol portion exerts an inotropic effect on isolated guinea pig atria.[50]

Migraines

Given its proposed anti-emetic action and the fact that the treatment of headaches is one of ginger's traditional uses, some have suggested that it may play a role in the management of migraines. The evidence to support this is limited to a single published paper reviewing one case history. In this case, 500-600 mg of powdered ginger was ingested by the patient at the first sign of an aura and then every 4 hours for 3 to 4 days thereafter. The development of the migraine was halted within thirty minutes. Subsequently the patient began adding ginger to her diet, which resulted in a decreased incidence of migraines over the next 13 months.[51]

Anti-Microbial Action

Certain constituents of ginger, notably the shogaols and zingerone, appear to exert an anti-microbial action against specific pathogens, including *Salmonella typhi, Vibrio cholerae,* and *Tricophyton violaceum in vitro.* The clinical relevance of this property is unknown.[52]

ADVERSE EFFECTS

Adverse effects of ginger appear to be so rare that the majority of Western European pharmacopoeias fail to mention any observed cases at all. In practice, unwanted side effects appear to be limited to gastric burning and dyspepsia.[7] This is found more often when unencapsulated preparations are taken and the individual lies down soon after taking the preparation.[30] While some have cautioned against the prolonged use of ginger due to its anticoagulant properties (see haemotology section), the use of ginger for culinary purposes or at therapeutic doses less than 1 g daily do not appear to be associated with any adverse affects.[17]

CAUTIONS/CONTRAINDICATIONS

The use of ginger in pregnancy has been questioned. This concern arises from two sources: 1) the use of ginger is "contraindicated" during pregnancy within the Traditional Chinese Medical (TCM) model; and 2) several animal studies performed in the 1980s suggested that large doses of the gingerol portion may exert a mutagenic action *in vitro.*[7,53,54] When considering the first source of concern, it should be noted that the doses given within TCM therapeutic protocols are normally far higher (approximately 9 g daily) than those suggested for therapeutic purposes in North America (1-2 g daily).[7] Regarding the second source, while it was shown that 6-gingerol possessed mutagenic properties, it should be noted that antimutagenic components were also found to be present in the total ginger extract.[54] In addition, in the only study in pregnant women (with hyperemesis gravidarum) no teratagenic effects nor increased rates of abortion were observed. Ginger has also been shown in animal studies to be devoid of any spermatoxic qualities.[55]

While the Commission E monographs does caution against the use of ginger in pregnancy, this concern is not shared by the other major pharmacopeias, such as the *British Herbal Compendium*.[7] Consequently, it is reasonable to conclude that ginger can be taken during pregnancy in doses within the North American standard therapeutic range for a limited period of time.[7]

Concerns have been raised over the possibility of increased bleeding time following surgery if the patient is taking ginger preparations due to the reported inhibition of thromboxane synthetase.[56] It appears unlikely that this presents a problem when the plant is taken in standard North American therapeutic doses as described in the management of post-surgical nausea.[17]

Given ginger's cholagogic properties some authors suggest against its use in cases of gall stones without medical supervision.[57]

DRUG INTERACTIONS
No specific interactions could be found between ginger and any conventional medications. Given the described pharmacological actions of ginger, it should be used with caution in situations of concurrent conventional cardiac, diabetic and anti-coagulant therapy.[1]

DOSAGE REGIMENS
General Use
❖ DRIED RHIZOME: 0.25-1.0 g taken orally as a capsule, tablet, powder or decoction three times daily.[6]

❖ WEAK GINGER TINCTURE BP (1:5, 90% ethanol): 1.5-3 mL three times daily.[6]

❖ STRONG GINGER TINCTURE BP (1:2, 90% ethanol): 0.25-0.5 mL.[6]

General Anti-Emetic
❖ POWDERED RHIZOME: 1-2 g single dose.[6]

Motion Sickness
❖ POWDERED RHIZOME: 2-4 g daily.[1,34]

Gingko
Ginkgo biloba L.

THUMBNAIL SKETCH

Common Uses
- ❖ Cerebral Insufficiency
- ❖ Intermittent Claudication
- ❖ Raynaud's Syndrome
- ❖ Memory Impairment/Dementia
- ❖ Tinnitus
- ❖ Vertigo

Active Constituents
- ❖ Ginkolides
- ❖ Bilobides
- ❖ Flavone Glycosides

Adverse Effects
- ❖ Extremely infrequent, but include: gastrointestinal disturbances and headache; very rarely spontaneous bleeding.

Cautions/Contraindications
- ❖ Pregnancy and Nursing (safety not established)

Drug Interactions
- ❖ May potentiate the effect of anti-coagulants (theoretical).

Doses
- ❖ *Standardized GBE (Gingko biloba Extract):* 40 mg three times daily
- ❖ *Dried Leaves:* 300 mg daily

  Note: Treatment for many conditions must be continued for 1-3 months before positive results can be expected.

Introduction

Family
* Ginkgoaceae[1]

Synonyms
* Maidenhair-tree[2-4]

Medicinal Forms
* Standardized Extracts
* Dried Leaves

Description

It has been estimated that the ginkgo tree has existed for more than 200 million years, making it the oldest known tree species on earth.[5,6] Charles Darwin is reported to have called the gingko tree a living fossil. A given tree may live for 1000 years, growing to a height of 30 meters or 100 feet and up to 120 centimeters or 40 inches in diameter. The fan-shaped leaves attach to short, horizontal branches. The foul-smelling fruit is inedible, but contains an edible seed which resembles an almond.[4] Ginkgo trees are now extensively cultivated to meet the growing medicinal demand and they continue to be favored by city planners because they flourish in adverse conditions in urban environments.[7]

Parts Used

The leaves of the gingko tree are the part used medicinally in Europe and North America. Products standardized to 24% flavone glycosides and 6% terpenoids have been available for several decades as non-prescription agents.[8] To date, the majority of the research has been conducted using one specific extract of ginkgo: EGb 761; however, several trials using a similar extract (LI 1370) are also reviewed here. Within Traditional Chinese Medicine, the malodorous fruits are used.

Traditional Use

Although ginkgo has been used in Traditional Chinese Medicine (TCM) for such indications as 'benefiting the brain', as an astringent to the lungs, and for the relief of asthma symptoms and coughs,[7-9] it is not generally regarded as a particularly important herb in TCM. However, ginkgo is considered a conventional drug in Europe, where annual sales are estimated at over US $500 million.

Current Medicinal Uses

Ginkgo biloba is one of the most widely used and best researched herbal medicines. While more evidence is needed, *Ginkgo biloba* products are used for a variety of conditions, many associated with aging, including: peripheral vascular disease, tinnitus, dementia, cases of trauma to the brain and "chronic cerebral insufficiency."[7,8] It is important to realize that the vast majority of research supporting the use of *Ginkgo biloba* refers to standardized extracts (*Ginkgo biloba* extract or GBE) made from the leaf. While many people take GBE to enhance memory, there is currently little scientific evidence that it will work unless you have significant memory impairment.

Relevant Research

Preventative and Therapeutic Effects

CONSTITUENTS [1-4, 9-14]

❖ TERPENES: diterpene ginkgolides (A, B, C, J and M); sesquiterpenes (bilobalides).

❖ FLAVONOIDS: ginkgo-flavone glycosides (e.g., bilobetin, gikgetin, isoginkgetin, sciadopitysin); glycosides of quercetin, and kaempferol; isorhamnetin derivatives.

❖ ORGANIC ACIDS: 6-hydroxykynurenic acid, kynurenic acid, shikimic acid, protocatechic acid, vanillic acid, p-hydroxybenzoic acid.

❖ ESSENTIAL OILS.

❖ TANNINS.

CARDIOVASCULAR EFFECTS

Mechanism of Action

Many studies have demonstrated the ability of extracts of ginkgo (EGb 761) to increase blood flow.[3,15-17] Egb 761 has been shown to: increase skin perfusion;[3] decrease blood viscosity;[3] decrease blood vessel elasticity;[3] increase blood flow in nail-fold capillaries;[15] decrease erythrocyte aggregation;[15] increase coronary blood flow (in isolated guinea pig heart);[18] and increase cerebral blood flow.[19] However, plasma viscosity;[3,15] packed cell volume;[15] haematocrit;[15] and thrombocyte aggregation[15] do not appear to be affected by this ginkgo extract. The specific compounds in the ginkgo extract responsible for these effects have not yet been identified, although much attention has been focused on the flavonoids and the ginkolides.[20,21]

Ginkgo extracts (e.g., EGb 761) appear to have the ability to relax blood vessels in spasm and constrict those that are abnormally dilated by increasing their tone.[22-25] Several authors have noted the ability of GBE (*Ginkgo biloba* extract) to produce dose-dependent relaxation of the aorta in animal models.[26] This relaxant effect appears to be at least partially mediated by a factor(s) that is released from endothelial cells.[26] Other studies report a dose-dependent contractile effect on rabbit isolated aorta[27,28] and vena cava.[29] It is suggested that ginkgo extracts cause contracted blood vessels to relax by prolonging the half-life of endothelium-derived relaxing factor.[30,31] The flavonoids are thought to be primarily responsible for this action.

Another important mechanism of action is the competitive antagonism of platelet activating factor (PAF).[10,21,32-45] Braquet and Smith provide excellent reviews of this action.[10,21] Ginkgo extracts have been shown to: decrease platelet aggregation;[39] decrease microvascular permeability; cause bronchodilation; and inhibit thromboformation *in vitro*[40,46] and *in vivo* to a degree comparable to ASA.[46,47] It is thought that the ginkgolides (especially ginkgolide B) are responsible for this action. However, several researchers have reported that ginkgo extracts do not affect coagulation or skin bleeding time.[39]

Interestingly, ginkgo seems to act preferentially at ischemic sites.[48-56] For example, administration of extracts of ginkgo in animals subjected to cerebral ischemia increased glucose consumption;[49] normalized mitochondrial respiration;[50] diminished cerebral edema;[50] preserved neurological function;[50] and decreased the accumulation of free polyunsaturated fatty acids.[55] In an animal study, *Ginkgo biloba* extract was found to be comparable to methylprednisone and more effective than thyroid releasing hormone at providing a protective effect against ischaemic spinal cord injury. This effect was thought to be due to its antioxidant actions.[52]

In addition, ginkgo has been shown to protect healthy volunteers from the effects of hypoxia.[57] Animal studies have confirmed this finding.[58-60] One study reported that both *Ginkgo biloba* extract and bilobalide alone were able to inhibit a hypoxia-induced decrease in ATP content and increase in total lactate production in endothelial cells *in vitro*.[61]

The flavonoid components of *Ginkgo biloba* extract are also reported to possess potent antioxidant activity.[62-68] Ginkgo's activity as an antioxidant is thought to play a role in many of its therapeutic actions, especially its postulated neuroprotective effect and its protection from ischemia-reperfusion damage.[64,66-71] Several studies have demonstrated that the ginkgo extract EGb 761 has both hydroxyl radical scavenging and superoxide dismutase-like activity.[30,71,72]

Cerebral Insufficiency

A variety of studies report the effectiveness of ginkgo in the treatment of "chronic cerebral insufficiency."[73-78] Symptoms typical of "cerebral insufficiency" include: memory loss; difficulty concentrating; confusion; fatigue; decreased physical strength; anxiety; dizziness; tinnitus; headache; and depressive mood. It is hypothesized that these symptoms may be associated with some impairment of the cerebral circulation.[3] Kleijnen and Knipschild reviewed 40 controlled trials studying the use of *Ginkgo biloba* in cases of "cerebral insufficiency,"[3] concluding that although only 8 trials were of "good quality,"[78-85] all the trials reviewed, except one,[86] showed clinically-relevant positive effects for ginkgo when compared with a placebo. For example, in an open trial of 112 patients suffering from symptoms of "chronic cerebral insufficiency" (mean age 71 years) taking 40 mg *Ginkgo biloba* extract three times daily for one year, significant improvements in short-term memory, alertness, mood disturbances, vertigo, headaches and tinnitus were reported.[78] A more recent double-blind, placebo-controlled trial of 90 patients suffering from "cerebral insufficiency" found that those taking ginkgo scored significantly higher on a variety of tests of cognitive function.[87]

Intermittant Claudication

Pittler and Ernst performed a meta-analysis to assess the efficacy of ginkgo extract for intermittent claudication based on the results of randomized, double-blind, placebo-controlled trials.[88] Eight trials met their inclusion criteria (which included using pain-free walking distance as a primary outcome measure).[89-96] The authors concluded that "*Ginkgo biloba* extract is superior to placebo in the symptomatic treatment of intermittent claudication. However, the size of the overall treatment effect is modest and of uncertain clinical relevance."[88] Kleijnen and Knipschild also reviewed 15 placebo-controlled trials which investigated the use of ginkgo extracts in the treatment of intermittent claudication.[3] They report that only two were of "acceptable" quality,[91,97] and that all fifteen indicated positive effects for treatment with ginkgo. Bauer's double-blind, placebo-controlled study of 79 patients given either ginkgo (40 mg) or placebo three times daily for 1 year reported reduction in pain that was four times greater in the ginkgo group (p<0.001).[91] Given the overall poor quality of trials in this area Kleijnen and Knipschild recommend further research into the use of ginkgo extract for this indication.[3] One additional randomized, double-blind study designed to compare two different doses of ginkgo (EGb extract 761 240 mg vs 120 mg daily) in patients with peripheral arterial occlusive disease Fontaine's stage IIb reported that both dosage regimens led to clinically relevant improvement in pain-free walking distance after 24 weeks of treatment and that the higher dose (240 mg) produced a statistically significantly superior effect.[98]

A double-blind, placebo-controlled trial investigated the use of ginkgo in 20 patients suffering from stage II claudicating arterial occlusive disease. Each patient ingested 160 mg *Ginkgo biloba* extract (EGb 761) or placebo twice daily for four weeks. The main outcome measure of this trial was measurement of the transcutaneous partial pressure of oxygen both at rest and after a treadmill test. The areas of ischemia decreased by 38% in the ginkgo group, but did not change in the placebo group (p<0.04). It should be noted that this trial used a much higher dose of ginkgo than most other reports in the literature.[99]

A double-blind, randomized study of 36 patients with arteritis found that those treated with *Ginkgo biloba* for 6 months experienced significantly greater pain relief and walking tolerance than those taking placebo. These benefits persisted when the ginkgo treatment was continued in an open trial for a total of 65 weeks.[100]

While these results are promising and GBE may be of use in the conditions listed above, more research is needed before a definitive conclusion can be reached.

Ischemic Heart Disease

It is suggested that *Ginkgo biloba* extract may have a protective effect against cardiac-reperfusion injury.[65,101] One study reports that EGb 761 improved cardiac mechanical recovery, suppressed leakage of lactate dehydrogenase and diminished the decrease of myocardial ascorbate during reperfusion.[64] It is hypothesized that this action of ginkgo may be attributed to its anti-oxidant properties.[65] In addition, ginkgolide B has been shown to have dose-related protection against dysrrhythmias induced by ischemia (comparable to diltiazem and superior to metoprolol) which the authors hypothesize may be related to an antagonism of an increase in slow calcium influx induced by PAF in myocardial cells.[102] This study noted that gingkolide B did not produce any changes in heart function, even in when given in high doses.

NEUROLOGY/PSYCHIATRY EFFECTS

Mechanism of Action

Animal studies have shown that extracts of *Ginkgo biloba* can influence neuron metabolism and have a positive effect on neurotransmitter disturbances.[23] It appears to increase the production of dopamine and noradrenaline, as well as increasing the number of acetylcholine and serotonin receptors.[103-107] In addition, one study demonstrated that chronic oral treatment with ginkgo prevented decline in muscarinic (cholinergic) receptor density in the hippocampus of rats as they aged.[108] *In vitro and in vivo* studies indicate that the *Ginkgo biloba* extract EGb 761 increases synaptosomal uptake of 5-hydroxytryptamine[109] and decreases the synaptosomal uptake of dopamine and serotonin.[106]

It has been suggested that the bilobalides may aid in the regrowth of damaged neurons in the central nervous system; however an exact mechanism of action has yet to be proposed.[9,110] *Ginkgo biloba* extract (EGb 761) was also reported to prevent dopaminergic neurotoxicity in an animal study.[111] Amri and colleagues suggest that the neuroprotective effects of ginkgo are caused by its effect on glucocorticoid biosynthesis: it appears to decrease glucocorticoid levels and increase ACTH release. They described this mechanism of action in detail.[112] Other possible mechanisms for the neuroprotective properties associated with ginkgo have been described by many other authors.[10,20,113-115]

The effect of ginkgo on cerebral glucose utilization continues to be controversial; some studies reporting increases in cerebral glucose utilization;[23,48,116-118] some reporting no change;[19] and others reporting decreases.[119]

Dementia

Over recent years, much attention has been focussed on the role of GBE in the management of various forms of dementia. A variety of studies indicate that ginkgo may be useful in the treatment of vascular dementia or dementia of the Alzheimer type.[75,77,82,120-126] One of the most convincing is a prospective, randomized, double-blind, placebo-controlled, multi-center trial of the efficacy of *Gingko biloba* extract (EGb 761) in which 216 outpatients diagnosed with mild to moderate pre-senile, senile primary degenerative dementia of the Alzheimer type and multi-infarct dementia ingested either EGb 761 or placebo for 24 weeks. Ginkgo was found to be more effective than placebo ($p<.005$). The three primary outcome measures in this study were: the Clinical Global Impressions (CBI) for psychopathological assessment; the Syndrom-Kurztest (SKT) for assessment of memory and attention and the Nurnberger Alters-Beobachtungsskala (NAB) for assessment of behavior during the activities of daily life.[122] These results confirm the findings of an earlier, smaller (n=40) double-blind, placebo-controlled trial.[124]

This finding is supported by another randomized, double-blind, placebo-controlled study that plans to follow patients who were mildly to severely impaired and diagnosed with uncomplicated Alzheimer's disease or multi-infarct dementia (n=244) for 52 weeks. In the interim analysis (after 26 weeks of data collection), ingestion of ginkgo (40 mg three times daily of EGb 761) was associated with a significant improvement on both the Alzheimer's Disease Assessment Scale-Cognitive Subscale (ADAS-Cog) (26% of patients achieved at least a 4 point improvement) and the Geriatric Evaluation by Relative's Rating Instrument (GERRI) (30% showed improvement) compared to placebo according to an intent-to-treat statistical analysis.[127]

Another North American multi-center, randomized, controlled trial that followed 309 out-patients who had been diagnosed with mild to severe Alzheimer disease or multi-infarct dementia for 52 weeks reported similar results. *Ginkgo biloba* extract (EGb 761) at a dose of 40 mg three times daily was compared with placebo on the following outcome measures: ADAS-Cog; GERRI; and the Clinical Global Impression of Change Scale (CGIC). The investigators used an intention-to-treat analysis and reported that the treatment group scored significantly higher on both the ADAS-Cog and the GERRI; however, there was no difference between the placebo group and the ginkgo group with respect to the CGIC scores. Although the changes in patients taking ginkgo were considered modest by the investigators, they were of sufficient magnitude as to be identified by the caregivers as measured by the GERRI.[126]

Another longitudinal, multi-center, double-blind, placebo controlled study (n = 166) of ginkgo extract for the treatment of a variety of cerebral disorders due to ageing found that those on ginkgo for more than 3 months showed significantly higher scores (as compared to the placebo group) on a specially designed geriatric clinical evaluation scale. This difference continued to increase in subsequent months.[82]

In addition, an article comparing placebo-controlled efficacy studies of cholinesterase inhibitors and ginkgo extracts that were at least six months in duration concluded that ginkgo extract Egb 761® and second-generation cholinesterase inhibitors (donepezil, rivastigmine, metrifonate) should be considered equally effective in the treatment of mild to moderate Alzheimer's dementia.[128]

Memory Enhancement Among Individuals with Memory Impairment
Studies on the effectiveness of *Ginkgo biloba* in the treatment of memory impairment and as an agent of memory enhancement have been conflicting.[85,123,129-136] Generally, ginkgo preparations appear to enhance memory in cases where significant memory impairment exists (often associated with increasing age), but to have no effect on those whose memory is unimpaired. For example, one study found that aged rats (22-24 months old) treated with 100 mg/kg of ginkgo extract EGb 761 daily for three weeks had improved short-term memory measured by avoidance latency after adverse stimulus (p<.05); however, no significant effects were seen in young (3-month- old) or middle-aged (12-month-old) rats.[135] In addition, in a study of 40 volunteers (57-77 years), those with initially low scores on tests of vigilance and reaction time showed significant improvement when taking ginkgo as compared to placebo, while those with initially normal scores on these tests showed no improvement when taking ginkgo when compared to the placebo group.[76] In another double-blind, placebo-controlled study, 31 patients over the age of 50 with mild to moderate memory impairment were given 40 mg of *Ginkgo biloba* extract or placebo three times daily for 6 months. The results indicate that those taking ginkgo had improved performance on

the Kendrick digit copying task, and the median reaction time for the classification task; however, no statistical difference was found with the Kendrick object learning task and a decrease in performance on the digit recall task was noted. The authors suggest that more significant results may be expected if the subjects had more severe memory impairment at baseline.[129] Finally, a double-blind, placebo-controlled, cross-over study of 18 elderly men and women diagnosed with slight age-related memory impairment suggests that ingestion of 320 or 600 mg of ginkgo (EGb 761) one hour before performing a dual-coding test is associated with an improvement in the speed of information processing.[130] It should be noted that this is considered a relatively large dose of *Ginkgo biloba*.

Memory Enhancement Among Individuals Without Memory Impairment
Although improvement of short-term memory,[131,132,137] simple reaction time,[76] attention,[138] speed of processing abilities,[139] and other neuropsychological tests[140,141] in healthy volunteers and improved retention of learned behavior in healthy rats[133,136,142] have been reported, the evidence supporting these effects remains controversial. This is because other studies have also reported negative results (i.e., that ginkgo did not have a beneficial effect on neuropsychological tests of learning, memory, attention, concentration or verbal fluency).[131,143] Several studies have also reported enhanced cognitive function in health volunteers who ingested combination products that included ginkgo and Asian ginseng.[141,144,145] The benefits attained from the ginkgo as compared to either the combination of herbs or the Asian ginseng alone is not known. Given the wide range of neuropsychological outcomes assessed it is difficult to compare the results of different studies. Additional research is required to determine if ingesting ginkgo will have any clinically significant effect on the cognitive function and memory of healthy individuals. This is particularly important since memory enhancement is a frequently the reason people take ginkgo.[131]

Depression
One randomized, placebo-controlled trial with 40 patients diagnosed with resistant depression (aged 51 to 78 years) found that *Ginkgo biloba* extract (EGb 761) was significantly more effective than placebo. Patients in the trial had shown insufficient improvement on tri- and/or tetracyclic antidepressants for a minimum of three months prior to being enrolled in the trial. During the trial, patients continued to take anti-depressant therapy, but were also given either EGb 761 (80 mg) or placebo three times daily. The main outcome measure was the sum score of the Hamilton Depression Scale (HAMD). After four weeks, a 50% decrease in the severity of depression for the EGb 761 group (compared to a 10% decrease in the placebo group) was noted ($p<.01$). A further decrease in the HAMD scores was noted after 8 weeks for the ginkgo group.($p<.01$).[146] However, another randomized, double-blind, placebo-controlled study of patients with seasonal affective disorder (n=27) did not support this claim. Treatment with ginkgo (1 tablet twice daily of ginkgo extract PN246, Bio-Biloba® brand) for 10 weeks starting in a symptom-free period about 1 month prior to the expected onset of symptoms did not prevent the development of the symptoms of seasonal affective disorder. No significant differences were found between the ginkgo and the placebo groups.[147]

Animal studies have suggested that ginkgo extracts may reduce the emotional and behavioural consequences of stress.[142,148] One study found that extracts of ginkgo leaves caused reversible inhibition of rat brain MAO-A and MAO-B, suggesting a mechanism for reported anti-stress and anxiolytic activities of *Ginkgo biloba*.[149]

Sudden Hearing Loss
Two studies have investigated the effects of ginkgo in patients with sudden hearing loss. One randomized, double-blind trial compared two doses (120 mg vs 12 mg twice daily over 8 weeks) of ginkgo extract EGb 761 in outpatients (n=106) with acute idiopathic sudden

hearing loss of at least 15 dB at one frequency within speech range occurring less than 10 days prior to inclusion in the study.[150] A majority of both treatment groups recovered completely. The authors conclude that a "higher dose of Egb 761 (oral) appears to speed up and secure the recovery." In this case, while promising, it is important to realise that without a placebo group it is difficult to determine if these results would be greater than those seen with placebo. The second randomized, double-blind study compared a non-oral ginkgo extract Egb 761 (200 mg IV infusion) to pentoxifylline (300 mg IV infusion) in patients with sudden deafness (n=72) for 10 days. The authors concluded that ginkgo extract Egb 761 given by IV was as effective a treatment for sudden deafness as pentoxifylline.[151]

Trauma to the Brain
Numerous animal studies have suggested that gingkolide B has a protective effect against neuronal damage following trauma, probably related to its PAF antagonist action.[55] A study with rats suggests that treatment with *Ginkgo biloba* extract (GBE) reduced the extent of brain swelling in response to injury (bilateral frontal cortex lesions) and was associated with less impairment following the injury.[152] In addition, it has been shown in rat experiments that EGb 761 treatment prior to electroconvulsive shock (ECS) treatment reduces the extent and duration of the remodelling of membrane phospholipids which traditionally results from seizures.[153]

Schizophrenia
There is one randomized, double-blinded, placebo-controlled study of ginkgo (360 mg EGb extract daily) as an adjunctive treatment to haloperidol (0.25 mg/kg/day) on the symptoms experienced by patients with treatment-resistant chronic schizophrenia (n=82) according to ICD-10 criteria. Both groups' scores on the Scale for the Assessment of Negative Symptoms improved compared to baseline, but only those taking ginkgo had improved scores on the Scale for the Assessment of Positive Symptoms. The authors conclude that these results suggest that ginkgo may "enhance the efficacy of the classic antipsychotic haliperidol in patients with schizophrenia, especially on their positive symptoms."[154] While promising, additional research is necessary to confirm the findings from this preliminary study.

OPHTHALMOLOGY EFFECTS
Ginkgo biloba extract is believed to protect the eye from damage by reducing free-radical damage to the retina.[155,156] Animal studies suggest that ginkgo may be useful in the prevention of retinal damage in diabetes,[155,157] and in cases of lesions, inflammations or degenerative insults of the retina.[158] Several small clinical studies provide preliminary evidence that ginkgo may be beneficial in the management of glaucoma. A double-blind trial (n =10) with senile macular degeneration, found ginkgo to be significantly better than placebo at improving long-distance visual acuity.[159] Another randomized, double-blind, placebo-controlled crossover study reported that ingestion of ginkgo (40 mg of Ginkoba® three times daily) for 2 days resulted in a significant increase in end diastolic velocity in the ophthalmic artery in 11 healthy volunteers. The authors suggest that ginkgo deserves further investigation as a possible treatment of glaucomatous optic neuropathy and other ischemic ocular diseases.[160] Finally, a third randomized, placebo-controlled, double-blind, crossover study assessed the effect of ginkgo (40 mg extract standardized to 24% flavinoid glycosides and 6% terpenes three times daily) for 8 weeks on pre-existing visual field damage in patients with normal tension glaucoma (n=27). In this study, ginkgo treatment resulted in significant improvement in visual field indices compared to baseline; no significant changes were noted in the placebo group.[161] Additional research in this area is necessary to confirm these preliminary findings.

OTOLOGY EFFECTS

The effects on the ear appear to be related to the ability of ginkgo to increase cochlear blood flow (CBF). One study of *Ginkgo biloba* extract (EGb 761) in guinea pigs demonstrated that after 4 to 6 weeks of treatment, EGb 761 partly counteracted sodium salicylate-induced decreases in CBF.[139] In a double-blind trial of ginkgo for the treatment of acute cochlear deafness, ginkgo was found to be more effective than nicergoline (an alpha-blocker), but significant improvement was seen with both treatments.[162]

Tinnitus

A review of randomized, controlled trials of ginkgo for the treatment of tinnitus found five trials which met the following inclusion criteria: performed on patients with a primary complaint of tinnitus (as opposed to cerebral insufficiency, hearing loss etc.); ginkgo was compared to placebo or another active medication; and ginkgo was tested as a monotherapy. [81,163-166] The authors concluded that "overall, the results of these trials are favourable to *Ginkgo biloba* as a treatment for tinnitus, but a firm conclusion about its efficacy is not possible.... More trials are needed to test the therapeutic value of *Ginkgo biloba* for relieving tinnitus."[167]

In addition, two studies have been published on this topic since this review that have conflicting results. One randomized, double-blind, placebo-controlled trial (n=1121, 978 had matched controls) reported that 12 weeks of treatment with ginkgo (50 mg LI 1370 extract three times daily) was no more effective at treating stable tinnitus than the placebo.[168] The other study of 60 patients with confirmed chronic tinnitus reported that ginkgo (200 mg IV daily for 10 days followed by 160 mg EGb 761 extract orally daily for 12 weeks) was effective in alleviating the patients' symptoms according to an intention to treat analysis.[169] Clearly, given these conflicting results, additional research in this area is needed.[81,170]

Vertigo

Several animal studies have demonstrated that the administration of ginkgo extract speeds vestibular compensation.[171,172] For example, accelerated postural, locomotor balance recovery, spontaneous neck muscle activity, vestibulo-collic reflexes, and spontaneous firing rates of vestibular units on the lesioned side were noted in unilateral vestibular neurectomized cats.[171] One clinical study of patients with recent-onset idiopathic vertigo found that ginkgo significantly decreased the intensity, frequency and duration of symptoms of vertigo when compared with placebo.[83]

UROLOGY EFFECTS

Impotence

Ginkgo biloba extract has been suggested in the treatment of impotence. One study of 60 patients with proven arterial erectile dysfunction who had not responded to papaverine injections were given 60 mg/day of ginkgo extract for 12-18 months. Improvement in blood flow (as measured by duplex sonography) was noted after 6 to 8 weeks and 50% of the men gained potency after 6 months. In another 20% of the sample, a new trial with papaverine proved successful.[173] This trial was not blinded, and given the large psychological component of impotence, additional studies are required to confirm these results.

These positive findings were not supported by another study of the use of ginkgo in the management of antidepressant-induced sexual dysfunction. In this randomized, double-blind, placebo-controlled study (n=37) ingestion of ginkgo (120 mg daily for 2 weeks followed by 160 mg for the second 2 weeks, followed by 240 mg daily for the final 4 weeks) was not associated with any significant improvement in sexual dysfunction compared to placebo, although both patient groups did improve from baseline (confirming the presence of a placebo effect).[174]

One laboratory study reported that fractions of *Ginkgo biloba* extract had a relaxing effect on corpus cavernosum tissue *in vitro*.[175] Further research in this area is needed to determine if ginkgo may provide some benefit to patients with sexual dysfunction.

RESPIROLOGY EFFECTS

Asthma

Several preliminary studies suggest that *Ginkgo biloba* extracts may have a beneficial effect in patients with asthma.[8,38,42] A study of the smooth muscle relaxant activity of *Ginkgo biloba* on the guinea pig trachea noted a concentration-dependent relaxation *in vitro* and an antagonism of bronchoconstriction induced by various agonists *in vivo*.[25] One single-blind, randomized cross-over study in 10 patients found that ingestion of 240 mg of *Ginkgo biloba* extract (BN 52063) 1 hour prior to induction of bronchoconstriction by hyperventilation with dry cold air did not result in any reduction in bronchoconstriction. However, an inhibition of PAF- induced platelet aggregation was noted after oral administration of BN 52063. On the third day of treatment with either BN 52063 or placebo, asthma was induced by exercise in these patients. There was no effect on the initial bronchoconstriction of those receiving ginkgo; however, the prolonged reduction of peak expiratory flow was attenuated. The rise in plasma concentrations of platelet factor 4 and beta-thromboglobin seen in the placebo group was inhibited in the group treated with ginkgo extract (p<.01).[36]

MISCELLANEOUS EFFECTS

Ginkgolide B (BN 52021) administered i.v. (120 mg twice daily for 4 days) was found to be useful as an adjunct to standard intensive care support in the treatment of patients with severe Gram-negative bacterial sepsis, as determined by a randomized, double-blind, placebo-controlled, multicenter phase III clinical trial. There was a significant reduction in mortality of patients treated with ginkolide B compared with those taking the placebo. The authors suggest that this was due to its ability to prevent a systemic inflammatory response to infection through platelet-activating factor (PAF) antagonism, inhibition of amplification of sepsis-induced tumor necrosis factor and thromboxane B_2 release, plasma trypsin-like activity and several other steps of the immuno-inflammatory cascade associated with gram negative bacterial sepsis.[45]

Persons irradiated (either for therapeutic reasons or accidentally) have clastogenic factors in their plasma. Thirty workers accidentally exposed to radiation were given 40 mg of *Ginkgo biloba* extract (EGb 761) three times daily for two months, at which time the clastogenic activity of their plasma had returned to the same level as controls. This effect persisted for at least 7 months.[176] This anti-clastogenic effect was also demonstrated *in vitro*.[177] Another study demonstrates the ability of ginkgo to protect microsomal fatty acids and proteins from UV-C radiation-induced peroxidative degradation.[178]

Ginkgo biloba extract was shown to inhibit cyclosporin A-induced peroxidation in human liver microsomes in a dose-dependent manner. Thus, it may have some use in the prevention of damage to human membranes caused by cyclosporin A.[179]

Several components isolated from *Ginkgo biloba* have been reported to have anti-tumor activity.[180]

Ginkgo is reported to have beneficial effects in cases of cyclic edema. The flavonoids are thought to normalize excessive capillary permeability and one clinical study found complete elimination of edema in 3 patients and partial elimination of the edema in 6 patients.[181] Ginkgo has also been reported to be effective against the "congestive" symptoms of PMS (esp. breast symptoms).[182]

One open-label, uncontrolled clinical trial (n=48) reported that ginkgo (extract GBE 761 ONC) administered i.v. once every three weeks in conjunction with 5-fluorouracil may enhance the response to treatment of patients with locally or metastatic advanced pancreatic cancer.[183] Additional studies are needed to confirm these preliminary findings.

ADVERSE EFFECTS

Most sources suggest that side effects from *Ginkgo biloba* are extremely infrequent, but include: gastrointestinal disturbances, headache, and allergic skin reactions.[1,8,9,23,88,184,185] Two systematic reviews report no serious side effects in any trial reviewed.[3,88] Headaches, although relatively rare, appear to be the most common side effect.[80] Some authors have suggested that these adverse effects may be decreased by slowly increasing to the therapeutic dose level. Skin reactions are thought to be caused only by direct contact with the fruit of the ginkgo tree,[184,185] which is not the part used medicinally. However, there is one case of a women who ingested 2 doses of a ginkgo preparation (brand and dose not known) as well as a ginkgo-containing product called "One-A-Day Memory and Concentration®" (Bayer Pharmaceuticals) prior to hospital admission for an exfoliative rash, blistering and other symptoms consistent with Stevens-Johnson syndrome. The content of the products ingested by the patient were not analyzed and the role of ginkgo in this case cannot be confirmed.[186]

Several cases of spontaneous bleeding associated with ingestion of ginkgo have been reported;[187-190] however, the role of ginkgo in these cases remains unclear. In one case report, a healthy 33-year-old women with a long term history of use of *Ginkgo biloba* (60 mg twice daily for 2 years) was reported to have an increased bleeding time and suffered bilateral subdural hematomas. Her bleeding times had returned to normal 35 days after discontinuation of ginkgo ingestion.[187] In another case, a 70 year old man presented with spontaneous bleeding from the iris into the anterior chamber of the eye one week after beginning treatment with 40 mg *Ginkgo biloba* extract daily. The patient had also been taking ASA (325 mg) daily for three years.[191] Given the large number of individuals ingesting *Ginkgo biloba* world-wide, this appears to be a relatively rare phenomenon; however, ginkgo has been shown to be a platelet-activating factor antagonist in *in vivo* and *in vitro* studies.

CAUTIONS/CONTRAINDICATIONS

Safety in pregnant and nursing mothers has yet to be established.[8,9,13]

DRUG INTERACTIONS

Most authors suggest that there are no known drug interactions.[3,8,9,78] Although there is little clinical evidence, theoretically *Ginkgo biloba* may potentiate the action of anti-coagulants.

DOSAGE

Almost all the research has been conducted using a standardized extract (SE): ginkgo-flavone glycosides (24%) and terpenoids (6%).[3] A recent pharmacokinetic study found no significant differences between the bioavailability of three different formulations of *Ginkgo biloba* (capsules, drops and tablets).[192] Sticher provides an excellent review of the quality control and standardization of ginkgo preparations.[12]

❖ STANDARDIZED EXTRACT GBE (Gingko biloba Extract standardized to 24% ginkgo-flavone glycosides and 6% terpenoids): 40 mg three times daily.[1,8]

❖ DRIED LEAVES: 300 mg daily.[9]

   Note: Treatment for many conditions must be continued for 1 to 3 months before positive results can be expected.[3,8,9]

Ginseng
(Asian and American/Canadian)
Panax ginseng C.A. Meyer; *Panax quinquefolius* L.

THUMBNAIL SKETCH

Common Uses
- Stress and Fatigue (both physical and mental)
- Exercise (increased endurance and performance)
- Immune System (strengthen the immune system in cases of inadequate resistance to infection and in convalescence)
- Hyperglycemia (as an adjunct in the treatment of mild conditions)

Active Constituents
- Ginsenosides
- Panaxans

Adverse Effects
- Insomnia (most common), Restlessness, Nervousness
- Euphoria
- Hypertension
- Diarrhea
- Skin Eruptions

Cautions/Contraindications
- Hypertension, Acute Illness, Premenopausal Women (with unstable hormonal cycles), Controlled Diabetics, Concomitant Use of Stimulants

- Children, Pregnancy, Lactation (safety not established)

Drug Interactions
- Possible with many centrally-acting drugs (e.g., phenalzine, pentobarbital and haloperiol) and stimulants, including caffeine.

Doses
- *Standardized Extract* (4% to 8% ginsenosides): 100-500 mg daily in two or three divided doses
- *Raw Root Decoction* (boiling in water or broth): 0.6-4.0 g usually taken in the morning

Notes: In cases of long-term administration, ginseng is usually taken for a period of 2-3 weeks, followed by a 2-week resting period.

Introduction

Family
❖ Araliaceae

Synonyms
PANAX GINSENG:

❖ Asian ginseng
❖ Chinese ginseng
❖ Ginseng
❖ Korean ginseng
❖ Panax schinseng
❖ Nees
❖ Asiatic ginseng
❖ Oriental ginseng

PANAX QUINQUEFOLIUS:

❖ American ginseng
❖ Canadian ginseng[1-3]

Description

Although many different kinds of 'ginseng' may be sold in Canadian and American retail outlets, two species are commonly seen in pharmacy practice: *Panax Ginseng* C.A. Meyer (also called Panax, Ginseng, Chinese ginseng, Korean ginseng or Oriental ginseng) and *Panax quinquefolius* L. (also called American or Canadian ginseng). Other closely related species include: *Panax pseudoginseng* Wallich var. *japonicus* (C.A. Meyer) G.Hoo & C. J. Tseng (Japanese ginseng), *Panax pseudoginseng* Wallich var. *notoginseng* (Burkill) G. Hoo & C.J. Tseng (Sanchi ginseng) and *Panax trilolius* L. (Canadian dwarf ginseng); however, these three species are rarely seen.[4,5] Another product widely available is *Eleutherococcus senticosus* (Rupr. & Maxim.) Maxim. (Siberian ginseng or eleuthero), which is in the same family (Araliaceae) but is not a true ginseng (member of the *Panax* genus). *Panax ginseng* (Chinese/Korean ginseng) and *Panax quinquefolius* (Canadian / American ginseng) will be discussed in this chapter, while *Eleutherococus senticosus* (Siberian ginseng) will be reviewed in the next.

Panax ginseng C.A. Meyer is the most widely used and most extensively studied species of ginseng.[6,7] Native to (and now widely cultivated in) both Korea and China, this herbaceous shrub grows to a height of 60 to 70 cm or 20 to 25 inches from a tap root and produces a cluster of small green-yellow flowers. The fully-grown tap roots are approximately 2 centimeters in diameter and 8 to 20 centimeters long. Many ginseng products available in North America are made from *Panax ginseng* grown in the Orient.

Panax quinquefolius is a smaller plant, growing to 30 centimeters or 1 foot, with oval leaflets, green flowers, and kidney-shaped red berries. Native to eastern North America, it is now cultivated to be sold primarily for medicinal products in the Orient. *Panax quinquefolius* tastes sweeter and is considered to be more 'yin' in the traditional Chinese medicine paradigm than *Panax ginseng*.[4]

Panax is derived from the Greek roots pan meaning "all" and akos meaning "cure" and refers to the "cure all" or "panacea" quality generally attributed to the herb.[4] The name ginseng means "essence of the earth in the form of a man," and refers to the resemblance of the root to a human form.[5]

Parts Used

For both Asian and American/Canadian ginseng, the roots from 4 to 6 year old plants are harvested in the autumn and used medicinally.

Traditional Use

Ginseng has been an important part of Traditional Chinese Medicine for over five thousand years. It is considered to be a bitter-sweet herb with a warming character. Within Traditional Chinese Medicine, ginseng was used to restore 'yang' quality and to treat general weakness, deficient qi (chi) patterns, anemia, lack of appetite, nervous agitation, thirst and impotence.[5] It is classified as an adaptogen, which is thought to increase non-specific resistance to adverse influences such as stress and infection. Traditionally it was used as a tonic to "increase strength, increase blood volume, promote life and appetite, quiet the spirit, and give wisdom."[5] It was generally thought to improve vitality.

Current Medicinal Use

As with its traditional uses, Asian ginseng is primarily used as a tonic in the treatment and prevention of stress and fatigue and in strengthening the immune system. While Asian ginseng has been the subject of many clinical trials, the quality of the trials has often been poor and the results often conflicting. American/Canadian and Asian ginseng may be useful in stabilizing blood sugar levels.

Medicinal Forms

For both Asian and American/Canadian ginseng, the roots are the part used medicinally. In North America, Asian ginseng is commonly sold in two forms: white and red, which represent different processing procedures. White ginseng is obtained by drying the root, often peeling the external skin in the process. In contrast, red ginseng root is steamed, which produces a caramel-like color.[7] According to Traditional Chinese Medicine philosophy, red ginseng is more 'heating' (more 'yang' in nature) than white ginseng.

Relevant Research

Preventative and Therapeutic Effects

CONSTITUENTS

Panax ginseng [6-9]

❖ TRITERPENOID GLYCOSIDES (SAPONINS)[10]:

ginsenosides Rb1, Rb2 = panaquilin B, panaxoside E

ginsenoside Rc = panaquilin C, panaxoside D

ginsenoside Rd = panaquilin D, panaquilin E_2, ganaxoside C, ginsenoside Re_2

ginsenoside Re = panaquilin E_3, panaxoside B, ginsenoside Re_3

ginsenoside Rg_1 = panaquilin G_1, panaxoside A

ginsenoside Rg_2 = panaquilin G_2

ginsenoside Ra = panaxoside F

❖ OTHER GINSENSIDES: Ra_1, Ra_2, Rb_3, Rf, Rh_1, Rh_4, Ro.

❖ PEPTIDOGLYCANS: panaxans.

❖ VOLATILE OIL: panacene.

❖ POLYSACCHARIDES.

❖ VITAMINS (e.g., thiamin, riboflavin, B12, nicotinic acid, pantothenic acid, and biotin).

Panax quinquefolius [4]

❖ TRITERPENOID GLYCOSIDES (SAPONINS) ❖ ginsenosides (also called panaxosides), including: Rb_1, Rb_2, Rb_3, Rc, Rd, Re, Rg_1, Rg_2, Ro, which produce 20-S-protopanaxadiol and 20-S-protopanaxatriol in alkaline conditions.

Note: There are both qualitative and quantitative differences in the ginsenoside content of various species and varieties, allowing easy verification of the identity and quality of commercial ginseng products by high performance liquid chromotography.

QUALIFICATIONS

Although hundreds of studies since the 1950s have attempted to separate factual therapeutic properties of ginseng from fictitious ones, there are many inconsistencies among the results (primarily due to different extraction procedures, use of different plants, adulterants and lack of quality control).[11,12] To compound this problem, few of the studies involve the use of human subjects.[12,13] A systematic review of 16 randomized clinical trials that assessed the efficacy of ginseng for a variety of different medicinal uses, including enhancing physical and psychomotor performance as well as congnitive function, immunomodulation, diabetes mellitus and herpes simplex type-II infections, concluded that the efficacy of ginseng is "not established beyond reasonable doubt for any of these indications."[14] Because many of the studies completed with ginseng are animal studies that often examine the effects of a single ginsenoside, it is not possible to extrapolate the results to the human ingestion of commercial ginseng products. Unless noted otherwise, all studies discussed here were completed with *Panax ginseng*, which is the most well-research Panax species.

ADAPTOGENIC ACTIVITY

Historically, ginseng has been used as a general tonic, relying on its adaptogenic action. An adaptogen works in a non-specific manner, drawing the patient toward normal function, irrespective of the direction of the pathologic state.[6,8] For example, ginseng has been found to increase blood pressure in cases of hypotension or shock, but restored blood pressure to normal in cases of hypertension.[15] Other researchers have noted that there are at least three components of *Panax ginseng* root which can depress CNS activity and at least two other constituents that stimulate the CNS.[8] It appears that different constituents of *Panax ginseng* have opposing action, generally stimulating or sedating, respectively.[15-17] Thus, different doses of ginseng can have opposite effects clinically and the same dose of ginseng given to individuals with differing physiological states can have different clinical actions. This is a defining feature of an adaptogenic herb.

Anti-Stress Activity

Ginseng has been reported to enhance one's ability to cope with various mental and physical stressors (e.g., exposure to heat or cold, environmental toxins, physical trauma and emotional responses to various stimuli).[11-18] One of the few double-blind clinical studies to date investigated the effects of taking a multivitamin and taking ginseng in addition to the same multivitamin on the quality of life of 501 city-dwellers. After 4 months, the study found that those ingesting the ginseng and multivitamin had a significant improvement in all 11 quality of life measures, while those ingesting the vitamins alone had no significant improvement.[19]

Ginseng's anti-stress effects have been linked primarily to its effects on the adrenal glands.[20-21] It has been suggested rather than a direct stimulation, ginseng influences the higher control centres including the hypothalamus and pituitary gland, which in turn influence the adrenals.[22] Studies suggest that *Panax ginseng* has the ability to increase both ascorbic acid and cholesterol stores in the adrenal gland, while decreasing the 17-ketosterol and increasing ACTH excreted in the urine.[15-17,21] An increase in plasma ACTH and corticosteroids following administration of ginseng is well-documented.[21,23,24] All of these effects are blocked by the administration of dexamethasone. It is hypothesized that the end-organ effects of the ACTH and related substances, whose release ginseng stimulates, can explain many of its antistress and antifatigue actions. However, another study reported that ingestion of ginseng (2 g daily) by competitive athletes for six weeks was not associated with any change in hormonal indices of stress such as cortisol and testosterone levels.[25]

Anti-Fatigue — Physical

An extensive review concludes that there is currently insufficient scientific evidence to demonstrate enhancement of physical performance by ginseng due to poor methodological quality, conflicting results and the use of 10 to 100 times the usual human dose in many animal studies.[8-14] Animal studies report mice who were shown to: swim longer;[26] run up a seemingly endless rope for a longer period of time;[27] and run on a treadmill longer[28] when taking ginseng. Other animal experiments found no significant anti-fatigue action for ginseng compared to placebo.[29,30] The majority of the animal trials in this area were not blinded or placebo-controlled.

Several clinical experiments with humans have also been published, most of which did not find ginseng to enhance physical performance significantly.[31-36] Early, often quoted studies, were small and negative. For example, one found that nurses (n=12) switching from day to night duty reported improvement in 11 of 16 mood variables and 8 of 14 somatic symptoms while taking 1.2 g of Korean ginseng as opposed to placebo; however contrary to the description of this study in many lay publications, none of these differences were statistically significant.[31] It has been suggested that the lack of significant results in this study was due to the relatively low dose and short study period. Another study comparing army cadets (n=11) ingesting 2 g of *Panax ginseng* daily for 4 weeks found no difference in performance during heavy, prolonged exercise when compared with cadets taking a placebo.[32] In contrast, a double-blind, placebo-controlled, cross-over study with 50 male sports teachers found that total work load, and maximal oxygen uptake were increased, while plasma lactate levels, carbon dioxide production and heart rate were all significantly lower when the individuals were ingesting ginseng than when they were taking the placebo.[33] Another double-blind, placebo controlled trial with 43 male triathletes taking either 200 mg of ginseng or placebo twice daily found no significant differences in the physical fitness of the two groups after 10 weeks; however, at a follow up 10 weeks later, the group taking the ginseng had significantly better maximal oxygen uptake which suggested that ginseng may retard the loss of physical fitness.[34]

A more recent randomized, placebo-controlled study of ginseng (200 mg, 7% standardized extract daily) for 3 weeks found that ginseng did not enhance peak aerobic exercise (nor did maximal oxygen uptake change) in 28 healthy young adults with moderate exercise capabilities.[35] To some extent these findings were supported by a subsequent randomized, double-blind, placebo-controlled trial of 350 mg ginseng daily for 6 weeks. This study found that while ginseng did not influence maximal oxygen uptake or lactate threshold, it did shorten multiple choice reaction time (a measure of psychomotor performance) in 15 soccer players.[36] Larger studies are needed to confirm any of the effects documented in these small studies.

Several mechanisms of action have been postulated for ginseng's anti-fatigue effects including: stimulation of nerve impulses;[15] an ability to affect the hypothalamus/pituitary/adrenal axis;[11,21,28] an ability to spare glycogen utilization in exercising muscle;[20,37] and improved oxygen utilization.[33] Biochemical studies have noted increased blood glucose levels and decreased levels of both lactic acid and pyruvic acid in ginseng-treated animals after exercise when compared to saline controls (no differences were noted at rest).[38] However, much of this work has been citicized due to lack of proper control animals and little attempt to guarantee the purity and quality of the ginseng products tested.[8]

Anti-Fatigue — Mental

Several much-quoted studies have reported that ginseng enhances mental activity and decreases mental fatigue. For example, radio operators who ingested ginseng extract were reported to transmit text faster and make fewer errors than those on placebo;[39] and university students in Italy were reported to perform better on a series of mental tests (including attention, mental arithmetic, logical deduction, integrated sensory-motor function and auditory reaction time) while taking ginseng in comparison to those on placebo.[40] However, a closer look at the second study reveals that although positive trends were noted in the some of the other tests, the only test in which the ginseng-treated group performed significantly (statistically) better than the control group was the mental arithmetic test and no difference at all was found between the placebo and the ginseng group on three other tests: pure motor function; recognition and visual reaction time. Animal studies have demonstrated the ability of ginseng to: modify brain-wave tracings;[41] improve metabolic activity in the brain;[42] affect the hypothalamus/pituitary/adrenal axis; and have favorable effects on learning and memory.[43]

Anti-Aging Effects
Ginseng's 'anti-aging' effects have yet to be proven; however, it does appear to exert an action on cellular function.[44] It appears to stimulate protein synthesis and decrease cellular destruction.[11] As well, it promotes Kupffer cell activity, which increases hepatic detoxification and thus may decrease cellular damage caused by external pollutants.[11]

Hepatic Effects
Many of the adaptogenic effects of ginseng appear to be related to its effects on the liver. Ginseng has been reported to: enhance the activity of the Kupffer cells (hepatic macrophages), which are primarily responsible for detoxification of the blood;[11] provide protection against carbon tetrachloride-induced hepatotoxicity in rats;[45,46] induce tyrosine aminotransferase gene expression *in vitro*;[47] and decrease AST and ALT levels in dexamethasone-treated rats.[48] Ginseng has been reported to increase protein synthesis in the liver of animal models.[49,50] This has yet to be confirmed in clinical trials. In addition, ginseng is thought to have a significant anti-hepatotoxic action.[51]

CARDIOVASCULAR EFFECTS
Blood Pressure
It appears that ginseng has a dose-related action on blood pressure. In low doses it slightly increases blood pressure and in high doses it appears to decrease blood pressure in animal models.[52,53] One study of dogs given 10-20 mg/kg of ginseng intravenously reported an initial increase in blood pressure, which was followed by slight decrease in blood pressure.[54] Another study of 40 mg/kg of ginseng extracts administered intravenously to dogs reported significant decreases in mean arterial pressure, cardiac output, stroke volume and central venous pressure.[55] Clinically, increased blood pressure has been reported as a side effect.[56] However, several clinical trials have reported that ginseng may decrease blood pressure.[57,58] One clinical trial of 26 participants with essential hypertension found that ingestion of 4.5 g of red ginseng daily in three divided doses for 8 weeks resulted in a significant reduction in mean systolic blood pressure, but only a trend toward a decline in diastolic blood pressure. However, in 8 participants with "white coat hypertension," no significant blood pressure change was observed.[57] Another clinical study suggests that Korean red ginseng can improve vascular endothelial dysfunction in patients with hypertension possibly through increasing synthesis of nitric oxide.[59] Additional research studies are needed to confirm these results.

Platelet Aggregation
Several *in vitro* and *in vivo* studies have noted ginseng's ability to decrease platelet aggregation.[60-64] Ginsenosides R_{g2} and R_0 were found to inhibit significantly the conversion of fibrinogen to fibrin induced by thrombin in experimental models.[62,64] Other studies suggest

that components of ginseng inhibit thromboxane A_2.[65] However, the clinical effects of oral ingestion of commercial ginseng products by humans is unknown. Prolonged thrombin time (TT) and activated partial thromboboplastin time (APTT) have been reported in animal studies.[64] Decreases in blood-clotting time in humans do not appear to have been reported in the literature.

Other Cardiovascular Effects

Ginseng has also been reported to cause vasodilation of the coronary vessels,[54] and to have a cardioprotective action against catecholamine tachycardia.[15,17] Under experimental conditions, *Panax ginseng* was found to delay induced heart miochondrial impairment and muscle contraction deterioration.[66] When administered to patients with hyperlipidemia, ginseng has been shown to increase serum HDL-cholesterol levels while at the same time decreasing total serum cholesterol, triglyceride and fatty acid levels.[67] Other studies have found that *Panax ginseng* may protect against myocardial ischemia/reperfusion damage[68] and cerebral damage caused by ischemia.[69,70] It has been suggested that the cardioprotective effects of ginseng may be mediated by the release of nitric oxide, a potent anti-oxidant.[68]

IMMUNOSTIMULATING EFFECTS

Ginseng appears to enhance antibody response;[71] increase natural killer cell activity;[71,72] stimulate macrophage activity;[73,74] stimulate lymphocytes *in vitro*;[75,76] stimulate the reticuloendothelial system (RES);[77,78] increase proliferation of T cells and B cells;[75] and increase the production of interferon.[79,80] In laboratory animals, ginseng has been shown to reduce the incidence of viral infections.[81] This finding has been confirmed by a multicenter, double-blind, randomized, placebo-controlled trial in 227 individuals.[71] Each participant was given 100 mg of Ginsana® daily for 12 weeks, while receiving an anti-influenza polyvalent vaccination at week 4. In the placebo group 42 cases of colds or flus were reported in the final 8 weeks of the trial in comparison with 15 reports in the ginseng group, which represents a statistically significant difference. In addition, the group receiving ginseng had significantly higher antibody titres, and natural killer activity levels.[73] However, at high doses there is *in vitro* evidence that ginseng may inhibit some immune functions including lymphocyte proliferation.[80,82-84]

NEUROLOGICAL EFFECTS

Treatment of Emotional Disorders

Although *Panax ginseng* has reportedly been used in the treatment of a variety of emotional conditions, this clinical application is supported by very little research. Ginsenoside R_{b1} has been shown to decrease aggressive behavior (between resident and intruder mice) when given to the resident mouse at doses of 25 to 100 mg of ginsenoside/kg intraperitoneally (IP). However, when ginsenoside R_{b1} was given to the intruder mouse, no change in activity was noted. In addition, ginsenoside R_{g1} produced no change in behavior when given to either mouse.[85] Another study reported that a crude extract of ginseng (50 and 100 mg/kg) and ginsenoside R_{b1} (2.5 and 5 mg/kg) given IP significantly decreased maternal aggression in female mice without causing motor dysfunction; however, ginsenoside R_{g1} appeared to increase maternal aggression.[86] None of these studies were blinded and there have been no studies reporting similar effects in humans.

A study of *Panax ginseng* 50 mg/kg showed that it was as effective as diazepam 1 mg/kg in decreasing experimentally-induced anxiety in mice.[87] However, another study using 50 to 100 mg/kg given orally to mice found no effect on the pentobarbital sleep of psychologically stressed mice.[88] This is supported by an additional study that also found no effect on pentobarbital sleep induction.[89]

Miscellaneous

Several animal studies have investigated the effects of ginseng on the development of tolerance to and dependence on a variety of narcotics, including morphine,[90,91] cocaine,[92,93] and methamphetamine.[92-94] Other *in vitro* studies have reported the ability of ginsenoside R_{b1} to potentiate nerve growth,[95] and of ginsenosides R_{g1}, R_{b2}, R_d, R_e and R_f to protect cerebellum growth *in vivo*.[96] Another *in vivo* study suggests that ginsenosides directly affect the activity-dependent synaptic plasticity in the brain.[97]

EFFECT ON DIABETES

Ginseng has had a long history of folk-use in the treatment of diabetes. Most of the recent studies have focused on *Panax quinquefolius* (Canadian or American ginseng). Overall, the findings from clinical trials are not consistent, but a number of studies have documented the hypoglycemic effects of American ginseng, in both healthy participants and individuals diagnosed with Type 2 diabetes mellitus.[98-101] However, not all studies have been positive. One study could not reproduce these findings and the authors suggest that this may have been because the extract they tested varied in its total ginsenoside content as well as in key ratios of different ginsensides when compared to another extract that was shown to have hypoglycemic effects.[102]

Other studies suggest that the hypoglycaemic effects of ginseng may depend on when the ginseng is taken in relation to food. One study reported that a single 3 g dose of American ginseng attenuated postprandial glycemia (blood sugar after eating) in both non-diabetic participants (n=10) and those diagnosed with type 2 diabetes mellitus (n=9) when the ginseng dose was ingested 40 minutes prior to the glucose challenge. When the ginseng dose was ingested at the same time as the glucose challenge, the hypoglycaemic effect was found only in those with Type 2 diabetes mellitus.[100] In another study, American ginseng reduced postprandial glycemia in type 2 diabetic individuals (n=10) irrespective of the dose (3 g ,6 g, or 9 g) or the time of administration (120, 80, 40 or 0 minutes before the glucose challenge).[99]

It appears that that ginseng may reduce serum cortisol (which antagonizes insulin) levels in patients with diabetes, but increase them in non-diabetic individuals. Another found that a fraction isolated from ginseng (DPG-3-2) stimulated insulin secretion, but only in diabetic mice and non-diabetic controls who had been loaded with glucose. There was no effect on insulin secretion in non-diabetic mice on a standard diet.[103] These findings reinforce the adaptogenic character of ginseng — and its ability to restore balance. Research suggests that the ginseng components responsible for these effects include: panaxans A, B,C,D,E; adenosine; and a fraction designated DPG-3-2.[103-106]

MISCELLANEOUS EFFECTS

Reproductive Effects

Although ginseng has a reputation as an aphrodisiac, no human studies support this belief. However, *Panax spp.* has been shown to: increase the formation of sperm and the growth of the testes in rabbits;[107] enhance ovulation and the growth of the ovaries in frogs; stimulate egg-laying in hens and increase the mating activity in male rats.[6,11] Ginseng has been shown to increase sperm count and motility in men, as well as increasing plasma total and free testosterone, DHT, FSH and LH levels.[108] An *in vitro* study suggests that extracts from *Panax ginseng* may relax the corpus cavernosum by releasing nitric oxide.[109]

In addition, the estrogenic action of ginseng has been demonstrated in post-menopausal women who experienced reduced atrophy and dryness of the vaginal epithelium.[110] It should be noted that breast tenderness has been reported in women taking ginseng.[111,112]

Anti-Cancer Properties

Ginseng has been reported to decrease the incidence of some human cancers and to have a protective effect against the adverse effects of radiation;[113,114] however, studies in humans were not found. Other studies have reported that components of *Panax ginseng* caused inhibition of lung metastasis of B16-BL6 melanoma and colon 26-M3.1 carcinoma in mice;[115,116] inhibition of the growth of human ovarian cancer cells in mice;[117] and induction of differentiation in teratocarcinoma cells *in vitro*.[118] Two case-control epidemiological studies and one prospective study in populations with high rates of ginseng use (70% users) suggested that oral ingestion of ginseng may decrease the incidence of some human cancers.[119] It has been hypothesized that the possible anti-cancer effects of ginseng may be due to its stimulating effects on the immune system.[75]

Symptoms of Menopause

A randomized, double-blind, placebo-controlled study that assessed the effects of ginseng (Ginsana® brand containing 100 mg G115 standardized extract) in 384 healthy postmenopausal women found a trend toward overall symptom improvement that was not statistically significant. Those ingesting ginseng scored significantly better on the depression, well-being and health sub-scales. However, no significant differences were seen between the ginseng and the placebo group on the Women's Health Questionnaire and visual analogue scales used to assess specific symptoms (i.e., hot flushes). The study also reported that physiological parameters such as Follicle Stimulating Hormone (FSH) and estradiol levels, endometrial thickness, maturity index and vaginal pH were also not affected by ginseng treatment.[120]

Quality of Life/Mood

A randomized, double-blind, placebo-controlled study of ginseng (200 mg or 400 mg; G115 extract daily) ingested for 60 days by 83 healthy volunteers reported that ginseng supplementation has no effect on positive affect, negative affect, or total mood disturbance. The authors concluded that their findings "do not support claims that chronic ginseng supplementation — at either its clinically recommended level or at twice that level — enhances affect or mood in healthy young adults."[121] In contrast, another randomized, double-blind, placebo-controlled study (n=30) reported that ingestion of ginseng (200 mg of Ginsana®) for 4 weeks was associated with an increase in mental health and social functioning (as measured by the Health-related Quality of Life questionnaire); however, these effects were attenuated after another 4 weeks of ginseng use so that no differences between the ginseng and placebo group were noted at the end of the 8 week study.[122]

HISTORICAL EVIDENCE

The review above is limited to the scientific/clinical evidence available within the biomedical model. However, it would be a disservice to this herb to discount its historical use within the Traditional Chinese Medical paradigm. In using this herb it is important to remember that extensive empirical evidence exists. This is reviewed thoroughly in several texts.[16,123]

ADVERSE EFFECTS

The most common adverse effect noted is insomnia.[71] Other reported effects included diarrhea, skin eruptions, vaginal bleeding,[56] and breast tenderness.[111,112] One case each of Stevens-Johnson syndrome,[124] mania,[125] and cerebral arteritis[126] possibly associated with ingestion of ginseng have been reported; however, the ginseng products were not tested for purity, thus these reactions may have been caused by adulterated products.[127] In addition, given the widespread use of ginseng products worldwide, such reactions are very rare indeed.

The term "Ginseng Abuse Syndrome" has been used to describe symptoms of over-stimulation, including hypertension, diarrhea, restlessness, nervousness, euphoria, insomnia and skin eruptions, which may occur in the overuse of the product.[128,129] However, this description has been criticized due to the fact that the majority of the individuals in this study were also ingesting high levels of caffeine.

CAUTIONS/CONTRAINDICATIONS

Ginseng should be used with caution in: hypertension, acute illness, premenopausal women with unstable hormonal cycles, controlled diabetics and concomitant use of stimulants.[56] As well, given that ginseng is considered a tonic, its use may not be appropriate in young, robust individuals.[3] The safety of *Panax ginseng* and *Panax quinquefolius* has not been established in children, pregnant and/or lactating women. Ginseng should not be ingested in the evening due to its ability to induce insomnia.

DRUG INTERACTIONS

Ginseng is generally considered to have an additive effect when used concomitantly with MAOIs.[130] This caution is derived from a case study describing symptoms of headache and tremulousness in a 64-year-old woman who was taking phenelzine and added ginseng to her regimen.[131] Three years later a re-challenge with ginseng in the same woman resulted in the same symptoms.[132] A second possible case of an interaction between ginseng (contained in an ingredient in a herbal tea) and phenelzine has also been reported.[133]

One study found that ginseng augmented the hypnotic effect of pentobarbital,[17] while others have found no effect.[88,89] However, potentiation of amphetamine-induced increase in motility and stereotypy as well as potentiation of haloperidol catalepsy have been reported in animal studies.[89] Caution with concomitant use of centrally-acting medications is recommended.

QUALITY OF DOSAGE FORMS

Premium ginseng root is extremely expensive, often costing thousands of dollars per kilogram, which leads one to question the quality of cheaper brands of the product. Commercially, ginseng is available in a wide range of forms including: teas, capsules, extracts, tablets, roots, chewing gum, cigarettes, and candies.[12] It is extremely difficult to determine the quality and quantity of ginseng present in some of these dosage forms. A study done in the late 1970s (and currently being repeated by the American Botanical Council) reported that 60% of the 54 North American ginseng products tested did not contain enough ginsenosides to be considered pharmacologically active and that 25% contained no ginsenosides at all.[134] Another study of 17 commercial ginseng products available in Sweden found that only one out of the five brands that listed their ginsenoside content on the label met the label claim.[135] In a follow up study of 50 ginseng products from eleven countries, the same team of researchers reported a range of 1.9% to 9.0% ginsenoside content, with six products (gathered from Sweden, the USA and the UK) that did not contain any ginsenosides.[136,137] Several cases of athletes consuming adulterated ginseng products (e.g., with ephedrine, psuedophedrine) that have resulted in doping charges have been reported.[136,138]

DOSAGE REGIMENS

❖ STANDARDIZED EXTRACT (4% to 8% ginsenosides): 100-500 mg daily in two or three divided doses.[11]

❖ RAW ROOT DECOCTION (boiling in water or broth): 0.6-4 g usually taken in the morning.[11]
   Note: In cases of long-term administration, ginseng is usually taken for a period of 2-3 weeks, followed by a 2-week resting period.[11,39]

Ginseng
(Siberian)
Eleutherococcus senticosus (Rupr. & Maxim.) Maxim

THUMBNAIL SKETCH

Common Uses
- ❖ Stress, Fatigue, General Debility
- ❖ Endurance/Performance (in work/sports)
- ❖ General Tonic (e.g., for long-term immune stimulation)

Active Constituents
- ❖ Eleutherosides

Adverse Effects
- ❖ Rare — most occur because of adulterated products

Cautions/Contraindications
- ❖ Pregnancy and Lactation
- ❖ Children

Drug Interactions
- ❖ May increase the duration of action of some sedatives

Doses
- ❖ *Dried Root:* 2-4 grams (in 1-3 divided doses) daily
- ❖ *Tincture* (1:5): 10-20 mL (in 1-3 divided doses) daily
- ❖ *Fluid Extract* (1:1): 2-4 mL (in 1-3 divided doses) daily
- ❖ *Solid Extract* (20:1): 100-200 mg (in 1-3 divided doses) daily

Introduction

Family
❖ Araliaceae

Synonyms
❖ Eleuthero
❖ Touch-me-not
❖ Devil's shrub
❖ Eleuthero
 ginseng
❖ Wild pepper[1]

Medicinal Forms
❖ Dried Root
❖ Tincture
❖ Fluid Extract
❖ Solid Extract

Description
Eleutherococcus senticosus is native to the Russian far east, as well as the parts of Korea, China and Japan north of the 38th latitude. This shrub grows to approximately 2 to 3 meters or 7 to 10 feet in height, with several leaflets in each stem.

Parts Used
The root, which is the part used medicinally, is normally harvested in the fall when the medicinally-active constituents are the most concentrated. The leaves can also be used medicinally.[2]

Traditional Use
Although historical documentation of the medicinal use of plants in the Araliaceae family (which also includes *Panax ginseng* C.A. Meyer and *Panax quinquefolium* L.) can be confusing,[3] it appears that *Eleutherococcus senticosus* was used within Traditional Chinese Medicine for over 4000 years to increase longevity, improve general health, improve appetite and aid memory.[2,4] Traditional Chinese Medicine indications for Siberian ginseng also include benefiting qi (chi) or the vital energy and treating 'yang' deficiency, especially of the spleen and kidney, as well as normalizing body functions.[1] Although documentation of *Eleutherococcus senticosus* in Russia dates back to 1855 when two Russian scientists began studying the plant,[2] interest in its medicinal use began only in the 1960s when researchers in that country became interested in its potential as a substitute for the more expensive and difficult to obtain *Panax* sp. (e.g., *Panax ginseng* and *Panax quinquefolium*). Although some of the adaptogenic properties of Siberian ginseng are thought to be similar to those of *Panax ginseng*, it is not the same botanical species, nor are the main active constituents the same. Marketing in North America under the common name Siberian ginseng only compounds the confusion surrounding these species.[1] Today, this species is becoming more commonly known by its abbreviated scientific name, eleuthero, in an attempt to reduce this confusion.[5,6]

Current Medicinal Use
Siberian ginseng, or eleuthro, is primarily used as a tonic in cases of stress and fatigue. Based on traditional evidence, eleuthro may be used in attempts to increase endurance and enhance sporting performance, but the majority of current scientific evidence suggests it will not work for this indication. While limited evidence exists in humans, preliminary research with rats indicates that eleuthro may decrease the adverse effects of radiation used in cancer therapy.

Relevant Research

Preventative and Therapeutic Effects

CONSTITUENTS [2,7,8]

The main active chemical constituents are a group of chemically-dissimilar compounds which have been called eleutherosides. Tyler argues that this was done to make eleuthro appear more similar to the true ginsengs from the *Panax* sp., whose active constituents are the ginsenosides – a group of triterpenoid saponins.[5] Eleuthero does not contain any of the ginsenosides found in *Panax* spp.

Roots

* COUMARINS: eleutheroside B1 (isofraxidin-7-0-alpha- L-glucoside, also known as beta-caly canthoside), isofraxidin, coumarin X.
* LIGNANS: eleutheroside B4 ((-)-sesamin), eleutheroside D ((-)-syringarsinol di-0-beta-D-glucoside), eleutheroside E (different crystal form of D, also known as acanthoside D).
* PHENYLPROPANOID: eleutheroside B (syringin), caffeic acid and caffeic acid ethyl ester.
* POLYSACCHARIDES: eleutheroside C (methyl-alpha-D-galactoside), eleutherans A-G.
* STEROLS: eleutheroside A (daucosterol).
* TRITERPENE: oleanolic acid.
* MISCELLANEOUS ELEUTHEROSIDES: eleutheroside B2, eleutheroside B3, eleutheroside F, eleutheroside G.

Leaves

* TRITERPENES: eleutheroside I (also known as mussenin B), eleutheroside K, eleutheroside L, eleutheroside M (also known as hederasaponin B), senticosides A to D (may be identical to eleutherosides I, K, L and M).

RESEARCH NOTE

Numerous *in vivo*, *in vitro*, and human clinical trials have been conducted on this species in Russia. Unfortunately, few have been translated into the English language. This monograph includes information from review articles (the review by Farnsworth is the most extensive encountered),[2] as well as any original articles available in English.

ADAPTOGENTIC ACTIVITY

Historically, Siberian ginseng has been used as a general tonic, relying on its adaptogenic action. An adaptogen is thought to work in a non-specific manner, drawing the patient toward normal function, irrespective of the direction of the pathologic state.[9,10] Fulder reports that eleuthero is widely used in Russia by such diverse populations as deep sea divers, mine and mountain rescue workers, soldiers, factory workers, cosmonauts, and athletes largely for its perceived ability to increase endurance and promote the body's ability to tolerate stressful conditions.[11]

Anti-Stress Activity

An early study suggested that eleuthero increases non-specific development of resistance to stress, as well as inhibiting the alarm-reaction to stress including decreasing the activation of the adrenal cortex.[12]

Anti-Fatigue – Physical

Perhaps the most common use of eleuthero in North America is its use to increase physical endurance and stamina. However, most of the Russian studies of this indication were neither double-blinded nor controlled adequately, making it difficult to assess its true clinical effect. Several animal studies found no significant difference between the length of time that mice ingesting eleuthero could swim in comparison with placebo.[13,14] One animal study also found no difference in plasma lactic acid, glucagon, insulin or liver glycogen levels in exercised rats who had ingested eleuthero.[14] Yet, in one single-blind, placebo-controlled study in healthy males (n=6), all four parameters of physical capacity (oxygen uptake, oxygen pulse, maximal work capacity and exhaustion time) were significantly increased in the group taking the eleuthero as compared to those taking placebo.[15]

In a more recent double-blind, placebo controlled study of 20 highly trained long distance runners, no significant differences were noted between the group who took the eleuthero extract daily for 6 weeks and the placebo group.[16] The authors caution that while eleuthero may not enhance the physical ability of highly-trained athletes, it may still provide some benefit to the average individual.

IMMUNOSTIMULATING EFFECTS

A placebo-controlled, double-blind study of healthy volunteers who were given 30 to 40 mL of an eleuthero extract (0.2% w/v eleutheroside B) reported that those ingesting eleuthero experienced a significant increase in total lymphocyte count with the most pronounced effect noticed with the T-lymphocytes. Granulocyte and monocyte levels were unchanged in these individuals.[17]

NEUROLOGICAL EFFECTS

Eleuthero has been reported to have both a sedative action and a stimulant effect in animal experiments.[2] One study found that mice given eleuthero exhibited significantly more aggressive behavior than those given distilled water.[13]

MISCELLANEOUS EFFECTS

Diabetes

Hypoglycemic activity has been reported in animal studies with some forms of induced-hyperglycemia;[18] however, another study found no effect of eleuthero on alloxan-induced hyperglycemia in rats.[2,19] Positive effects appear to be due to the polysaccharide components also known as eleutherans A-G.[18]

Platelet Aggregation

An anti-aggregatory compound, 3,4-dihydroxybenzoic acid (DBA) has been identified in eleuthero, which is reported to be as potent as ASA in inhibiting collagen- and adenosine-induced platelet aggregation, but less potent at inhibiting arachidonic acid-induced platelet aggregation.[20]

Anti-Cancer Properties

Several Russian *in vitro* and *in vivo* studies suggest that eleuthero may have direct cytostatic activity as well as metastasis-preventing effects. These studies are briefly reviewed by Hacker and Medon, who reported that aqueous extracts of eleuthero in combination with cytarabine provided additive antiproliferative effects against L1210 murine leukemia.[21] No human clinical trials could be found for this indication.

Protection from Radiation

Siberian ginseng is noted for its ability to provide protection in animals subjected to both single exposure and long-term X-ray radiation. In one study, rats given *Eleutherococcus senticosis* survived twice as long as control rats when exposed to long term radiation (total dose 1620 to 7000 rads). When the rats were given both eleuthero and antibiotics and exposed to radiation (total dose 3000 rads over 60 days), they survived three times as long.[2] An *in vitro* study noted only slight radio protective effects of eleuthro on the survival of cultured mammalian cells, while *Panax ginseng* was found to have significant effects in the same test system.[22] Although no human trials were available for review, Siberian ginseng is thought to be useful as an adjunctive treatment for those undergoing radiation treatment for a variety of cancerous conditions.

ADVERSE EFFECTS

Two reviews of clinical trials in which over 6000 individuals ingested eleuthero for up to 60 days reported no incidences of serious toxicity.[2,7] In addition, no long-term toxicity was reported in mice at a dose of 5.0 mL/kg of fluid extract.[2] Another comprehensive review of the literature concluded that unlike *Panax ginseng*, eleuthero never produces excitation or a stress-like syndrome in patients.[23] However, the Farnsworth review cites one study in which an unspecified proportion of 64 atherosclerotic patients (taking 4.5 to 6.0 mL of an ethanolic root extract daily for 25 to 30 days, repeated 6 to 8 times with 3 to 4 month intervals) experienced hypertension, cardiac problems (e.g., extrasystole, shifts in cardiac rhythm, tachycardia) and insomnia.[2] This review cites a second study in which 2 of 55 patients with rheumatic heart lesions reported headaches, hypertension, pericardial pain and palpitations.[2]

Eleuthero products have been commonly misidentified or adulterated in the past, most commonly with a plant known as *Periploca sepium* Bunge, Asclepiadaceae (the bark of silk vine). The Chinese name for eleuthero is "Ci-wu-jia", while the Chinese name for *Periploca sepium* is "Wu-jia", which may explain the original source of confusion.[1] *Periplocia sepium* is known to contain cardiac glycosides and chemicals with steroidal bases which may explain many of the side effects which have previously been attributed to eleuthero products. The most famous Canadian case is one of maternal-neonatal androgenization attributed to "Siberian ginseng."[24] The "Siberian ginseng" product, was later determined to contain no *Eleuthercoccus senticocus*, but almost certainly *Periploca sepium* instead.[25] However, oral administration of the original adulterated material to rats in a bioassay for androgenization failed to produce positive results. Thus, either the androgenizing effects noted in mother and infant were not due to the implicated herbal product, or the effects were specific to humans or idiosyncratic to the individuals involved.[26]

Tyler reports another Canadian incident in which an eleuthero product, adulterated with 0.5% caffeine, provided a stimulant effect to the user.[5]

Clinically, ingestion of true eleuthero products is associated with very few adverse effects.

CAUTIONS/CONTRAINDICATIONS

Some authors suggest that eleuthero should not be given to individuals with hypertension (greater than 180/90 mmHg); asthma or emphysema; diabetes; cardiac disorders; or those receiving anxiolytic or sedative treatment.[2] Baldwin also suggests caution when treating individuals with acute illness or fever; suffering from mania, schizophrenia or in pre-menopausal women.[7] Safety has not been established for use in children, and pregnant or lactating women.[8]

Clinically, eleuthero appears significantly less likely to cause problems in most individuals than *Panax* spp. (e.g., *Panax ginseng* and *Panax quinquefolium*).

DRUG INTERACTIONS

Some authors suggest caution with concomitant use of eleuthero and a variety of other therapies, including: cardiac, anti-coagulant, hypoglycemic, and hypo/hypertensive agents.[2] Eleuthero has been reported to both increase and decrease barbiturate sleeping time in *in vitro* and *in vivo* experiments.[2,27,28] In addition, a recent Canadian case study reported that eleuthero may be responsible for elevated serum digoxin levels in a 74-year-old man who presented with elevated serum digoxin levels at a routine check up with no signs of toxic effects. The authors suggested that there were three possible explanations for this finding: (1) some chemical constituent of eleuthero was converted to digoxin *in vivo*; (2) some component of eleuthero interfered with digoxin elimination; or (3) the eleuthero caused a false serum assay result.[29] Dennis Awang, a Canadian expert on herbal products, argues that the eleutherosides are in no way chemically similar to cardiac glycosides such as digoxin and have not been observed to have any cardiotonic effects. He argues that the case reported by McRae is most likely another case in which *Periploca sepium* is substituted for *Eleutherococcus senticosus* because the former contains several cardiac glycosides which provide a more rational explanation for the rise in serum digoxin noted in the patient.[30] It should be noted that the "Siberian ginseng" product in this case has never been tested for eleutheroside content.

DOSAGE REGIMENS [2]

❖ DRIED ROOT: 2-4 grams (in 1-3 divided doses) daily.
❖ TINCTURE (1:5): 10-20 mL (in 1-3 divided doses) daily.
❖ FLUID EXTRACT (1:1): 2-4 mL (in 1-3 divided doses) daily.
❖ SOLID EXTRACT (20:1): 100-200 mg (in 1-3 divided doses) daily.
Note: Most human studies involving long-term administration of eleuthero have involved eleuthero-free periods of 2-3 weeks every 30-60 days.[27]

Goldenseal
Hydrastis canadensis L.

THUMBNAIL SKETCH

Common Uses
❖ Infections and Inflammation (mucous membranes of the digestive tract, upper respiratory tract and genitourinary tract)

Active Constituents
❖ Isoquinoline Alkaloids (including hydrastine and berberine)

Adverse Effects
❖ Few at therapeutic doses, but there is a potential of poisoning.

Cautions/Contraindications
❖ Pregnancy
❖ Hypertension

Drug Interactions
❖ None noted in clinical practice

Doses
❖ *Dried Root and Rhizome:* 0.5-1.0 g dry or as decoction, three times daily

❖ *Hydroalcoholic Tincture* (1:10 in 60% ethanol): 2-4 mL three times daily

❖ *Liquid Extract* (1:1 in 60% ethanol): 0.3-1 mL of three times daily

❖ *Solid Extract* (4:1): 250 mg three times daily

❖ *Standardized Extract* (to 5% hydrastine): 250-500 mg three times daily

Introduction

Family
❖ Ranunculaceae

Synonyms
❖ Hydrastis
❖ Yellow root
❖ Orange root
❖ Indian turmeric
❖ Eye root
❖ Jaundice root
❖ Indian dye
❖ Yellow puccoon
❖ Ground raspberry
❖ Turmeric root[1-3]

Medicinal Forms
❖ Dried Root and Rhizome
❖ Tincture
❖ Liquid, Solid and Standardized Extracts

Description
The perennial goldenseal is a member of the buttercup family that stands up to 30 centimeters or 1 foot in height and produces a single white/green flower. While it was once found commonly throughout the woodlands of the central and eastern United States and southern Ontario, over-collection has now seriously diminished its numbers.[1,4] Goldenseal is now considered an endangered species. The berberine alkaloid found in goldenseal is common to several related plants that are used medicinally, including Bayberry (*Berberis vulgaris* L., Berberidaceae) and Oregon Grape/Trailing Mahonia (*Mahonia aquifolium* (Pursh) Nutt., Berberidaceae).

Parts Used
The knotty, distinctively yellow rhizome is used medicinally.[4]

Traditional Use
Goldenseal has enjoyed a long medicinal history, originally used by the First Nations peoples for a variety of conditions, including skin diseases, ulcers, liver conditions, digestive conditions and infections.[1,5] While herbalists use goldenseal for many conditions, it is considered especially useful in the management of infections and conditions of mucous membranes. Given its bright yellow color, it was also used commonly as a dye.[1,2] The early Eclectic physicians continued to use goldenseal into the beginning of the 20th century. Goldenseal is now mentioned in most of the world's herbal pharmacopoeias.

Current Medicinal Use
Goldenseal has astringent action which may be of use in managing a variety of inflammatory and infectious conditions of the gastrointestinal tract (gastritis, digestive problems, infectious diarrhea), upper respiratory tract, eyes and genitourinary system. Based primarily on traditional evidence, goldenseal is used to treat the common cold, either alone or in combination with other herbal medicines, notably echinacea.

Relevant Research

Preventative and Therapeutic Effects

CONSTITUENTS [1,3,4,6-10]

❖ ALKALOIDS: isoquinoline alkaloids (berberine, hydrastine, canadine), canadaline, hydrastidine, isohydrastidine, berberastine.

❖ MISCELLANEOUS: meconin, saturated and unsaturated fatty acids, chlorogenic acid, carbohydrates (D-fructose, D-galactose, sucrose).

COMMON USES

Astringent Action

Goldenseal is often referred to by herbalists as the 'king of the tonics of the mucous membranes'.[11] Goldenseal has been used for a variety of indications, including inflammatory and infectious conditions of the gastrointestinal tract (gastritis, digestive problems, infectious diarrhea),[1] upper respiratory tract, eyes and genitourinary system. As a bitter and a cholagogue, it is used to aid digestion and treat dyspepsia.[12,13]

Given its astringent action, goldenseal is also used to treat menorrhagia and post-partum hemorrhage (see cautions/contraindications).[12,13] Externally it has been suggested useful in the treatment of various skin conditions such as eczema, ringworm, athlete's foot, impetigo and pruritis.[12,14]

Common Cold

Goldenseal is often used to treat the common cold, either alone or in combination with echinacea. Bergner has recently questioned its effectiveness in the management of this condition. Firstly, the active anti-microbial agent (berberine) is poorly absorbed following oral administration and secondly because of the lack of historical data to support this indication. Its popularity in this situation is more likely due to an inappropriate transposition of modern antibiotic protocols.[15] It has been suggested that goldenseal acts in these cases not as an 'antibiotic-like' agent but rather as an alterative, aiding the body's inherent defensive processes.[15]

Excretion

Goldenseal has often been used to mask detection of illegal substances, such as marijuana and heroin, by urinalysis.[16] However, there is no data to support this use. It has been shown that even large doses of goldenseal have no influence on the excretion of narcotics.[17,18] In a review article, Foster concludes that this myth originated from a fictional novel written by a prominent 19th-century Eclectic physician.[19]

ANTI-MICROBIAL EFFECT

Most of the evidence used to support the anti-microbial action of goldenseal is actually taken from information relating to the use of berberine salts (especially sulfate). *In vitro* studies have shown berberine to be effective against a large number of bacteria including members of *Bacillus* sp., *Streptococcus* sp., *Staphylococcus* sp., *Klebsiella* sp., *Proteus* sp., *Corynebacterium diptheria*, *Enterobacter aerogenes*, *Salmonella typhi*, *Vibrio cholerae*, *Shigella boydii*, *Pseudomonas aeruginosa*, *Mycobacterium tuberculosis*, *Escherichia coli* and *Xanthomonas citri*.[5,6,15,20] In addition it is active against a wide variety of fungi (including *Candida albicans*, *Cryptococcus neoformans*, *Saccharomyces cerevisiae*, *Trichophyton mentagrophytes*, *Sporothrix schenkii*) and parasites (including *Giardia lamblia*, *Entamoeba histolytica*, *Leishmania donovani*).[5,6,20-23] Using chick embryos, berberine at a dose of 0.5 mg per egg offered protection from *Chlamydia trachomatis*. This action was comparable to that afforded by a dose of 1 mg of sulphadiazine per egg.[24]

Berberine sulfate has been shown to prevent the adherence of streptococci to host cells and this could in part explain its 'anti-biotic' properties.[25] *In vitro* experiments have shown that the pH of the medium influences the anti-microbial action of berberine salts,[20] with the action increasing with the basic nature of the medium used (e.g., when pH=8 anti-microbial activity is 2-4x greater than when the medium has a pH of 7.5) Both berberine sulfate and berberine hydrochloride appear to have similar anti-microbial properties.[20]

In a randomized controlled trial, a single dose of berberine sulfate (400 mg) was shown to decrease the mean stool volume and duration of diarrhea when given to adult individuals (n=165) suffering from acute diarrhea due to *Escherichia coli*. In patients with diarrhea caused by *Vibrio cholerae*, the decrease in stool volume was slight and was not additive to the effects of tetracycline.[26] In another randomized, placebo-controlled, double-blind clinical trial of adults (n=400) presenting with acute watery diarrhea, the effects of berberine hydrochloride (HCl) (100 mg 4x daily), berberine HCl (100 mg 4x daily) plus tetracycline (500 mg 4x daily) and tetracycline (500 mg 4x daily) alone were studied. In the subgroup suffering from cholera (n=186), a significant reduction in duration, frequency and need for rehydration fluid was noted in the tetracycline and tetracycline/berberine group. Berberine HCl by itself was shown to have no antisecretory action (a reduction of stool volume by 1L which was not clinically significant) but did decrease the number of excreted vibrios in the stool. The authors suggest that an antisecretory action may not have been demonstrated because the dose given was too low. Both berberine HCl and tetracycline were shown to be ineffective in patients (n=215) suffering from non-cholera diarrhea.[27]

An uncontrolled study showed that berberine administered orally in children (n=137, aged 5 months to 14 yrs) was comparable to other medications in the management of giardiasis. The author suggested that it could be of use in this situation especially due to the ease of administration and lack of unpleasant adverse effects. It should be noted that there was an increased rate of relapse after one month when compared to conventional treatments such as metronidazole.[28]

In determining the use of goldenseal for its reputed anti-microbial properties it must be remembered that the above information comes from the use and applications of berberine salts. Some authors have suggested that the claims made for this botanical medicine are exaggerated.[16]

CARDIAC ACTION

In vitro studies have produced contradictory results. While hydrastine has been shown to have a vasoconstrictive and thus hypertensive action,[9] it has also been noted that berberine and hydrastine have a hypotensive action.[6,9] In addition, berberine has been shown to: have ant-icoagulant properties in human blood;[6] have a dose dependant action on cardiac function;[6] increase coronary blood flow;[6] and to exert a protective effect in dogs following ventricular failure.[1]

ANTI-CANCER ACTIVITY

Berberine sulfate has been shown to inhibit the tumor promoting action of 12-0-tetradecanoylphorbol-13-acetate and telecodin *in vitro*.[29] In addition, berberine was shown to have anti-neoplastic activity *in vivo* against malignant human and rat brain tumors cell lines.[30]

HEPATIC ACTIVITY

The historical choleretic action of berberine has been demonstrated in a number of clinical trials.[5] Berberine has been shown to decrease elevated tyramine levels commonly associated with liver cirrhosis by inhibiting tyrosine decarboxylase produced by gut flora.[5]

MISCELLANEOUS EFFECTS

While not exhibiting a hypoglycemic effect, goldenseal has been shown to decrease polydipsia in streptozotocin-induced diabetic mice.[31]

ADVERSE EFFECTS

As for the therapeutic action, possible adverse effects are due to the isoquinoline alkaloids, notably hydrastine and berberine. In high doses (details not given), goldenseal has been noted to cause: oral and pharyngeal irritation, nausea, vomiting, diarrhea, parasthesia, convulsions, weak pulse, hypotension and death from respiratory or cardiac paralysis.[32] Given the lack of cases of adverse reactions, some authors suggest the dangers posed by the use of this herb medicinally have been exaggerated.[15] Some authors argue that the trials mentioned above support this position;[26,28] however, most were conducted using berberine alone, and not whole goldenseal products (which are those normally seen in clinical practice).

Contact ulceration has been noted when goldenseal root is applied externally to mucous membranes, such as in the form of vaginal douches.[6] In addition, drying of the mucous membranes has been noted after the oral administration of goldenseal, even at doses within the therapeutic range.[15] High doses of plants rich in berberine may cause functional vitamin B problems due to altered metabolism.[33]

The administration of a plant rich in berberine (*Coptis chinensis* Franch., Ranunculaceae) to neonates suffering from glucose 6 phosphate dehydrogense deficiency has resulted in jaundice and hemolytic anemia. While the exact mode of action is yet unknown, berberine appears to exert a bilirubin displacing action. These reported adverse effects have, in part, led to a restriction of sale of berberine rich herbs in general.[34] The applicability of these cautions to the use of goldenseal has been questioned.[15]

The risk of complications due to the destruction of gut flora commonly seen with conventional antibiotics has yet to be completely determined. Many authors suggest this to be unlikely,[5,15] a possible explanation being that berberine salts are also active against opportunistic fungi such as *Candida albicans*.[5]

CAUTIONS/CONTRAINDICATIONS

Due to the fact that the isoquinoline alkaloids are reputed to have a stimulant action on the uterus, goldenseal is contraindicated in pregnancy.[35] Goldenseal should also be used with caution in cases of hypertension.[11] Bergner cautions that the myth that goldenseal is a 'natural antibiotic' has led to the herb being used inappropriately in a large number of cases.[15]

Liquid products containing goldenseal are bright yellow in color and will stain clothing if spilled accidentally.

DRUG INTERACTIONS

While no specific drug interactions could be found for goldenseal, berberine has been noted to increase the sleeping time induced by barbiturates in rats.[6]

DOSAGE REGIMENS

❖ DRIED ROOT AND RHIZOME: 0.5-1 g dry or as decoction, three times daily.[3]
❖ HYDROALCOHOLIC TINCTURE (1:10 in 60% ethanol): 2-4 mL three times daily.[3]
❖ LIQUID EXTRACT (1:1 in 60% ethanol): 0.3-1 mL of three times daily.[3]
❖ SOLID EXTRACT (4:1): 250 mg three times daily.[5]
❖ STANDARDIZED EXTRACT (to 5% hydrastine): 250-500 mg three times daily.[36]

Hawthorn

Crataegus laevigata (Pois) DC.,
Crataegus monogyna (Jacq)

THUMBNAIL SKETCH

Common Uses
- ❖ Congestive Heart Failure (mild)
- ❖ Hypertension (mild)

Active Constituents
- ❖ Triterpene Glycosides
- ❖ Oligomeric Procyanidins

Adverse Effects
- ❖ Nausea, Dizziness, Headache (rare)

Cautions/Contraindications
- ❖ Pregnancy and Lactation

Drug Interactions
- ❖ Heart Conditions Medications

Doses
- ❖ *Standardized Extract* (2.2.% flavonoids or 18.75% oligomeric procyanides): 900 mg daily
- ❖ *Dried Fruit:* 0.3-1.0 g taken as an infusion
- ❖ *Liquid Extract* (1:1 in 25% alcohol): 0.5-1.0 mL of three times per day
- ❖ *Solid Extract:* ¼–½ teaspoon of daily
- ❖ *Tincture* (1:5 in 45% alcohol): 1-2 mL three times daily
- ❖ *Syrup:* 1 teaspoon two to three times daily

Introduction

Family
❖ Rosaceae

Synonyms
❖ Whitethorn
❖ Haw
❖ Mayherb
❖ Hagadorn[1-3]

Medicinal Forms
❖ Dried Fruit
❖ Standardized
  Extracts
❖ Liquid and
  Solid Extracts
❖ Water Ethanol
  Extract
❖ Tincture
❖ Syrup

Description
Hawthorn is a thorny deciduous tree, native to Europe, where it was often grown as a hedge, reaching a height of 25 feet or 8 meters. Clusters of white flowers bloom in the spring and the berries turn bright red in the autumn.

Parts Used
While flowers, leaves and even bark have been used medicinally, the bright red berries are the part most commonly used.

Traditional Use
Various species of hawthorn have been used traditionally for their healing powers by many different cultures.[4] In Ancient Britain, the hard wood of hawthorn and the berries were thought to have magical powers. Many Christians believe that the crown of thorns worn by Christ was made of hawthorn.[5] In Europe, hawthorn is considered to be one of the most important medicinal herbs, used to treat heart, blood, kidney, and memory disorders. Its universal appeal is evident when you consider that it is also consumed as a food in the form of jams, preserves and syrups.[3]

Current Medicinal Use
Under the supervision of a trained health-care provider, hawthorn products are used for cardiovascular conditions, notably mild congestive heart failure and hypertension.

Relevant Research

Preventative and Therapeutic Effects

CONSTITUENTS [2,3,5-7]
❖ TRITERPENE ACIDS: flavonoglycosides, vitexin, isovitexin, crataegolic acid.
❖ OLIGOMERIC PROCYANIDINS: procyanidins B-2, epicatechin, catechin
❖ MISCELLANEOUS: fatty esters, amines.

TRADITIONAL USES
Traditionally, hawthorn is considered to be one of the most important cardiac tonics. It is used to treat conditions resulting from heart or circulation problems. It has also been used as to treat such conditions as asthma, diabetes, nervous tension, anxiety and kidney stones.[3,5,6,8] While many different forms of hawthorn have been used traditionally, in Western herbalism *C. laevigata and C. monogyna* are the most common species used.

CARDIOVASCULAR EFFECTS
Hawthorn contains a number of medicinally active constituents, but most attention has been focused on the triterpene acids and oligomeric procyanidins and their cardiovascular properties. While specific actions differ depending on the constituent investigated, in general it is safe to say that hawthorn products appear to increase the force of heart contractions

(inotropic) and have little or a slightly negative effect on heart rate (chronotropic).[3,6,8,9] Specific extracts of hawthorn and its constituents have been shown to increase the force of contraction and blood flow to the heart muscles, protect the heart muscle from decreased blood flow, increase the refractory time between heart beats and decrease the potential for arrhythmia.[2,9,10]

It appears likely that the way hawthorn products exert their action is similar to several conventional heart medications. By decreasing the action of a group of enzymes called phosphodiesterases, the amount of a cell messenger called cyclic AMP is increased.[2,9,11] This increases the ease with which calcium can enter the cells which in turn causes increased action of the myocardium and vasodilation of the coronary blood vessels as well as vasodilation in peripheral blood vessels.[10,12] In addition to this, the antioxidant properties of the oligomyeric procyanidins and triterpene glycosides such as vitexin, protect the cells from oxidative damage.[9,10]

Congestive Heart Failure

There is a growing amount of evidence from studies of various designs including systematic reviews, randomized clinical trials, observational studies and case series that show hawthorn products are effective in treating mild cases of congestive heart failure (New York Heart Association levels I and II). Improvements are reported in a number of different outcome measures, including exercise performance, quality of life measures, symptom severity and EKG readings.[5,12,13] Individuals ingesting hawthorn have experienced these benefits when compared with others ingesting placebos and/or using conventional care, including drug therapy such as digitalis, nitrates and angiotensin converting enzyme (ACE) inhibitors such as captopril.[3,6,10-14]

One of the most detailed systematic reviews published to date included the placebo-controlled double-blind trials published between 1983 and 1994. In that period, eight trials were identified with a total of 433 patients suffering from mild congestive heart failure (NYHA II).[14] All these studies identified an improvement in both objective and subjective signs among those ingesting hawthorn. An analysis published in 2003 identified 13 clinical trials evaluating the effectiveness of monopreparations of hawthorn extracts in the treatment of congestive heart failure. This analysis identified that patients taking hawthorn had an improvement in dyspnoea, fatigue and heart rate.[15]

Evidence from a randomised controlled trial suggested that an extract of hawthorn may be effective in NYHA level III congestive heart failure. Long-term, multicenter, randomized, controlled trials are currently underway, including one with 2300 patients suffering from class II and class III congestive heart failure comparing standardized extracts of hawthorn to conventional care.[9]

While this evidence appears compelling, there is still a need for longer-term studies and research investigating the role of hawthorn products in more severe cases of congestive heart failure as well as more information on precise mechanisms of action.[13,16]

Hyperlipidemia

Evidence from animal studies suggests that hawthorn berry products may reduce blood cholesterol.[17] Additional research in humans is necessary to confirm these findings.

Anti-Oxidant

While hawthorn's antioxidant activities have been demonstrated in animal models, no evidence in humans was found to support the use of hawthorn products as a long-term antioxidant supplement.

Hypertension

Extracts of hawthorn have been to reduce blood pressure; however, evidence is still preliminary in humans. Results from one small pilot study of 36 mildly hypertensive patients found some beneficial results associated with ingesting hawthorn. After taking baseline anthropometric, dietary assessment, blood pressure measurements at rest, as well as after exercise and a computer 'stress' test, volunteers were randomly assigned to receive magnesium 600 mg, a 500 mg extract of hawthorn, a combination of both magnesium and hawthorn or placebo. While no statistically significant differences were seen between the four groups, a trend toward lowered systolic and diastolic blood pressure as a well as toward decreased anxiety was noted in the groups taking hawthorn.[18]

MISCELLANEOUS EFFECTS
Psychological Problems
The fact that many of the oligomeric procyanidins found in hawthorn are also found in other herbal medicines with CNS properties have led many to think that hawthorn may be useful in mental illness. Results from one small placebo-controlled, double-blind trial of 182 patients comparing a proprietary herbal combination product (Euphytose®) containing hawthorn to placebo over a 28-day period showed a significant improvement in the Hamilton Anxiety Rating scale. Since Euphytose contained more than one herb, it is not possible to determine how much of the effect noted in the trial can be attributed to hawthorn. More research is definitely needed in this area.[18]

ADVERSE EFFECTS
A series of reviews of the acute toxicity of commercial hawthorn products in animals found the LD50 to fall between 18-24 mL/Kg following intravenous administration and 1.5-33.8 mL/Kg when taken orally. The LD50 for various hawthorn constituents following oral and intravenous administration was found to fall between 6 g/Kg and 50-2600 mg/Kg, respectively.[19-21]

Hawthorn appears to be quite well tolerated with adverse effects rare. Results from one post-marketing surveillance of 3664 patients with congestive heart failure (NYHA I and II) taking a commercial hawthorn extract showed that only 22 patients suffered side effects which could be attributed with certainty to the herbal products.[5] When adverse effects do occur they are largely limited to nausea, palpitations, fatigue, sweating and skin irritation of the extremities.[2,5,8]

The most recent meta-analysis found that nausea, dizziness and digestive disorders were the most common adverse effects.[15]

CAUTIONS/CONTRAINDICATIONS
Since constituents found in hawthorn have been shown to effect uterine muscle in animal models, hawthorn berry products should be avoided in pregnancy and lactation.[2] Hawthorn should only be taken on the advice of a health care provider if it is being taken for cardiac conditions.[2] Given the fact that hawthorn products are not appropriate for self medication, hawthorn should not be used without the supervision of a healthcare provider.

DRUG INTERACTIONS
The potential exists for hawthorn berry products to potentiate the effects of cardiac glycosides, nitrates and other drugs used to treat cardiovascular conditions.[3] Although the evidence from clinical trials suggests a potential beneficial role for hawthorn in patients taking cardiovascular drugs, they should only be taken together on the advice of an appropriately trained health care provider.[5] Procyanidins in general may augment the coronary dilating action of a number of common drugs including caffeine and theophylline.[3]

DOSAGE REGIMENS [3,8,22,23]

- ❖ DRIED FRUIT: 0.3-1.0 g taken as an infusion three times daily.
- ❖ LIQUID EXTRACT (1:1 in 25% alcohol): 0.5-1.0 mL three times daily.
- ❖ TINCTURE (1:5 in 45% alcohol): 1-2 mL of three times daily.
- ❖ SOLID EXTRACT: ¼–½ teaspoon of daily.
- ❖ SYRUP: 1 teaspoon two to three times daily.
- ❖ WATER ETHANOL EXTRACT OF FLOWERS AND LEAVES (equivalent to 3.5-19.8 mg of flavonoids): 160-900 mg two to three times per day.
- ❖ STANDARDIZED EXTRACT (2.2% flavonoid or 18.75% oligomeric procyanides): 900 mg daily in divided doses.

Hops
Humulus lupulus L.

Common Uses
- ❖ Insomnia
- ❖ Agitation
- ❖ Nervous Tension Ailments (such as irritable bowel syndrome, poor digestion)

Active Constituents
- ❖ Volatile Oil
- ❖ Resinous Components
- ❖ Flavonoid Glycosides

Adverse Effects
- ❖ Contact Dermatitis and Respiratory Difficulties (following exposure to the herb itself)
- ❖ Menstrual Cycle (disruption)

Cautions/Contraindications
- ❖ Depression
- ❖ Pregnancy

Drug Interactions
- ❖ May potentiate the action of hypnotics and alcohol.

Doses
- ❖ *Dried Strobiles:* 0.5-1.0 g three times daily and before bed
- ❖ *Liquid Extract* (1:1 in 45% ethanol): 0.5-1 mL three times daily and before bed
- ❖ *Tincture* (1:5 in 60% ethanol): 1-2 mL three times daily and before bed

Introduction

Family
* Cannabaceae

Synonyms
* Humulus
* Lupulus
* Common hops
* European hops[1-3]

Medicinal Forms
* Dried Strobiles
* Liquid Extract
* Tincture

Description
Hops is a climbing perennial herb standing up to 6 meters or 20 feet in height found in marshy areas throughout North America, Europe and Asia.[2,4] It produces a yellowish-green male flower and a 'catkin-like' cone-shaped female flower or strobile.[5] These strobiles have glandular hairs that are rich in volatile oils producing a characteristic 'heavy' aroma.

Parts Used
The strobiles are the parts used medicinally.[5]

Traditional Use
Hops is an essential plant in the brewing of beer, making it arguably one of the most commonly used herbs. Hops has a long medicinal history, used primarily as a mild sedative. In addition to being taken orally, 'hops pillows' are also often used to aid sleep with the aroma allegedly having a calming action.[5] Hops is also said to influence both male and female sexual function. In female hop-pickers it was noted that menarche often occurred early and in men a decrease in 'sexual excess' was seen.[4]

Current Medicinal Use
Hops is used primarily for its hypnotic and anti-anxiety properties in the treatment of insomnia, nervous tension and conditions with a psychological component, such as irritable bowel syndrome. These uses are primarily supported by traditional evidence and a few clinical trials of combination herbal products that contain hops along with other active ingredients.

Relevant Research

Preventative and Therapeutic Effects
CONSTITUENTS [1-3,5-8]
* VOLATILE OILS: including: humulene, myrcene and beta-caryophyllene.
* CHALCONES: including: xanthohumol and xanthohumol.
* RESINOUS COMPONENT: alpha-bitter acids including humulone, cohumulone and adhumulone; beta-bitter acids including lupulone, colupulone, adlupulone; 2-methyl-3-buten-2-ol*.
* FLAVONOID GLYCOSIDES * including: astargalin, quercetin and rutin.
* MISCELLANEOUS * condensed tannins, 'estrogenic substances'.
  Note: While 2-methyl-3-buten-2-ol exists in small amounts in the plant, the amount is thought to increase on storage from the auto-oxidation of other resinous components.[7] This component is thought to be one of the active sedative constituents.[7,9,10]

COMMON USES

Hops is considered to be a mild sedative and is indicated in the management of insomnia and agitation/restlessness.[1,2,5,11-13] It has also been used in the treatment of conditions related to nervous tension such as irritable bowel syndrome, palpitations and nervous coughs.[4,5,11] Given the bitter nature of the resinous material, it is used as a digestive aid and to help stimulate appetite.[1,2,4,5,12,13]

ANTI-MICROBIAL ACTIVITY

Components of hops have been shown to exert anti-bacterial action primarily against Gram-positive bacteria.[2,3,14,15] Humulone and lupulone appear to be particularly responsible for this action.[2,15] The activity against Gram-negative bacteria is low due to the presence of a phospholipid rich membrane leading to an increased inactivation of the active principles.[15]

Clinically, aqueous extracts of hops have been used to treat various infections, including acute bacterial dysentery and pulmonary tuberculosis.[2] However, no clinical trial investigating these uses could be found.

Activity against a number of fungi and yeasts, including *Trichophyton*, *Candida*, *Fusarium* and *Mucor* spp, has been demonstrated.[3,14,16] The action of one component, 3-isopentenylphlorisovalerophenone, was compared favorably to griseofulvin in potency against *Trichophyton* spp.[16] A more recent evaluation noted no action against the yeast *Candida albicans*.[14]

SEDATIVE ACTION

A sedative/hypnotic action has been attributed to 2-methyl-3-butene-2-ol *in vivo*.[7,10,17,18] The sedative action of commercial products containing hops could be due to the in vivo formation of 2-methyl-3-butene-2-ol.[7,17] This volatile product can induce an hypnotic effect when inhaled,[9] and exists in relatively high concentrations in bath products,[7] giving possible credence to the use of items such as 'hops pillows'. However, Tyler questions whether enough 2-methy-3-buten-2-ol exists in most commercial products to support its use as a sedative.[9]

Oral administration of a commercial product (Seda-Kneipp®), which contains valerian in addition to hops, has been shown to decrease the impact of noise on sleep patterns (both slow-wave and REM).[19] Combination products containing both valerian and hops have been shown not to cause morning 'hangover' effects but may impair performance a few hours after ingestion.[20] In both the above scenarios it should be noted that valerian (*Valeriana officinalis* L. Valerianaceae) has been shown to possess hypnotic characteristics of its own.[21,22]

MISCELLANEOUS EFFECTS

Metabolism

Both colupulone and 2-methyl-3-buten-2-ol have been shown to induce cytochrome P4503A in mice and rats[23-26] and cytochrome P4502B in rats.[26]

Anti-Inflammatory

Humulone has been shown to possess anti-inflammatory properties, reducing 12-O-tetradecanoylphorbol-13-acetate induced inflammatory ear edema in mice.[27] The mechanism of action suggested is an inhibition of arachidonic acid metabolism.[28]

Oncology

Hops has been used historically in the treatment of cancer.[2] Humulone has been shown to inhibit the tumor-promoting effect of 12-O-tetradecanoylphorbol-13-acetate on skin tumor formation in mice.[28]

Endocrine

Using the uterine-weight assay of immature female mice as a determinant, no estrogenic properties could be shown for various components of hops, including the essential-oil fraction and bitter acids.[8] This finding contradicts others which have stated that hops has 'appreciable estrogenic activity',[5] and could aid in the treatment of hot flushing resulting from hormonal imbalance.[29] A disruption of menstrual cycle in female-hop pickers and decrease in male libido has been documented.[5]

ADVERSE EFFECTS

Components of hops are known to have allergenic potential resulting in instances of contact dermatitis as well as respiratory allergy and distress following frequent contact with hops.[3,30,31] The parenteral administration of large doses of hops has proved fatal *in vivo*.[3] The implication for clinical practice is unknown.

CAUTIONS/CONTRAINDICATIONS

Products containing hops should not be taken by individuals diagnosed with depression.[1,3,5,11]

Given its possible 'estrogenic' action, hops may disrupt menstrual cycles,[5] and the documentation of *in vitro* uterine anti-spasmodic activity suggests that hops should be avoided during pregnancy.[3,5]

DRUG INTERACTIONS

While no clinical instances were found, caution is prudent when herbal products containing hops are used with hypnotic medications and alcohol.[3] The implication of induction of components of the cytochrome P450 system on concurrent drug therapy has yet to be evaluated.

DOSAGE REGIMENS [1]

❖ DRIED STROBILES: 0.5-1.0 g of three times daily and before bed.
❖ LIQUID EXTRACT (1:1 in 45% ethanol): 0.5-1 mL three times daily and before bed.
❖ TINCTURE (1:5 in 60% ethanol): 1-2mL of three times daily and before bed.

Horsechestnut

Aesculus hippocastannum L.

THUMBNAIL SKETCH

Common Uses
❖ Chronic Venous
Insufficiency

Active Constituents
❖ Escin (or asecin)

Adverse Effects
❖ Horse Chestnut Seed Extract
or HSCE: Gastrointestinal
Upset, Calf Spasm, Headache,
Nausea, Itchy Skin
❖ Cream/gel: none reported

Cautions/Contraindications
❖ Pregnancy and Lactation
❖ Kidney and Liver Disease

Drug Interactions
❖ Diabetic Drugs and
Anti-Coagulants (potentially)

Doses
Orally
❖ *Extract* 5:1 (40 mg escin):
200 mg two to three
times daily
❖ *Escin:* 50-75 mg every
12 hours
❖ *Dried Seed:* 1-2 g of daily.
❖ *Fresh Seed:* 0.2-1.0 g seed
three times daily

As a cream or gel
❖ *HSCE gel* (2% escin):
3-4 times daily

Introduction

Family
❖ Hippo-
   castanaceae

Synonyms
❖ Aesculus
❖ Aesucule
❖ Eschilo
❖ Buckeye[1-3]

Medicinal Forms
❖ Standardized
   (to escin)
   Extract
❖ Fresh and
   Dried Seed
❖ Gel or Cream

Description
Native to the Balkans, the horsechestnut tree now grows throughout Europe and North America. Standing up to 25 meters or 80 feet in height with a characteristic domed shaped, it is found commonly in the grounds of English stately homes and in ornamental gardens.[4] The tree has 5 to 7 oval leaflets comprising the leaf, with clusters of white-to-pink flowers, bearing a spiny-hulled fruit encasing several shiny brown seeds. In the United Kingdom, the hard fruits are referred to by many small boys as 'conkers' and used in a traditional game. Unlike chestnut, the fruit is not edible, though it can be used as fodder for animals.

Parts Used
Medicinally, the seeds and the bark, rather than the fruit, are used.

Traditional Use
While horsechestnut products are not sold widely in North American market, they are very popular in Europe, especially Germany, where in 1996 it was the third best-selling herbal product, with estimated sales of $51 million US.[5] Most of these sales are made up of horsechestnut seed extract (HSCE), typically standardized to escin content. In Europe, horsechestnut seed products have been used orally for liver, prostate, kidney and bladder conditions. It has been applied in creams to treat bruising and arthritis pain.

Current Medicinal Use
Horsechestnut is now primarily used to treat conditions of cardiovascular insufficiency, notably varicose veins and, potentially, hemorrhoids.

Relevant Research

Preventative and Therapeutic Effects
CONSTITUENTS [2,4,5]
❖ TRITERPENE SAPONINS: aescin (or escin).
❖ COUMARINS: aesculetin, fraxin.
❖ FLAVONOIDS: kaempferol, quercetin.
❖ MISCELLANEOUS: tannins, allantoin, amino acids.

TRADITIONAL USES
Horsechestnut seed products have historically been used medicinally for a number of conditions, including liver conditions, benign prostatic hypertrophy, bladder conditions, applied as a cream for bruising, osteoarthritis, tinnitus, ulcers and upper respiratory conditions.[2,5]

CHRONIC VENOUS INSUFFICIENCY

Even though horse chestnut has been used traditionally for a number of conditions, almost all the modern research has investigated the use of HSCE in chronic venous insufficiency or CVI. CVI is a common condition that is due to decreased blood flow in the veins, most notably those in the leg. This can cause a number of problems such as leg pain, itchiness, swelling of the leg and even generalized fatigue.[5]

HSCE and escin have been shown to inhibit the inflammation associated with the onset of chronic venous insufficiency (CVI). By inhibiting the production of inflammatory mediators produced by the body, leakage from the blood capillaries is decreased.[1,5] This leads to a decrease in the localized swelling and edema seen with CVI. While escin is thought to be the primary constituent responsible for this action, the effects appear to be enhanced by the antioxidants found in HSCE.[2] In addition to this anti-inflammatory effect, HSCE also appears to increase the muscle tone of the veins found in the leg and increase blood flow and pressure in the femoral vein.[5,6]

HSCE has also been shown to reduce the breakdown of proteoglycans, substances found in the walls of blood vessels that effect vessel stability and permeability. Elevated levels of the enzymes known to cause the breakdown of proteoglycans have been found in patients with varicose veins.[7]

HSCE as a whole and some of the individual constituents of the plant have been also shown to influence blood sugar.[8] One constituent, esculin, found in Horse Chestnut but generally not in available extracts of the plant has been shown to have anti-thrombin activity.[5] Aescin has been shown to bind with blood proteins.[8]

To date, there have been 14 randomized clinical trials, some comparing HSCE to conventional care and others to placebo, investigating the effectiveness of oral HSCE in the treatment of CVI.[5,9,10] While these studies are typically small with some methodological challenges, a systematic review of all the quality studies concluded that oral administration of HSCE decreases a number of signs and symptoms of CVI, including ankle swelling, lower leg edema, pain, pruritis, fatigue and leg tenseness.[10] Though still preliminary, results from one study showed that HSCE may be as effective as compression therapy, such as medical stockings.[9] Most of these clinical trials used HSCE at a daily dose equivalent to 50-100mg of escin daily.

While HSCE creams and gels are often reputed to be of use in CVI, the evidence supporting these claims is limited. Based largely on the horse chestnut's pharmacological properties and the results from small studies, HSCE creams and gels (usually standardized to 2% escin) are also claimed to useful in bruising, sports injuries, varicose veins and hemorrhoids.[1-3,5,11] At this moment, the evidence supporting the use oral dosage forms of HSCE (e.g., tablets) is significantly stronger than that for topical applications such as gels and creams.

ADVERSE EFFECTS

Consumption of horse chestnut leaves, twigs and raw seeds can be potential harmful and even in some cases fatal.[5] Symptoms of horse chestnut poisoning include headache, vomiting, diarrhea, coma and paralysis.[12]

In contrast, side effects of HSCE are quite rare and are thought to occur in approximately 0.6% of people taking the products.[13] When adverse effects associated with HSCE do occur, they typically included gastrointestinal upset, calf spasm, headache, nausea and itchy skin or pruritis when HSCE is applied to the skin.[1,5,13-15] More serious adverse effects have been noted following the use of injectable HSCE or escin. Most notable amongst these are cases of hepatitis and damage to the tubular system in the kidneys. One case of anaphylaxis has been reported following intravenous administration of a horsechestnut product.[5]

CAUTIONS/CONTRAINDICATIONS

Until more is known, horsechestnut products should not be used in pregnancy or lactation. Given the potential for serious adverse effects, horsechestnut products should not be used in patients with liver or kidney conditions.[1]

DRUG INTERACTIONS

While no cases could be found, theoretically horse chestnut products may interact with anti-coagulants, drugs which are highly protein bound and anti-diabetic drugs.[5]

For more information, an excellent, a clinical review of horse chestnut can be found in the *Journal of Herbal Pharmacotherapy*.[5] We would like to thank the authors of this paper for their help with this chapter.

DOSAGE REGIMENS

Orally

❖ ESCIN: 50-75 mg every 12 hours.[5]

❖ EXTRACT 5:1 (40 mg escin): 200 mg two to three times daily.[2]

❖ DRIED SEED: 1-2 g of daily.[2]

❖ FRESH SEED: 0.2-1 g seed three times daily.[1]

Juniper
Juniperus communis L.

THUMBNAIL SKETCH

Common Uses
- ❖ Genitourinary Tract Infections (minor, including cystitis)
- ❖ Chronic Arthritic Conditions
- ❖ Digestive Upset

Active Constituents
- ❖ Volatile Oils (monoterpenes and sesquiterpenes)

Adverse Effects
- ❖ *Internal:* 'Kidney Pain', Urination, Hematuria, Albuminuria, Tachycardia, Hypertension
- ❖ *External:* Burning, Blistering, Erythema, Inflammation

Cautions/Contraindications
- ❖ Pregnancy
- ❖ Chronic or Acute Kidney Disease (disputed)

Drug Interactions
- ❖ Avoid with conventional hypoglycemic and diuretic therapy.

Doses
- ❖ *Dried Fruit:* 1-2 g three times daily
- ❖ *Liquid Extract* (1:1 in 25% alcohol): 2-4 mL three times daily
- ❖ *Tincture* (1:5 in 45% alcohol): 1-2 mL three times daily

Introduction

Description

Juniperus communis is an evergreen shrub native to Northern and Central Europe.[3,4] The tree itself can stand up to 6 meters or 20 feet, with whorls of needles, and produces a distinctive round, deep purple fruit.[3,4] While the fruits are often referred to as berries, they are in fact fleshy cone scales.[3-5] For best effect, the berries should be harvested in the second year when they are dark blue/purple in color.[5] Many adults will be familiar with its distinctive odor and taste since juniper berries are the principal flavoring agent in gin. However, gin contains insufficient amounts of the essential oil to afford it any medicinal properties.[6]

Parts Used

The dried or expressed 'berries' are rich in essential oils.

Traditional Use

Juniper berries have been used for centuries not only for culinary but also for medicinal purposes as a urinary tract antiseptic for treating cystitis and as digestive aid for colic, flatulence, and loss of appetite.[6] In the Middle Ages, it was thought that burning juniper branches in a fire would ward off evil spirits and the plague.

Current Medicinal Use

Based on traditional evidence, juniper is primarily used to treat minor uncomplicated (no kidney involvement) genitourinary tract infections such as cystitis. When applied as a lotion, it is also used to treat certain arthritic conditions.

Relevant Research

Preventative and Therapeutic Effects

CONSTITUENTS [2-4,7-10]

❖ VOLATILE OIL: monoterpenes (including 1,4-cineole, terpin-4-ol, sabinene, limonene, myrcene), sesquiterpenes (including caryophyllene, cadinene and elemene).
❖ TANNINS: proanthocyanins and gallotannins.
❖ FLAVONOID GLYCOSIDES: including rutin, isoquercitin and quercetin.
❖ MISCELLANEOUS: sugars, junionone, resin, vitamin C, diterpene acids, glucuronic acid.

COMMON EFFECTS

While juniper has many medicinal uses, it is primarily considered to be useful in the treatment of conditions of the genitourinary tract and musculoskeletal system.[5,11-14] It is also considered a 'urinary antiseptic' and diuretic and is used in conditions such as cystitis.[5,11] Weiss considers it useful both internally and externally in chronic arthritis, chronic gout, neuralgia and other rheumatic conditions.[5,12]

Given its aromatic quality, it is also classified as a bitter and carminative and used for digestive upset and colic as well as to stimulate appetite.[5,12]

MISCELLANEOUS EFFECTS

Most of the evidence supporting the therapeutic usefulness of juniper is empirical, and what little research there is, is often not available in English. The diuretic action of juniper is attributed to the terpinen-4-ol portion which is purported to stimulate glomerular filtration.[6] Juniper has also been demonstrated to have a hypoglycemic action in both rats and mice.[15,16] This action appears to be primarily extrapancreatic in origin.[15] In a variety of *in vitro* and *in vivo* models, juniper has been shown to have anti-fungal, anti-viral (against herpes simplex virus 1) and anti-inflammatory properties.[2] Finally, oral administration of an extract of juniper berries was seen to decrease experimentally-induced foot edema in rats.[17]

ADVERSE EFFECTS

Adverse effects have been reported following consumption or topical application of the oil. External application has been seen to result in burning, erythema, inflammation, blistering and edema. Internally, lower back pain in the kidney area, urination, discolored urine, hematuria, albuminuria, tachycardia and hypertension have been reported.[2] Positive patch test reactions following the topical application of an extract of juniper resulting in a dermatitis have also been noted.[18]

CAUTIONS/CONTRAINDICATIONS

Juniper berries are generally considered to be contraindicated in cases of chronic and/or acute kidney disease,[2,6,12] because of the high concentration of the irritant terpene hydrocarbons, such as alpha and beta pinenes, relative to the diuretic terpenin-4-ol.[19] A recent review article has challenged this opinion, suggesting that this warning arises from the administration of high doses of juniper and terpentine oil in veterinary medicine. In addition, the author argues that the clouding of urine seen following administration of high doses of the oil probably results from the excretion of juniper oil metabolites and is not an indication of kidney irritation.[20] Oil distilled from the needles, branches and unripe fruit may be particularly high in the irritant components and should still be of concern to the practitioner.[21] Given the present situation, the oil should be administered only under medical supervision.[2]

Juniper has been shown to have uterostimulant, anti-implantation and possible anti-fertility properties and should not be used in pregnancy.[2,22]

DRUG INTERACTIONS

Juniper should be used with caution in cases of concomitant conventional hypoglycemic and diuretic therapy.[2]

DOSAGE REGIMENS [2]

❖ FRUIT (BERRIES): 1-2 g of three times daily.
❖ TINCTURE (1:5 in 45% alcohol): 1-2 mL of three times daily.
❖ ESSENTIAL OIL (1:5 in 45% alcohol): 0.03-0.2 mL three times daily.

Kava

Piper methysticum G.Forst

THUMBNAIL SKETCH

Common Uses
❖ Anxiety, Tension, Restlessness
❖ Muscle Tension/Spasm and Pain

Active Constituents
❖ Kavalactones (kavapyrones)

Adverse Effects
❖ Liver Toxicity (including cirrhosis, hepatitis and liver failure)
❖ Vision Disturbances (photophobia, diplopia and oculomotor paralysis)
❖ Skin Conditions (yellowing and pruritic skin condition and allergy)
❖ Equilibrium (dizziness and stupor)
❖ Gastrointestinal Discomfort

Cautions/Contraindications
❖ Liver Conditions (pre-existing)
❖ Pregnancy and Lactation
❖ Not recommended for prolonged use (> 3 months)

Drug Interactions
❖ May potentiate the action of other centrally acting drugs

Doses
❖ *Standardized Extract* (70% kavalactones): 100 mg two to three times daily
❖ *Dried Rhizome:* 1.5-3.0 g daily in divided doses
❖ *Alcoholic Extract* (1:2): 3-6 mL daily in divided doses

Note: Generally the duration of use should not exceed 3 months.

Introduction

Family
❖ Piperaceae

Synonyms
❖ Kawa
❖ Kava-Kava[1,2]

Medicinal Forms
❖ Standardized Extract
❖ Dried Rhizome
❖ Alcoholic Extract

Description

Kava is a perennial shrub found throughout Polynesia and the Pacific islands.[1,3] The plant grows to 3 meters or 10 feet in height, with fleshy stems and few leaves, from a knotty, pithy root stock that has lateral roots extending to 3 meters or 10 feet.

Parts Used

The substantial, juicy rootstock (rhizome) is the part used medicinally.[1,3,4]

Traditional Use

Kava was first described in the West by the British explorer, Captain James Cook, in the 18th century during his exploration of the South Pacific.[4] It has been used as an aphrodisiac, narcotic, and antiseptic, as well as a tonic for pain relief from arthritis, toothache, and other chronic pain conditions.

In addition to its importance as a medicinal agent, kava plays an important role in many social and religious customs of the Polynesian indigenous peoples. Consumption of a beverage made from kava is used during funeral and marriage ceremonies as well as to honor visiting guests and dignitaries. The preparation of the beverage made from kava was a deeply orchestrated procedure, often involving the chewing of the root to aid extraction. Kava beverage (kava-kava) is considered to be a social beverage which causes numbness of the mouth followed by a pleasant mellow and relaxed state when consumed.[4,5] Hangovers do not seem to be a common occurrence.[4]

Current Medicinal Use

Though a significant amount of both traditional and scientific evidence supports the use of kava in the treatment of anxiety, concerns about liver toxicity need to be addressed before it can be widely recommended. Kava may also be useful in treating muscle spasms and pain.

Relevant Research

Preventative and Therapeutic Effects

CONSTITUENTS [1,3,4,6,7]

❖ KAVALACTONES: including the pyrones: kavain (kawain), dihydrokavain, methysticin, dihydromethysticin, and yangonin.
❖ ALKALOIDS: cepharadione A (an isoquinoline), pipmethystine (a pyridone, in the leaf only).
❖ MISCELLANEOUS: flavonoids and benzyl-ketones.

COMMON USES

Kava is considered by many to be one of the most effective herbal medicines for the treatment of anxiety.[4,5,8,9] As a muscle relaxant it is used in conditions associated with muscle tension such as headaches.[4,8] It is also reputed to be effective in the management of mild insomnia and pain;[4,8] stress and restlessness;[10] the treatment of urinary tract infections;[11] and arthritic conditions.[8] Application of the raw herb has been reported to ease dental pain and canker sores.[8,12]

MECHANISM OF ACTION

Most interest and investigation has been focused on the resinous pyrones or kavalactones. Their affinity for various GABA and benzodiazepine binding sites is debatable, with conflicting evidence being found on investigation.[13,14] Kavalactones are very poorly soluble in water, so for medicinal use they must be placed in colloidal solution or at least converted to a finely divided form to promote absorption of the suspension from the gastrointestinal tract.[15,16] Kava, or its constituents, have been reported to exhibit neuroprotective effects against ischemia;[17] produce EEG changes similar to those exhibited by diazepam;[18] block the voltage dependent sodium ion channel;[19] exert an anticonvulsive action;[4,20-22] possess antifibrillatory properties;[6] exert an analgesic effect;[4] relax skeletal smooth muscle;[6] inhibit conditioned reflexes in a number of animal models;[23] have local anaesthetic properties;[4-6] and possess antispasmodic and tranquilizing characteristics.[4-6]

EFFECT ON ANXIETY AND TENSION

A number of clinical trials, published primarily in German, have shown that kava extracts may prove beneficial in the management of anxiety and tension of non-psychotic origin.[4,5,9] A systematic review and meta-analysis assessing kava as a symptomatic treatment for anxiety identified 7 high-quality randomized controlled trials, all of which found kava to be superior to placebo. The meta-analysis of the results from three trials indicated that there was a significant difference in the reduction of the total score on the Hamilton Rating Scale for anxiety in favor of kava extract.[9] One double-blind placebo controlled trial found that administration of 100 mg of kava extract standardized to 70% kavalactone to patients with anxiety (n=58) three times daily for 4 weeks resulted in a significant improvement as measured by the Hamilton anxiety scale. Improvement was noted within the first week and no significant adverse effects were noted.[24]

Another randomized, double-blind, placebo-controlled study of kava in the management of patients (n=37) diagnosed with generalized anxiety disorder reported that 4 weeks of treatment with kava (extract standardized to 70% kavalactones, 70 mg twice daily for 1 week followed by 140 mg twice daily for the next three weeks) did not result in a statistically significant difference between the kava and placebo groups at the end of the study. However, differences in baseline anxiety levels between the two groups make these results difficult to interpret.[25]

In contrast to benzodiazepines, experience with the therapeutic use of kava preparations has shown no evidence that there is any potential for physical or psychological dependency. Nine double-blind studies have been done with the isolated compound DL-kawain, comparing it to reference drugs and placebo, with results similar to kava extract.

MISCELLANEOUS EFFECTS

Anti-fungal activity[4] and anti-mycobacterial activities[7] have been noted *in vitro*. A number of other excellent reviews in English of this plant's medicinal action and historical/cultural importance exist.[3,4,6,26]

ADVERSE EFFECTS

Kava has recently been removed from the food and supplement market in a number of countries, including Canada, due to concerns about kava-related liver toxicity.[27,28] The reports to date have all been case reports of varying degrees of quality that describe liver toxicity, including cirrhosis, hepatitis and liver failure in patients ingesting kava.[27-30] It is not clear if these effects are dose-related or related to long-term use or specific extracts of kava only. In addition, there has been much criticism over the thoroughness of some of the actual case reports as well as the fact that many of the patients were taking drugs with potential hepatotoxic properties at the same time as the kava.[31] Health Canada has determined that kava is currently not sufficiently safe to be sold as a food.[28] This decision may be revisited in the future if any new evidence becomes available.

There is a single case report of a women who experienced a delayed hypersensitivity reaction to kava that presented as a generalized rash and severe itching. A patch test with kava was strongly positive, suggesting an allergic reaction to kava.[32]

Excessive consumption can result in disturbances of vision (photophobia, diplopia and oculomotor paralysis), yellowing of the skin, problems with equilibrium, dizziness and stupor.[1,4-5] These effects are seen with consumption of the beverage and it is unlikely that they are of any particular concern in practice.[4] Kava does not adversely affect cognitive function, mental acuity or coordination in comparison to oxazepam, as measured by event-related potentials during cognitive testing.[33]

Chronic administration can result in a characteristic scaling of the skin on the extremities associated with intense itching.[1,3,4] It has been hypothesized that this was due to a deficiency in vitamin B3 but symptoms are not improved following administration of nicotinamide (100mg daily for 3 weeks).[4] It is now considered to be an allergic skin reaction.[16]

CAUTIONS/CONTRAINDICATIONS

Due to its dopaminergic properties, kava should be used with caution in cases of Parkinsons disease.[34] Use is contraindicated in pregnancy, lactation, depression[35] and patients with liver conditions or other risk factors for liver disease.

DRUG INTERACTIONS

Concomitant administration of kava with barbiturates and centrally acting conventional medication may result in a potentiation of their action.[1,4] Administration of dihydromethysticin is known to potentiate the action of hexobarbital in animal models.[6] While large doses of alcohol are known to potentiate the action of kava in mice, there does not seem to be such as problem in humans. Excessive alcohol consumption is still best to be avoided in people taking kava.[36]

A possible interaction between kava and a benzodiazepine (alprazolam) has been noted in a 54-year-old man. The individual was admitted to hospital in a 'lethargic and disorientated' state after recently introducing kava to his supplement regimen. The patient was also taking cimetidine and terazosin.[37]

DOSAGE REGIMENS

❖ STANDARDIZED EXTRACT (70% kavalactones): 100 mg two or three times daily.[5]
❖ DRIED RHIZOME: 1.5-3 g daily in divided doses.[4]
❖ ALCOHOLIC EXTRACT (1:2): 3-6 mL daily in divided doses.[4]
   Note: Generally the duration of use should not exceed 3 months.[16]

Lemon Balm

Melissa officinalis L.

Common Uses

Internal

❖ Insomnia, Anxiety,

❖ Nervous Tension
(including digestive
and cardiac conditions,
pediatric conditions)

Topical

❖ Cold Sores

Active Constituents

❖ Volatile Oils

❖ Tannins

❖ Flavonoids (rosmarinic acid)

Adverse Effects

❖ None reported

Cautions/Contraindications

❖ Thyroid Conditions
(existing)

Drug Interactions

❖ Potential exists for
interactions with
concomitant thyroid
medications

Doses

Oral

❖ *Dried Leaves:* 1-4 g taken
three times daily, as an
infusion or in a comparable
dosage for a tincture or
fluid extract

Topical

❖ *Concentrated Extract* (70:1):
applied 2-4 times daily
in the management of
cold sores

Introduction

Family
* Lamiaceae (also known as Labiatae)

Synonyms
* Melissa
* Common balm
* Bee balm
* Balm
* Honeyplant
* Sweet balm
* Cure-all[1-3]

Medicinal Forms
* Fresh or Dried Leaves Infusion
* Tincture
* Fluid Extract
* Concentrated Extract
* Essential Oil

Description
Native to Mediterranean Europe, North Africa and Western Asia but now widely distributed, lemon balm is a perennial herb standing up to 1 meter or 40 inches in height, with light green leaves and flowers ranging in color from light yellow to rose and blue-white.[2] Like most members of the mint family, it is aromatic, producing a characteristic lemony scent when bruised or crushed.[1,2] The name "Melissa' derives from the Greek for bee, referring to the attraction the plant holds for bees.

Parts Used
The aerial parts, fresh and dried, have many reputed actions.

Traditional Use
Lemon balm has enjoyed a long medicinal and culinary history, with references to it found in Roman, Arabic, and British herbal lore. Brewed as a tea, lemon balm has been enjoyed for its flavor and as a relaxing tonic. It has been used as a mild sedative for anxiety and nervous conditions, and as an aid to longevity. Lemon balm is also a key component of perfumes and cosmetics.

Current Medicinal Use
Lemon balm is one of the primary nervines, and based on traditional evidence, it is commonly used for conditions arising from nervous tension.[1,4] Given its traditional reputation as a gentle herbal product, it is considered particularly well-suited to pediatric conditions. Results from clinical trials suggest that creams made from lemon balm may also be of use in treating cold sores.

Relevant Research

Preventative and Therapeutic Effects

CONSTITUENTS [1-3, 5]
* VOLATILE OILS (0.1-0.2%): citral a and b, caryophyllene oxide, citronellal, geraniol, linalool, nerol.
* FLAVONOIDS: including isoquercetrin, apigenin-7-O-glucoside, rhamnocitrin, luteolin-7-O- Glucoside.
* HENYLPROPANOIDS: including triterpenoids, rosmarinic acid.
* MISCELLANEOUS: tannins, ursolic acid, caffeic acid, and polyphenolic agents.

COMMON EFFECTS

Lemon balm is reputed to have sedative;[1,6,7] anti-spasmodic;[1,2,6-8] carminative;[1,6-8] anti-emetic;[4,7] anti-microbial;[4] and anti-hormonal; and diaphoretic properties.[1,4,7]

Oral consumption is considered useful in the treatment of anxiety, insomnia, colds/fevers and digestive upset (bloating). It is considered by many to be especially useful as a children's remedy.[1,4] Topically lemon balm is claimed to be effective in the treatment of cold sores. One randomized, double-blind, placebo-controlled trial (N=66) reported that lemon blam cream may prolong the intervals between periods of herpes in patients diagnosed with herpes simplex labialis.[9] Inhalation of the essential oil is reputed to have a direct influence on the nervous system, instilling calmness and improving mood.[4,7] It is particularly well-suited to the management of conditions, often cardiac or digestive, where the etiology has a psychological component.[1,6]

NERVOUS SYSTEM ACTION

A lyophilized hydroalcoholic extract of *Melissa officinalis* has been shown to exert hypnotic and peripheral analgesic activity in mice.[10] A German trial demonstrated that a combination herbal product containing valerian (160mg/tablet) and lemon balm (80mg/tablet) promoted sleep (1 tablet at bedtime) as effectively as triazolam 0.125 mg (Halcion®) at a similar regimen.[11] It should be noted that valerian has a long established hypnotic action of its own. This combination product did not influence concentration or induce daytime sedation,[11,12] and did not potentiate the effects of alcohol.[12]

ANTI-MICROBIAL EFFECTS

The essential oil fraction of *Melissa officinalis* exerts an anti-microbial action *in vitro* against a variety of bacteria and fungi.[2,13] In addition, antiviral properties of *Melissa officinalis* have been demonstrated on many occasions.[14-17] The active constituents appear to be primarily the polyphenols and tannins present.[17,18] Most interest has been focused on the action of *Melissa officinalis* in the management of herpes simplex infections. In a recent multi-center clinical study (n=115) and subsequent placebo controlled double-blind study (n=116), the topical application of 1% dried extract of lemon balm appeared effective in the management of herpes simplex. Improvement of symptoms was noted by day 2 of the treatment and the test agent was considered superior to placebo by both physicians and patients. For optimum results the authors suggest that treatment be started at the onset of the infection.[16]

ENDOCRINE EFFECTS

Extracts of *Melissa officinalis* have long been documented to possess anti-thyrotropic activities.[2,19,20] Aqueous extracts contain components, notably certain phenolic agents, that inhibit the extrathyroidal metabolism of both T3 and T4 in a dose related manner.[19] *In vitro* studies have demonstrated that a freeze-dried extract of *Melissa officinalis* inhibits the binding, in a dose dependent manner, of thyroid stimulating hormone (TSH) to thyroid membrane. It is hypothesized that components present in the freeze-dried extract interact with TSH preventing its binding to the membrane bound TSH receptor.[21] In addition, components of the freeze-dried extract of *Melissa officinalis* inhibit the binding immunoglobulin G found in Grave's disease to TSH receptors.[22] This may in part support the historical use of lemon balm in the management of certain thyroid conditions.[22]

Freeze dried extracts of *Melissa officinalis* that demonstrate the above anti-thyrotropic properties also possess anti-gonadotropic characteristics preventing the binding of human chorionic gonadotrophin (HCG) to rat testis *in vitro*.[21]

MISCELLANEOUS EFFECTS

Anti-Oxidant

Hydroalcoholic extracts of *Melissa officinalis* have been shown to possess anti-oxidant properties, thought in part to be due to the presence of rosmarinic acid.[23]

Anti-Inflammatory

Rosmarinic acid isolated from *Melissa officinalis* has been shown to influence complement activity. This may be explained in part by its ability to inhibit the action of C3-convertase [24] and C5 convertase.[25] Studies in animal models suggest that rosmarinic acid also exerts an anti-inflammatory action in complement-dependent inflammatory processes.[24]

ADVERSE EFFECTS

No examples of unpleasant side effects could be found for this phytomedicine.

CAUTIONS/CONTRAINDICATIONS

While no specific examples could be found, lemon balm should be used cautiously in patients with thyroid conditions. Safety in pregnancy has not been established. Lemon balm appears to have no mutagenic properties.[26]

DRUG INTERACTIONS

While no clinical examples could be found, products containing lemon balm may interact with conventional thyroid medications. A lyophilized hydroalcoholic extract of *Melissa officinalis* has been noted to promote the hypnotic action of pentobarbital in mice.[10]

DOSAGE REGIMENS

Oral

❖ DRIED LEAVES: 1-4 g taken three times daily, as an infusion or in a comparable dosage for a tincture or fluid extract.[1]

Topical

❖ CONCENTRATED EXTRACT (70:1): applied 2-4 times daily in the management of cold sores.[15]
  Note: Since lemon balm is rich in volatile oils, infusions should be made in a closed container.[6]

Licorice
Glycyrrhiza glabra L.

THUMBNAIL SKETCH

Common Uses
- ❖ GI Tract Inflammation (e.g., peptic and duodenal ulcers, gastritis)
- ❖ Skin Inflammation (e.g., oral herpes lesions, canker sores)
- ❖ Coughs (productive) and Bronchitis
- ❖ Adrenocorticoid Insufficiency (e.g., due to stress and overwork)
- ❖ Sweetening and Flavoring Agent

Active Constituents
- ❖ Glycyrrhizin
- ❖ Glycyrrhetinic acid

Adverse Effects
- ❖ Pseudoaldosteronism (which presents as hypernatremia, hypokalemia, hypertension, headache, edema, lethargy, and can lead to congestive heart failure)

Cautions/Contraindications
- ❖ Cardiovascular Disease (pre-existing)
- ❖ Liver or Kidney Dysfunction
- ❖ Pregnancy (safety not established)

Drug Interactions
- ❖ Increases the half-life of hydrocortisone and prednisolone; possible interactions with medications whose action is closely linked to potassium levels, including cardiac glycosides, and both loop and potassium-sparing diuretics.

Doses
- ❖ *Powdered Root:* 1-4 g daily in three divided doses
- ❖ *Solid* (dry powdered) Extract (4:1): 250-500 mg daily in three divided doses
- ❖ *Deglycyrrhizinated Licorice Tablets:* 380-1,140 mg (1-3 chewable tablets) three times daily
- ❖ *Licorice Extract:* 0.6-2 g daily.
- ❖ *Decoction:* 2-4 g (1 teaspoonful) of herb to 120 mL (1/2 cup) of boiling water, three times daily after meals
- ❖ *Lozenges/Candies:* as an expectorant and cough suppressant (make sure they actually contain real licorice)

Introduction

Family
- ❖ Fabaceae (also known as Leguminosae)

Synonyms
- ❖ Liquorice
- ❖ Glycyrrhiza
- ❖ Sweet wood
- ❖ Liquiritiae
- ❖ Glycyrrhizae radix[1-4]

Medicinal Forms
- ❖ Powdered Root
- ❖ Fluid and Solid Extracts
- ❖ Decoction
- ❖ Tablets and Candies/ Lozenges
- ❖ Deglycyrrhizinated Form (DGL)

Description

Licorice is a small perennial shrub native to temperate regions, growing to 1 to 2 meters or 3 to 6 feet in height, with dark green leaves, mauve flowers, and a long, round taproot and root branches and runners. Licorice is extensively cultivated as a medicinal herb and as a distinctively flavored sugar for use in making candy and in flavoring botanical formulations because of its distinctive flavor and its sweetening action: glycyrrhizin is 50 to 100 times sweeter than sucrose.[5-8] The amount of licorice in products varies dramatically.[9,10] Most of the licorice candy available in North America is flavored not with licorice, but with anise oil.[11] One study found that authentic licorice candy contained between 0.26 mg/g and 7.9 mg/g of glycyrrhizin; while medicinal products ranged from 0.30 mg/g to 47.1 mg/g of glycyrrhizin.[9] In addition, licorice flavored chewing tobacco contained between 1.5 mg/g to 4.1 mg/g of glycyrrhizin.[9]

Parts Used

The roots and underground horizontal stems, called rhizomes or stolons, are the parts used medicinally.[3,5]

Traditional Uses

Licorice has been used medicinally for over 4000 years,[1] as an expectorant, an anti-tussive and a mild laxative.[5] It is also a very important herb within Traditional Chinese Medicine, where its uses include treating peptic ulcers, asthma, and malaria.[6] Within Traditional Chinese Medicine, licorice (*Glycyrrhiza uralensis* Fisch. In DC.) is considered to be a sweet, neutral herb that clears phlegm and tonifies the spleen.[7]

Current Medicinal Use

Licorice is arguably the most common herbal medicine because it is frequently added to natural health products as a sweetening agent. Based primarily on traditional evidence, licorice is used as an adrenal tonic in cases of stress and fatigue, and as an expectorant in coughs and bronchitis. As an anti-inflammatory, licorice is applied topically to treat conditions such as cankers, cold sores and minor skin abrasions. A growing amount of scientific evidence supports the use of deglycyrrhizinated licorice in the treatment of peptic and duodenal ulcers.

Relevant Research

Preventative and Therapeutic Effects

CONSTITUENTS [1,3,5,12,13]

❖ TERPENOIDS: glycyrrhizin (also called glycyrrhizic or glycyrrhizinic acid) which yields glycyrrhetinic acid (also called glycyrrhetic or glycyrretic acid) and glucuronic acid after hydrolysis; glycyrrhetol, glabrolide, licoric acid, liquiritic acid.

❖ FLAVONOIDS AND ISOFLAVONOIDS: including isoflavonol, kumatakenin, licoricone, glabrol, for-mononetin, chalcone and chalcone derivatives including isoliquiritigenin, licochalcone A and B.

❖ COUMARINS: umbelliferone, herniarin, glycyrin, liqcoumarin.

❖ VOLATILE OILS: including anethole, benzaldehyde, cumic alcohol, eugenol, fenchone.

❖ MISCELLANEOUS: acetylsalicylic acid, salicylic acid, methylsalicylate.

METABOLIC EFFECTS

The pharmacology of licorice has been extensively studied and several good reviews discuss this in detail.[1,4,14-18] In summary, glycyrrhizin inhibits three enzymes: two (15-hydroxy-prostaglandin dehydrogenase and delta13 - prostaglandin reductase) are involved in the metabolism of two prostaglandins (E and F2a) and the third, which is found primarily in the kidneys and liver (11 beta-hydroxysteroid dehydrogenase) catalyzes the production of cortisone (inactive) from cortisol (active).[2,19,20] Thus, corticosteroid receptors become increasingly activated by cortisol, which may result in hypertension. In addition, gly-cyrrhizin and glycyrrhetinic acid bind weakly to mineralocorticoid and glucocorticoid receptors;[14,20,21] influences aldosterone secretion and elimination;[14,22] suppress plasma renin activity;[17,23] and decrease angiotensin levels.[16] Licorice has also been shown to increase atrial natriuretic peptide (ANP) and decrease vasopressin levels.[24]

Licorice is considered a "phytoestrogen," that is, the steroid-like configuration of several of the components of licorice, including the isoflavones and glycyrrhetinic acid, have the ability to influence estrogen metabolism. Generally, if estrogen levels are high, these constituents inhibit estrogen action by binding to the estrogen receptors and blocking the binding of endogenous estrogen. However, if estrogen levels are low, they appear to potentiate the action of estrogen. For this reason it is often referred to as being "amphoteric" (partial agonist) in nature. Phytoestrogens have between 1/20 and 1/100 the action of estrogen.[5,12]

Pharmacokinetics

Peak serum concentration of glycyrrhizin occurs approximately 4 hours after ingestion, but varies widely among individuals ingesting the same amount of glycyrrhizin. In contrast, gly-cyrrhetinic acid levels peak at approximately 24 hours. Glycyrrhizin serum concentration decreases quickly and is no longer detectable by 96 hours. Glycyrrhetinic acid levels decrease more slowly.[3,25] Consumption of 100 to 200 g licorice daily will result in plasma concentrations of glycyrrhetinic acid of 80 to 480 ng/mL.[19] It appears that the bioavailability (i.e. intestinal absorption) of glycyrrhizin is higher when it is consumed alone than when it is consumed as a constituent of licorice root or licorice root extract,[26-28] but it does not appear to be influenced by the presence of food.[3,29] Glycyrrhizin is excreted mainly (80%) by the liver into the bile by a process which can become saturated.[30]

GASTROINTESTINAL EFFECTS

Perhaps one of the most well-known uses for licorice is its use in gastrointestinal conditions. Licorice has been used to treat dyspepsia for centuries. In fact, two pharmaceutical products, deglycyrrhizinated licorice and carbenoxolone, have been available since the mid-1960s, both of which enhance the body's ability to protect the gastrointestinal lining in a variety of ways including: "increasing the number of mucous-secreting cells (thereby increasing the amount of protective mucosubstances secreted); improving the protective nature mucous produced; increasing the life span of the surface intestinal cells; and enhancing the microcirculation of the gastrointestinal tract lining." This mechanism of action is described in detail elsewhere.[31]

Carbenoxolone

This derivative of glycyrrhetinic acid has been marketed for the treatment of both duodenal and gastric ulcers. Although its exact mechanism of action has not yet been elucidated, it appears to increase synthesis and secretion of mucus. Although efficacy studies have reported conflicting results, one study showed that maintenance therapy of carbenoxolone decreased the recurrence rate of gastric ulcers significantly more than either antacids or a placebo.[1] Several randomized, double-blind, controlled trials have demonstrated that carbenoxolone is also more effective than placebo in the treatment of duodenal ulcers.[1] No information could be found comparing the effects of carbenoxolone with standard combination antibiotic therapy used in the management of peptic ulcer disease. Carbenoxolone is rarely used today because its adverse effects include water retention, as well as increased blood pressure. This will be discussed in detail in the Adverse Effects section.

DEGLYCYRRHIZINATED LICORICE (DGL)

Deglycyrrhicinated licorice or DGL was developed in an attempt to reduce the adverse effects that are largely caused by the glycyrrhizin content of licorice products. DGL has a glycyrrhizin content of < 3%[1] and no known adverse effects.[5] Although the active constituent of DGL has not been identified, it is believed to be a spasmolytic agent.[1] The majority of randomized, placebo-controlled trials of DGL tested a specific product currently only available in Europe called Caved-S®, which is a chewable tablet. Another European brand, Ulcedal®, which was available in capsule form (it has since been removed from the market) appeared to be ineffective, leading some researchers to hypothesize that DGL must mix with saliva to be effective.[5] One study (n=100) reported that DGL (760 mg three times daily between meals) had comparable efficacy to cimetidine (200 mg three times daily and 400 mg at bedtime) in its ability to increase the healing rate of gastric ulcers.[32] This study also found no significant difference in ulcer recurrence after one year when they compared maintenance therapy of DGL (760 mg twice daily) and cimetidine (400 mg at bedtime).[32] In addition, DGL has been shown to be equivalent to ranitidine in treatment of gastric ulcers.[33]

Several studies also report the effectiveness of DGL in the treatment of duodenal ulcers.[34,35] One (n=40) showed that both 3 g DGL daily for 8 weeks and 4.5 g daily for 16 weeks provided substantial improvement in most patients within 5 to 7 days; however, the higher dose was reported to be significantly more effective.[34] A second study (n=874) reported no significant difference in the rate of healing at 12 weeks between patients treated with DGL (380 mg three times daily), antacids (15 mL suspension of aluminum-magnesium hydroxide equivalent to 3 g/day) or cimetidine (200 mg three times daily and 400 mg at bedtime).[35]

ANTI-INFECTIVE AGENT

Anti-Viral

Several studies have found evidence of licorice's anti-viral activity.[36,37] In vitro studies document the ability of glycyrrhizin to directly inhibit the growth of several different viruses, including herpes simplex;[36,38,39] herpes genitalis and herpes zoster;[40] influenza virus A;[2,37] hepatitis A virus;[41] and HIV.[38,42,43] In addition, both glycyrrhizin and glycyrrhetinic acid have been reported to induce the production of interferon.[44]

A few clinical studies have been conducted which indicate that the topical application of glycyrrhetinic acid or its derivatives decreases the pain and increases the rate of healing of oral and genital herpes lesions.[45-47]

Anti-Bacterial/Anti-Fungal

Extracts of licorice have been shown *in vitro* to inhibit the growth of a variety of bacteria and fungi, including *Candida albicans*, *Staphylococcus aureus*, *Streptococcus mutans* and *Mycobacterium smegmatis*.[48] The isoflavonoid components appear to be the components responsible for this action. One study found that they had *in vitro* activity comparable to streptomycin against *Staphylococcus aureus*, *Mycobacterium smegmatis* and *Candida albicans*.[1]

Anti-Parasitic

Licochalcone A, a component of licorice, has been shown to inhibit both chloroquine-susceptible and chloroquine-resistant strains of *Plasmodium falciparum*[49] and *Leishmania major* and *Leishmanian donovani* promastigotes and amastigotes *in vitro*.[50,51]

ANTI-INFLAMMATORY AND ANTI-ALLERGIC ACTIVITY

The cortisol-like action of licorice confers an ability to inhibit the formation and secretion of inflammatory compounds. A recent study suggests that glycyrrhetinic acid may also have a direct anti-inflammatory action by selectively inhibiting the classical complement cascade (it has no affect on the alternative pathway).[52] In addition, a recent study reported that glycyrrhizin is a selective inhibitor of thrombin (however it did not effect the clotting activity of thrombin), which may be another mechanism of action for its anti-inflammatory activity.[53] Glycyrrhizin has been shown to inhibit allergenic reactions produced under controlled experimental conditions.[5]

HEPATOPROTECTIVE ACTIVITY

The role of licorice in liver disease is reviewed in detail by Hikino and Kiso.[54] Intravenous administration of glycyrrhizin is used in the treatment of hepatitis in Japan.[55,56] This indication is supported by several double-blind, controlled studies which have reported that glycyrrhizin is an effective treatment in the management of viral hepatitis.[57] It has been hypothesized that glycyrrhizin may bind to hepatocytes, modifying the expression of hepatitis B virus (HBV) antigens on their surface, thus suppressing their sialylation.[55,58]

In addition, several *in vitro* studies indicate that glycyrrhizin may protect the liver from damage caused by chemical toxins such as CCl4 (carbon tetrachloride).[59] The mechanism of action for this is hypothesized to be an inhibition of the cytochrome P-450 system conversion of CCl4 to CCl3.

MISCELLANEOUS EFFECTS

Premenstral Syndrome (PMS)

PMS symptoms have been associated with an increased estrogen:progesterone ratio. Phytoestrogens such as licorice are thought to be useful in decreasing the symptoms associated with PMS.[5]

Canker Sores

Licorice has been reported to decrease the pain and speed the healing rate of canker sores in the mouth.[5] One double-blind, crossover trial (n=24) reported that a mouth wash containing glycyrrhetinic acid reduced the pain associated with mouth ulcers, as well as significantly decreasing the number of new ulcers which developed.[60]

Expectorant/Anti-Tussive

Although the mechanism of action has not yet been elucidated, licorice has a long historical use as an expectorant and anti-tussive.[3,61] Its use for these indications continues to be widespread in North America today.[2,6]

Protection from Diabetic Complications

Many diabetic complications improve with the addition of inhibitors of aldose reductase (the first enzyme in the polyol pathway) to the therapeutic regimen.[12,62,63] Isoliquiritigenin, a component of licorice has been shown *in vitro* and *in vivo* to inhibit aldose reductase, thus decreasing the conversion of glucose to sorbitol and inhibiting sorbitol accumulation.[12,62,63]

Burn Victims

Glycyrrhizin has been shown to decrease the generation of burn-associated suppressor T cells (BTs cells) in thermally injured mice. Other reports have found an increasing incidence of septic infections with an increased number of BTs cells. The authors hypothesize that glycyrrhizin may play a role in the future treatment of burns.[64,65]

Anti-Cancer

A variety of compounds in licorice have been shown to have anti-mutagenic activity and to decrease the growth of some cancer cell lines *in vitro*.[66,67] The clinical significance of these findings is unknown.

Anti-Fatigue

Licorice is considered by some medical herbalists to be an adrenocorticotrophic agent (tonic to the adrenal glands). Consequently, it is used in the management of stress and fatigue.

ADVERSE EFFECTS

Licorice is considered safe in low doses; however, adverse effects are common at doses of more than 20 g of licorice root daily. Adverse symptoms have also been seen in doses significantly lower than this.[3] Because the adverse effects appear at widely differing doses in different individuals,[12,14,68] it is important to monitor patients. The adverse effects most commonly experienced are mineralocorticoid-related including: headache, lethargy, sodium and water retention, excessive excretion of potassium, hypokalemic myopathy,[12,69,70] and high blood pressure.[2,12] Because of the low serum potassium, cardiac arrhythmias and ECG abnormalities may also occur.[3] Together these constitute what has been called pseudo(hyper)aldosteronism. Spironolactone will reverse these adverse effects.[3] Amenorrhea and hyperprolactemia (possibly resulting in infertility) have also been reported.[71,72]

Several deaths have resulted from the ingestion of licorice products.[3,73] Most often these adverse effects are caused by the consumption of large amounts of licorice candy and/or in those with pre-existing cardiovascular or renal impairment.[3,74] One much-quoted case of severe congestive heart failure and pulmonary edema occurred when a 53-year-old man ate 700 g of licorice candy over 8 days.[75] Another study reports on the successful treatment of a 63-year-old patient with severe postural hypotension.[76]

Chandler suggests that a maximum of 10 mg of glycyrrhizin (approximately 5 g of authentic licorice candy) can be safely consumed daily over long periods.[3] The Dutch Nutrition Information Bureau suggests that no more than 200 mg of glycyrrhizin should be consumed daily.[3]

Deglycyrrhizinated licorice (DGL) does not appear to cause the adverse effects described above.[3]

CAUTIONS/CONTRAINDICATIONS

Caution should be used in patients with high blood pressure or any other existing cardio-vascular disorders, renal failure, and liver disease.[3-5,12] Safety in pregnancy has been questioned.[3,4,12]

DRUG INTERACTIONS

Licorice may interfere with hormonal therapy or hypoglycemic therapy.[12] For example, Chandler hypothesizes that glycyrrhizin may combine with insulin to cause increased electrolyte disturbances.[3] Newall suggests that potential for interaction exists with any drugs with a narrow therapeutic index or mechanism of action dependent upon potassium levels (e.g., cardiac glycosides, loop diuretics and potassium-sparing diuretics).

Glycyrrhetinic acid increases the half-life of hydrocortisone applied topically,[77] and also potentiates the action of hydrocortisone in lung tissue.[78] There are also several reports that oral administration of glycyrrhizin inhibits the metabolism of prednisolone, thus increasing plasma concentrations.[79]

DGL (deglycyrrhizinated licorice) has been reported to increase the bioavailability of nitrofurantoin over 50% if they are administered together; however, it also appears to decrease feelings of nausea associated with nitrofurantoin ingestion.[3]

DOSAGE REGIMENS

❖ POWDERED ROOT: 1-4 g daily in three divided doses.[5,12]

❖ FLUID EXTRACT (1:1): 4-6 mL daily in three divided doses.

❖ SOLID (DRY POWDERED) EXTRACT (4:1): 250-500 mg daily in three divided doses.

❖ DEGLYCYRRHIZINATED LICORICE TABLETS: 380-1,140 mg (1-3 chewable tablets) three times daily.[5]

❖ LICORICE EXTRACT: 0.6-2 g daily.[12]

❖ DECOCTION: add 2-4 g (1 teaspoonful) of herb to 120 mL (1/2 cup) of boiling water and simmer for 5 minutes. Strain and drink this quantity three times daily after meals.[2]

❖ LOZENGES/CANDIES: as an expectorant and cough suppressant (make sure they actually contain real licorice).[2]

Note: Commission E has approved the indication for ulcer treatment (200-600 mg of glycyrrhizin daily) for a maximum of 4 to 6 weeks.[80]

Lobelia
Lobelia inflata L.

THUMBNAIL SKETCH

Common Uses
- ❖ Respiratory Conditions (such as bronchial asthma and bronchitis)
- ❖ Tobacco Addiction

Active Constituents
- ❖ Piperidine Alkaloids (notably (-)- lobeline)

Adverse Effects
- ❖ Nausea, Vomiting, Diarrhea
- ❖ Coughing and Dizziness
- ❖ Administration of high doses may result in more severe symptoms such as convulsions, hypothermia, coma and even death.

Cautions/Contraindications
- ❖ Nicotine (situations where nicotine is contraindicated)
- ❖ Cardiovascular and Respiratory Disease

Drug Interactions
- ❖ None found

Doses
- ❖ *Dried Herb:* 0.2-0.6 g three times daily
- ❖ *Liquid Extract* (1:1 in 50% alcohol): 0.2-0.6 mL three times daily

Note: Given its potential for adverse effects, it is questionable whether lobelia is appropriate for self-medication.

Introduction

Family
❖ Campanulaceae

Synonyms
❖ Indian tobacco
❖ Wild tobacco
❖ Asthma weed
❖ Gagroot
❖ Emetic herb
❖ Vomit wort
❖ Puke weed[1-4]

Medicinal Forms
❖ Dried Leaves
❖ Liquid Extract

Description
Lobelia is a hairy annual or biennial, indigenous to the western parts of North America, that is often found in acidic soils. The plant grows from 6-36 inches or 30-100 centimeters tall, with pale blue flowers and a milky sap. While *Lobelia inflata* L.[2] is the plant most common to herbal practice in North America and Western Europe, other members of this genus have a medicinal reputation in many other traditional healing models.[5] For example, in the Chinese Pharmacopoeia, *L. chinensis* Lour. is specified.[6]

Parts Used
The aerial parts are dried for use.

Traditional Use
Lobelia has a rather infamous medical history. This herb was used by peoples of the First Nations primarily for respiratory conditions and as an emetic. It later became popular among the early European settlers.[4,5] Lobelia was smoked in a similar fashion to tobacco, hence one of the synonyms, Indian tobacco.[5] The New England healer Samuel Thomson (1769-1843) used it as one of his primary botanical medicines, naming it 'Old #1.'[7] When one of his patients died after taking the herb, Thomson was charged with murder but later acquitted. Many still consider lobelia to be a poison rather than a medicine.[4]

Current Medicinal Use
As with its traditional use, lobelia is primarily used for respiratory conditions such as asthma and bronchitis. Lobelia and lobeline (a constituent found in lobelia) products are often used in treating tobacco addictions because lobeline is chemically similar to nicotine.

Relevant Research

Preventative and Therapeutic Effects

CONSTITUENTS [1, 2, 8, 9]

❖ ALKALOIDS: ≥14, notably of the piperidine type including (-)- lobeline (main one at 0.36-2.25% dry wt), lobelanine, norlobelanine, lobelanidine, norlobelanidine, lelobanidine, lobinine and isolobinine.
❖ MISCELLANEOUS: lobelacrin (a bitter glycoside), chelidonic acid, beta- amyrin palmitate, resins and gums.

TRADITIONAL USES

Lobelia is considered to have expectorant,[5] diaphoretic,[5,10] emetic,[5,10] antispasmodic,[5,10] sedative,[10] and respiratory stimulant properties.[5,10] It is primarily used for conditions of the respiratory tract, such as bronchial asthma and bronchitis.[5,10,11] Expectorant and decongestant drugs containing lobelia are available in Canada.[12] External applications of lobelia have been used to relieve muscle spasm and tension.[5] Indian tobacco is also used in the treatment of tobacco addition.[5] Commercial cigarette smoking deterrents containing lobelia herb are available in Canada[12] and Europe,[6] while the purified alkaloidal salts, lobeline hydrochloride or lobeline sulphate, are marketed for this purpose in several other countries (but not in Canada).[6,12] Its use as an emetic seems primarily to be an historical one.

MISCELLANEOUS EFFECTS

The medicinal action of lobelia appears to be primarily due to lobeline's nicotinic properties. The exact action of lobeline at the nicotine receptor site appears complex and novel.[13,14] Lobeline is known to cause stimulation of the central nervous system followed by severe respiratory depression. Administration in a number animal studies has resulted in bronchoconstriction, while bronchodilation was also reported in guinea pigs.[15] A proposed explanation for these differing results is that guinea pigs are particularlly sensitive to adrenergic bronchodilating agents.[15] Bronchodilation resulting from adrenal stimulation has also been reported.[16]

Animal studies suggest that lobeline acts as a cardiovascular stimulant, causing sympathetically mediated hypertension as well as parasympathetically mediated bradycardia.[17] Lobeline has also been shown to inhibit intestinal motility in dogs.[15] Vomiting commonly seen with lobeline use is centrally mediated.[16] An antidepressant action has been reported in mice following administration of beta-amyrin palmitate extracted from *Lobelia inflata* L.

A number of human clinical trials of lobeline, either alone or combined with other substances, have reported that it is effective in the treatment of tobacco addition.[18-21]

No clinical trials could be found in which the action of the herb lobelia, rather than the alkaloid lobeline, was investigated.

ADVERSE EFFECTS

Adverse effects are similar to those of nicotine and include nausea, vomiting, diarrhea, coughing and dizziness. Administration of high doses may result in more severe symptoms, such as convulsions, hypothermia, coma and even death.[1] Many practitioners comment that the plant's emetic properties limit the potential for serious adverse effects.[22] Tyler does not recommend use of the crude herb due to the lack of standardized products and the relatively high risk to benefit ratio.[23]

A case of death following inhalation of an herbal asthma product containing lobeline (together with stramonium) in a 48-year-old asthmatic female has been documented.[24] It should be noted that stramonium (*Datura stramonium* L., Solanaceae) is a plant rich in alkaloids with a very high potential for toxicity.

CAUTIONS/CONTRAINDICATIONS

Lobelia should be used with caution by patients with cardiovascular disease, respiratory conditions and where nicotine is contraindicated. It should be considered contraindicated in pregnancy and lactation.[1]

DRUG INTERACTIONS

No clinical cases of drug interactions could be found. Given the pharmacological action of lobeline, this herb should be used cautiously with conventional medication in general.

DOSAGE REGIMENS

❖ DRIED HERB: 0.2-0.6 g three times daily.[1]
❖ LIQUID EXTRACT (1:1 in 50% alcohol): 0.2-0.6 mL three times daily.[1]
  Note: Given its potential for adverse effects, it is questionable whether lobelia is appropriate for self-medication.

Ma Huang
Ephedra sinica Stapf.

Common Uses
❖ Respiratory Tract Diseases (including asthma and bronchitis)

Active Constituents
❖ Alkaloids (including ephedrine and pseudoephedrine)

Adverse Effects
❖ Dizziness and Headache
❖ Insomnia
❖ Decreased Appetite and Gastrointestinal Distress
❖ Tachycardia, Sweating, Hypertension
❖ Psychosis
❖ Stroke, Seizures and Death

Cautions/Contraindications
❖ Heart Disease, Hypertension, Thyroid Disease, Diabetes, Prostate Conditions, Anxiety, Glaucoma
❖ Impaired Cerebral Circulation, Pheochromocytoma, Thyrotoxicosis
❖ Pregnancy and Lactation

Drug Interactions
❖ Similar precautions should be applied as for conventional medicines containing ephedrine and pseudoephedrine, including anti-hypertensives and antidepressants.

Doses
❖ *Dried Herb:* Maximum: 8 mg of ephedrine every six hours up to a maximum of 24 mg per day for no more than 7 days

Note: It is highly questionable whether ma huang products containing appreciable amounts of alkaloids are appropriate for self-medication. Consultation with an appropriately trained healthcare provider is advisable.

Introduction

Family
- ❖ Ephedraceae

Synonyms
- ❖ Ephedra
- ❖ Chinese Ephedra
- ❖ Herba Ephedraa
- ❖ Cao mahuang[1,2]

Medicinal Forms
- ❖ Dried Stems
- ❖ Tincture

Description
Many members of the genus *Ephedra* are reputed to have medicinal properties. This monograph will concentrate primarily on ma huang, which is the one most often encountered in North America. Other members of this genus with medicinal applications include: *Ephedra intermedia* Shrenk ex C. A. Mey. (Intermediate ephedra), *Ephedra equisetina* Bunge (Mongolian ephedra), *Ephedra geradiana* Wallich ex Stapf (Pakistani ephedra) and *Ephedra nevadensis* S. Wats (Mormon tea).[1,3,4]

Ma huang is a fragrant perennial shrub growing to 20 inches or 50 centimeters, with long stems and tiny leaves, native to many parts of Asia.[5] It is one of the smallest members of the genus, with greenish herbaceous stems, producing small white flower-like cones.[1,5]

Parts Used
Usually the aerial parts of the plant, including the stems, are used medicinally.[1,6]

Traditional Use
Ma huang has a long medicinal history within Traditional Chinese Medicine, where it is used for a number of conditions, most notably of the respiratory system, including asthma, colds and coughs.[3,7] This herb, or more correctly one of the alkaloids found in it (ephedrine), was probably the first Traditional Chinese herbal product to receive acceptance in the West.[3] Ephedrine was first synthesized in the 1920s and has been used widely in cold and allergy remedies. Ephedra species native to North America, such as *Ephedra nevadensis* S. Wats, do not contain any alkaloids.[3]

Current Medicinal Use
While ephedrine has been shown to be effective in promoting weight loss, the potential for serious adverse effects makes it very questionable whether this is a legitimate use for ma huang. Within Traditional Chinese Medicine, under the supervision of an appropriately trained healthcare provider, ma huang is used for respiratory conditions, including asthma, allergies and bronchitis.

Relevant Research

Preventative and Therapeutic Effects

CONSTITUENTS [1,2,8-10]
- ❖ ALKALOIDS OF THE PROTOALKALOID CLASS: including (-)- ephedrine (L-ephedrine, major portion), (+)-pseudoephedrine, (+)- norpseudoephedrine, and (-)- norephedrine.
- ❖ TANNINS: catechin, gallic acid, condensed tannins.
- ❖ MISCELLANEOUS: including ephedrans (glycans), ephedradine, volatile oil and flavonoid Glycosides.

ROOTS ❖ macrocyclic spermine alkaloids (e.g. ephedradine) and L-tyrosine betaine (maokonine).

Note: The alkaloid content may vary from 0.5% to 2.5% (dry wt.), 30% to 90% of which is ephedrine, depending on the species.[10] *E. sinica* contains approximately 1.3% alkaloids, with ephedrine making up 60% of this amount.[1]

TRADITIONAL USES

As has already been mentioned, ma huang is considered an herb of particular importance within many Asian healing models.[1,7] Ma huang is considered to be particularly useful in the treatment of respiratory conditions associated with fever;[7,8] asthma;[4,7,8,11] allergic rhinitis;[6-8] and bronchitis.[6,8] It is also considered to be a stimulant and hypertensive agent.[6,7] Ma huang is often included in weight loss formulas because of its stimulant action.[4]

MEDICINAL ACTION

The alkaloids, especially ephedrine and pseudoephedrine, are the main constituents responsible for this plant's medicinal action. Ephedrine acts primarily in the periphery as an indirect adrenomimetic agent, causing an increased release of norepinephrine. While it has a longer duration of action than norepinephrine, its peripheral action is limited since tachyphylaxis occurs. It is less potent than norepinephrine but is effective after oral administration.[12]

Ephedrine and pseudoephedrine are known to cross the blood brain barrier resulting in a stimulant action.[1,12] Administration of ephedrine results in direct bronchodilation.[12] Pseudoephedrine appears to work in a similar manner but is generally considered less potent than ephedrine.[4]

Localized anti-inflammatory properties have been demonstrated for both ephedrine and pseudoephedrine in a number of animal models.[13]

RESPIRATORY SYSTEM ACTIVITY

As mentioned above, ephedrine has bronchodilating properties, causing prolonged relaxation of smooth muscles upon oral administration.[12] Constriction of the blood vessels in the mucosa of the respiratory system results in decreased mucous production, providing a decongestant action.[14] Health Canada has published a labeling standard for ephedra-containing products as nasal decongestants,[15] an indication for which approximately 20 ma huang products have been registered as non-prescription drugs. There are also 3 commercial products containing ma huang registered in Canada as vasoconstrictors, 7 as sympathomimetics, and 4 as homeopathic products.[16]

The presence of the 'drying' astringent tannins and aromatic volatile oils may also be playing a part in the treatment of bronchial asthma and bronchitis.[1,8] While ephedrine was once used to treat asthma, the fact that its action is selective to beta-2 adrenoreceptors is a significant disadvantage. It has now been superceded by more selective agents such as salbutamol/albuterol, which have fewer adverse effects.[17]

CARDIOVASCULAR EFFECTS

Administration of ephedrine results in vasoconstriction as well as increased systolic and diastolic blood pressure, force of cardiac contraction and cardiac output.[12,14] Pseudoephedrine appears to have a weaker hypertensive action than ephedrine.[1] A number of medical herbalists comment that the hypertensive action of plant extracts seem to be less pronounced that those seen with ephedrine alone.[8,18]

Paradoxically, parenteral administration of mahuangen (the roots of Ma huang) has been reported to cause vasodilation in a number of animal models.[1] A variable effect on blood pressure may be observed depending on the relative concentrations of hypotensive ephedradines (ganglionic blocking agents) versus hypertensive maokonine, due to phyto-chemical differences between the various *Ephedra* species.[10]

EFFECT ON OBESITY

A number of clinical studies have shown that supplementation with ephedrine, normally combined with other agents, can result in significant weight loss in both animals[18-20] and humans.[21-30] This action appears to be more pronounced when combined with other methylxanthines, notably caffeine and theophylline. Addition of aspirin to the protocol has been shown to potentiate this effect further.[31,32]

Ephedrine appears to act as a thermogenic agent, increasing the ability of the body to produce heat from food. It has been suggested that this action is deeply influenced by adrenoreceptor stimulation and that ephedrine can influence all the receptor sub-types. The increased action of ephedrine/methylxanthine and ephedrine/aspirin combinations over ephedrine alone could be due to inhibition of feed-back mechanisms.[33] The thermogenic action appears to be more pronounced with chronic administration.[34] Ephedrine also appears to reduce appetite.[34] The ephedrine/caffeine combination also seems to be protective against reducing HDL-cholesterol during weight loss.[35]

While ma huang may be of use in the treatment of obesity, there is no reason to believe that it will offer any preferential benefits over ephedrine alone. Obesity is not generally considered a traditional indication for ma huang and therefore there is no significant empirical evidence to support its use. Tyler comments that the both the safety and effectiveness of ma huang is open to debate (see Adverse Effects section).[3] Claims for use of ephedra-containing products as stimulants or diet aids for weight loss are not allowed by Health Canada under the Herbs and Natural Products drug category.[16]

ATHLETIC PERFORMANCE

In a review article, Clarkson and Thompson conclude that there is very little evidence to support the use of ephedrine or pseudoepherine to improve sporting performance. While some athletes may take ephedrine to reduce body fat and promote muscle mass, there is no evidence to support this indication in individuals who are not overweight. It should also be noted that products containing ephedrine or pseudoephedrine are prohibited by a number of sporting authorities.[36]

Most of the evidence purported to support the use of ma huang for the indications described above comes from work carried out using ephedrine or pseudoephedrine alone and not the herb ma huang. While a substantial amount of historical and empirical evidence exists regarding this herb's medicinal usefulness, it is primarily restricted to the treatment of asthma, bronchitis and conditions of the upper respiratory tract.

ADVERSE EFFECTS

Numerous concerns have been voiced regarding the increased popularity of 'natural' commercial products containing ma huang. These products include sports supplements, diet aids and products intended to induce euphoria and increase sensory acuity.[37,38] While consumption does provide central nervous system stimulation, high amounts can lead to hallucinations, paranoia, and psychosis.

A number of fatalities have resulted from consumption of these products in the United States.[39-42] A review designed to evaluate possible cardiovascular effects associated with ma huang found 926 cases of possible ma huang toxicity that were reported to the Food and Drug Administration (USA) from 1995 to 1997. The authors concluded that: "(1) ma huang use is temporally related to stroke, myocardial infarction, and sudden death; (2) underlying heart or vascular disease is not a prerequisite for ma huang-related adverse events; and (3) the cardiovascular toxic effects associated with ma huang were not limited to massive doses. Although the pathogensis of the cardio toxic effects of ma huang remains incompletely defined, available observational and circumstantial evidence indicates that use of the substance may be associated with serious medical complications."[43] In one case, a 23-year-old healthy male died of 'patchy myocardial necrosis' after taking a commercial product containing ma huang and caffeine for approximately 6 weeks. The individual appears to have followed the instructions appearing on the product label.[44]

Products containing ma huang intended for weight loss have been implicated in cases of both mania and psychosis.[45,46] Other adverse effects seen following consumption of ephedrine products include dizziness, headache, decreased appetite, gastrointestinal distress, irregular heart beat, tachycardia, sweating, insomnia, hypertension, stroke and seizures.[47-48]

In response to these concerns, Health Canada has warned consumers not to use products containing ma huang unless the product label carries a Drug Identification Number and the consumer follows strictly the dosage directions and precautions.[49] The Food and Drug Administration (FDA) of the United States has proposed that products containing ephedrine should contain no more than 8 mg per unit dose; daily intake should not exceed more than 24 mg; duration of treatment should be limited to a maximum of 7 days; proper contraindications should appear on labels; and ephedrine should not be combined with other stimulants such as caffeine.[47]

While another case exists of acute hepatitis resulting from administration of ma huang, given the lack of cases of hepatotoxicity associated with this botanical medicine, the authors conclude that an adulterant in the product was probably responsible rather than the ma huang itself.[50]

Concerns have also been expressed that prolonged administration of products containing ma huang may result in a 'weakening' of the adrenal gland. Subsequently some practitioners may combine it with 'adrenal tonics' such as licorice.[4]

DRUG INTERACTIONS
Concomitant administration with stimulants, any centrally acting medication such as antidepressants and anti-hypertensives should be avoided. It would seem prudent to apply the restrictions associated with ephedrine to that of ma huang. The action of ephedrine is known to be affected by antacids and agents which alter the pH (acidity) of the urine.[51] Ephedrine is also known to interact with corticosteroids and theophylline.[51] The German Commission E monograph further warns of possible interactions with cardiac glycosides or halothane, resulting in disturbance of heart rhythm: guanetjidine resulting in enhancement of the sympathomimetic effect; monoamine oxidase inhibitors resulting in greatly increased sympathomimetic action of the ephedrine; and secale alkaloid derivatives or oxytocin, resulting in development of hypertension.[52]

CAUTIONS/CONTRAINDICATIONS
Products containing ephedrine should not be taken by people suffering from heart disease; hypertension; thyroid disease; diabetes; conditions associated with enlarged prostate;[4] anxiety;[6] glaucoma; impaired circulation of the cerebrum; pheochromocytoma; or thyrotoxicosis.[52] Since ephedrine has uterostimulant properties, ma huang should be avoided in pregnancy and lactation.

DOSAGE REGIMENS
❖ DRIED HERB: FDA guidelines suggest a maximum dose of 8 mg of ephedrine every 6 hours up to 24 mg per day for no more than 7 days.
  Note: Given the above concerns, it is highly questionable whether ma huang products containing appreciable amounts of alkaloids are appropriate for self-medication. Consultation with an appropriately trained health-care provider is advisable.

Meadowsweet
Filipendula ulmaria (L.) Maxim

THUMBNAIL SKETCH

Common Uses
- ❖ Digestive Upset (including ulceration, dyspepsia and hyperacidity)
- ❖ Rheumatic Conditions and Pain

Active Constituents
- ❖ Salicylate-rich Volatile Oil
- ❖ Flavonoids
- ❖ Tannins

Adverse Effects
- ❖ None noted

Cautions/Contraindications
- ❖ Salicylates (classic ones applicable to salicylates in general, e.g., aspirin)

Drug Interactions
- ❖ Salicylates (classic ones applicable to salicylates in general, e.g., aspirin)

Doses
- ❖ *Dried Herb:* 4-6 g three times daily
- ❖ *Fluid Extract* (1:1 in 25% alcohol): 1.5-6.0 mL three times daily
- ❖ *Tincture* (1:5 in 45% alcohol): 2-4 mL three times daily

Introduction

Family
❖ Rosaceae

Synonyms
❖ Filipendula
❖ Queen of the Meadow
❖ *Spiraea ulmaria* L.
❖ Bridewort[1-3]

Medicinal Forms
❖ Dried Herb
❖ Fluid Extract
❖ Tincture

Description

Meadowsweet is a perennial native to Europe, growing 1.5 meters or 5 feet tall, with a thick, pink aromatic root and elongated stems leading to creamy white flowers that have a distinctive sweet almond scent. The English herbalist Gerard described the aroma produced by this plant with the following phrase, "for the smell thereof makes the heart merry, delighteth the senses; neither doth it cause headache, or loathsomeness to meat, as some other sweet smelling herbs do."[4] The term "Spiraea," used in a former binomial name, comes from the fact that the fruits have a twisted appearance.[3] Established growths of meadowsweet often completely dominate the marshy areas in which they grow, making another common name, Queen of the Meadow, very appropriate.[3]

Parts Used

The aerial parts of the plant (fresh flowering tops and leaves) are used medicinally.

Traditional Use

Salicylic acid was first extracted from the flowering buds of this medicinal herb. The term aspirin (acetylsalicylic acid) means "from Spiraea."[3] Meadowsweet was used to reduce inflammation and relieve pain, especially arthritis pain. It was also used as a remedy for indigestion and diarrhea, even in children.

Current Medicinal Use

As with its traditional uses, meadowsweet products are primarily used as analgesics in treating arthritic pain and for digestive upset and hyperacidity.

Relevant Research

Preventative and Therapeutic Effects

CONSTITUENTS [1,2,5-8]

❖ VOLATILE OILS: salicylates (including salicylaldehyde, gaultherin, salicin and salicylic acid), vanillin, benzaldehyde.
❖ FLAVONOIDS: rutin, hyperoside, spireoside and kaempferol.
❖ MISCELLANEOUS: hydrolysable tannins, coumarins, mucilage, ascorbic acid.

COMMON USES

Meadowsweet is considered by many herbalists to be an important medicinal herb for the management of conditions of the digestive system.[9] It is reputed to have a soothing and healing action and is frequently used to treat such conditions as hyperacidity,[9,10] indigestion,[9,10] peptic ulcer disease,[9,10] nausea,[9,10] and pediatric diarrhea.[1,9]

The other primary use of meadowsweet is as an analgesic and anti-inflammatory and it has been suggested that it is useful in the management of pain and rheumatic conditions.[1,9,11] It may also act as an antipyretic.[9] While these properties are generally considered to be due to the presence of salicylates in the volatile oil portion, these applications easily predate the identification of these components.

MISCELLANEOUS EFFECTS

Various extracts of meadowsweet have been reported to: lower vascular permeability; increase bronchial tone in cats; increase the bronchospasm induced by histamine in guinea pigs; increase tonus in vitro in guinea pig intestine and rabbit uterus; decrease rectal temperature; and potentiate narcotic action.[1,2,6] In addition, an anti-ulcer action has been noted in various animal models, especially with aqueous extracts of the flowers.[1,6,12] In contrast, the ulcerogenic nature of histamine was potentiated by an extract of meadowsweet in the guinea pig.[12]

Extracts of meadowsweet have also been shown to possess bactericidal and bacterostatic properties.[1,2] The flowers and seeds have been shown to exert an anticoagulant and fibrinolytic effect both in vitro and *in vivo*.[13] Topical administration of a decoction made from meadowsweet flowers has been shown to decrease the frequency of experimentally induced squamous cell carcinoma of the cervix and vagina in mice. Application of an ointment was shown to increase regression of cervical dysplasia in 32 patients.[14]

ADVERSE EFFECTS

No instances of adverse reactions could be found for this herb.

CAUTIONS/CONTRAINDICATIONS

Given the lack of objective information, the presence of salicylates and the fact that meadowsweet effects uterine smooth muscle *in vitro*, it has been suggested that meadowsweet should be avoided during pregnancy and lactation.[1] While no clinical examples could be found, it has been argued that the classic precautions applicable to salicylates in general are applicable to products containing meadowsweet. Consequently, it should be used with caution in individuals sensitive to aspirin, asthmatics, gout, diabetes, hemophilia, active peptic ulcer disease, hypoprothrombinemia, kidney and liver disease.[1] Although salicylates are generally considered contraindicated in patients with active peptic ulcer disease, it is important to balance this caution with the empirical uses mentioned previously.

DRUG INTERACTIONS

While no clinical examples could be found, there is every reason to believe that classic drug interactions with salicylates in general (e.g., concomitant oral anti-coagulants) are relevant here.[1]

DOSAGE REGIMENS [1,15]

❖ DRIED HERB: 4-6 g three times daily.
❖ FLUID EXTRACT (1:1 in 25% alcohol): 1.5-6.0 mL three times daily.
❖ TINCTURE (1:5 in 45% alcohol): 2-4 mL three times daily.
  Note: Meadowsweet is often combined with other 'digestive' herbs such as chamomile, licorice, marshmallow and peppermint. Many herbal painkillers also contain meadowsweet, often combined with black or white willow bark.

Milk Thistle
Silybum marianum (L.) Gaertner

THUMBNAIL SKETCH

Common Uses
* Liver Disorders (including hepatitis and cirrhosis)
* Psoriasis

Active Constituents
* Silymarin

Adverse Effects
* Very Rare — Diarrhea (mild)

Cautions/Contraindications
* Pregnancy and Lactation (safety not yet established)

Drug Interactions
* None known, but may affect the liver metabolism of some medications

Doses
* *Standardized Extract (70% silymarin):* 200 mg three times daily

Introduction

Description

Although milk thistle originally grew wild throughout much of Europe, it is now naturalized to the east coast of North America, California and South America.[1] This biennial grows up to 1 meter or 40 inches in height with spiny leaves that are marked with white along the veins.[2] The plant is crowned with a bright pink-to-red flower head that produces numerous small seeds.

Milk thistle is sometimes confused with Blessed thistle (*Cnicus benedictus* L., Asteraceae). Although they are members of the same botanical family, their medicinal actions are quite different.

Parts Used

The flowerheads, fruit, and seeds are used medicinally.

Traditional Use

The specific name "marianum" refers to the legend that the leaves have a white mottling because a drop of the Virgin Mary's milk landed on them. In keeping with this legend, milk thistle has traditionally been used as a galactogogue (i.e., to stimulate milk production in lactating women).[1] Fresh milk thistle flowerheads were boiled and eaten like artichokes as a spring tonic. The herb has also been used in treating jaundice and other liver-related conditions. Milk thistle has been used medicinally for several thousand years. Both the Greeks and the Romans noted its hepatoprotective effects; however, current interest in this product did not begin until the late 1960s when silymarin, a combination of flavonolignans believed to be responsible for the hepatic activity, was first isolated from the ripe seeds.[1]

Current Medicinal Use

Milk thistle is primarily used for its hepato-protective properties. While more evidence is needed, results from clinical trials using standardized extracts of milk thistle are promising, suggesting that it may be useful in protecting the liver from environmental toxins and drugs (e.g., acetaminophen). It may also be useful in cases of hepatitis and cirrhosis.

Relevant Research

Preventative and Therapeutic Effect

CONSTITUENTS [1,3,4]

❖ FLAVONOLIGNANS: including silybin (silibin), silydianin (silidianin), silychristin (silichristin).

❖ MISCELLANEOUS: apigenin, silbonol, fatty acids.

Note: Silymarin, the component to which most milk thistle products are standardized, is a mixture of silybin, silydianin and silychristin

MEDICINAL ACTION

Silymarin, the active constituent isolated from the ripe seeds of milk thistle, has been extensively studied. Its actions on the liver are believed to result from three primary mechanisms of action:[1,5-7]

1. Stimulation of RNA polymerase A (also known as polymerase I) and DNA synthesis.[3,8,9] Silybin stimulates this enzyme which in turn increases the synthesis of ribosome proteins and thus stimulates cell development, ultimately increasing the regenerative capacity of the liver.

2. Competitive binding with some toxins.[3] Silymarin appears to compete with alpha-amanitin and phalloidin (two toxins from the deathcap mushroom) for a receptor on the cell membrane.

3. Anti-oxidant action via increasing hepatic contents of glutathione (both oxidized and reduced).[3,10-15] Glutathione is a powerful antioxidant which detoxifies a wide variety of substances in the liver, stomach and intestines; silymarin is reported to be a 10x stronger anti-oxidant than vitamin E; it may also increase the enzyme superoxide dismutase (SOD).[16]

Other mechanisms of action which have been hypothesized include: inhibition of lipoxygenase, which catalyses a reaction between polyunsaturated fatty acids and oxygen to produce leukotrienes which may cause liver damage;[17] inhibition of neutrophil function;[18] and inhibition of Kupffer cell functions.[19]

HEPATO-PROTECTIVE ACTIVITY

Currently, milk thistle is known primarily for its ability to protect the liver from damage and to restore its function following damage. Tyler feels that animal studies have "shown conclusively that silymarin exerts a liver protective effect against a variety of toxins ...[and] human trials have also been encouraging for conditions including hepatitis and cirrhosis."[20] In addition, the German Commission E has approved milk thistle as supportive treatment of cirrhosis and chronic inflammatory liver conditions.[21] A systematic review and meta-analysis to determine the efficacy and safety of milk thistle as a treatment of liver disease found 14 clinical trials which met their inclusion criteria. The authors concluded that although milk thistle appears to be safe and well-tolerated, there was no reduction in the death rate, improvement of biochemical markers assessed by liver function tests or changes in the liver as assessed by biopsy among patients with chronic liver disease who ingested milk thistle compared to placebo. However, the information available was too limited to exclude any substantial benefit or harm associated with milk thistle.[22]

Protection from Chemical Toxins

A variety of animal studies have demonstrated the ability of milk thistle preparations to protect the liver from a variety of toxins, including alpha-amanitin and phalloidin (both from the extremely poisonous Deathcap mushroom);[3,23-26] carbon tetrachloride; thioacetamide; DL-ethionine;[3] and acetaminophen.[15] In addition, silymarin has been shown to provide significant protection to animals against liver damage typically caused by ethyl alcohol.[3] One double-blind, placebo-controlled trial of "toxic liver damage" (alcohol in most cases) in 33 patients reported that AST, and ALT values were all significantly improved in the silymarin group in comparison with the control group.[3] This was confirmed in a second double-blind, placebo-controlled study of 106 patients with mild liver disease (most caused by alcohol). AST, and ALT serum levels were significantly improved in the group who took 420 mg of silymarin daily when compared with the controls and there was a positive trend in the concentrations of total and conjugated serum bilirubins in the silymarin group when compared with the control group. Due to the outpatient setting, alcohol consumption was not monitored in this study.[27]

Another double-blind, placebo-controlled trial (n=60) investigated the effect of silymarin in patients who were suffering from hepatotoxicity due to long term treatment with phenothiazines or butyrophenones. All patients taking silymarin (800 mg daily) were reported to have significantly decreased serum levels of malondialdehyde (MDA). Those who stopped taking their psychotropics during the 90 day study experienced the most pronounced, decrease; however, those continuing on their psychotropic medication also experienced a decrease which was significant in comparison to the placebo group.[28]

Hepatitis

A variety of studies report the effectiveness of silymarin in treating both acute and chronic hepatitis.[3,29,30] One double-blind, placebo-controlled study of patients with acute viral hepatitis (n=28) found that the group taking silymarin had significantly better bilirubin and AST values and a trend toward better ALT values than the control group.[3] Another double-blind, placebo-controlled trial with 20 patients suffering from chronic hepatic diseases showed that silymarin significantly improved seralbumin as well as improving the histopathological outcomes measured including focal necrosis and fibrosis when compared with the placebo group.[3] A more recent double-blind, placebo-controlled study of 20 patients with chronic viral hepatitis reported that those taking silybin-phosphatidylcholine (IdB1016) (two capsules twice daily which was the equivalent of 240 mg of silibinin) experienced significant decreases in AST, ALT and GGT when compared with the levels of the control group.[29] However, two other double-blind, placebo-controlled studies in patients with chronic hepatitis (n=24 and n=12) found no significant difference between the silymarin and placebo groups.[3] To date the majority of clinical trials have tested i.v. silymarin. The applicability of these findings to the ingestion of oral silymarin has been questioned.

Cirrhosis

A double-blind, placebo-controlled trial of 170 individuals with cirrhosis of the liver reported that those taking silymarin (200 mg of milk thistle standardized to 70% silymarin three times daily) had a significantly lower mortality rate over the 2 years of the study period and an additional 2 years of follow-up. Patients with mild alcohol-induced cirrhosis appeared to have received the most benefit from the silymarin treatment. No significant difference in serum concentrations of liver enzymes were noted between the two groups.[31] While these results appear promising, results from another randomised, double-blind, placebo-controlled study that assessed the effects of silymarin (450 mg daily in three divided doses) in 200 patients identified as alcoholics with liver cirrhosis were not as promising. In this study, silymarin did not have any significant effect on the course of the disease, nor on survival during the two year study period.[32] Additional research in this area is required.

Psoriasis

Some researchers have suggested that milk thistle may also be useful in the management of psoriasis. This may be secondary to its ability to improve liver function or directly due to its ability to decrease leukotriene synthesis by inhibiting lipoxygenase.[2,33]

ADVERSE EFFECTS

Adverse effects of silymarin appear to be very rare. Because it increases bile flow, it may cause mild diarrhea in some individuals.[2,5,20] There is one case report of a 57-year-old woman who presented with a two-month history of intermittent episodes of sweating, nausea, colicky abdominal pain, fluid diarrhea, vomiting, weakness and collapse with episodes lasting up to 24 hours. It appears that the herbal product was responsible for these effects since they stopped when the therapy was ended and returned quite violently when the milk thistle was started again.[34]

CAUTIONS/CONTRAINDICATIONS

Long-term safety and safety in pregnant and lactating women has not been established to date.

DRUG INTERACTIONS

Although no drug interactions could be found in our review of the literature, theoretically the fact that milk thistle increases liver function suggests that it may influence the metabolism of some medications. An open-label study investigating the effect of co-administration of milk thistle and inidinavir (a drug found to interact with other herbal medicines) reported no effect on overall exposure of indinavir. The authors concluded that milk thistle should not interfere with indinavir therapy in patients infected with HIV.[35]

DOSAGE REGIMENS

❖ STANDARDIZED EXTRACT (70% silymarin): 200 mg three times daily.[5]

Note: Most products on the Canadian market are standardized to 70% silymarin content; thus, a 200 mg tablet contains 140 mg of silymarin. Silymarin is not very water soluble; thus, this herb should not be taken as a 'tea'.[20]

Nettle

Urtica dioica L., *U. urens* L.

Common Uses

Leaf

- ❖ Rheumatism and Gout
- ❖ Hay Fever
- ❖ Nutritive Supplement

Root

- ❖ Micturition Disorders (associated with benign prostatic hyperplasia)

Active Constituents

Leaf

- ❖ Flavonoids
- ❖ Amines
- ❖ Carboxylic Acids (in stinging hairs)

Root

- ❖ Sterols
- ❖ Lectins

Adverse Effects

- ❖ Skin Irritation
- ❖ Gastric Distress

Cautions/Contraindications

- ❖ Pregnancy (safety not established)

Drug Interactions

- ❖ Root should be used with caution in cases of concomitant administration with conventional anti-hypertensives, diabetes and diuretic medication.

Doses

Aerial Parts

- ❖ *Dried Herb* (normally as an infusion): 3-6 g three times daily
- ❖ *Liquid Extract* (1:1 in 25% alcohol): 3-4 mL three times daily
- ❖ *Tincture* (1:5 in 45% alcohol): 2-6 mL of three times daily

Root

- ❖ *Dried Root:* 4-6 g daily
- ❖ *Liquid Extract* (1:1 in 45% ethanol): 1.5-7.5 mL daily
- ❖ *Tincture* (1:5 in 40% ethanol): 5 mL of daily

Introduction

Family
❖ Urticaceae

Synonyms
❖ Stinging nettle
❖ Urtica
❖ Common nettle (*Urtica dioica* L.)
❖ Small nettle
❖ (*Urtica urens* L.)[1-3]

Medicinal Forms
DRIED LEAVES
❖ Liquid Extract
❖ Tincture
DRIED ROOT
❖ Fluid Extract
❖ Tincture

Description

Nettle is a perennial standing up to 1.5 meters or 60 inches in height, with lanced leaves and green and yellow flowers. Different members of the genus *Urtica* grow naturally throughout most of Europe and North America.

Parts Used

The aerial parts and the roots/rhizomes of two species, *U.dioica* L. and *U. urens* L., are used medicinally.[4-6]

Traditional Use

Nettle has been used in cleansing tonics, teas and soups for detoxification, skin conditions, and allergies. While it has enjoyed a long medicinal history in many different models of traditional herbalism, it is considered by many members of the public to be a noxious weed, causing a characteristic pruritic rash on contact with the skin. Stinging nettle is also a common homeopathic remedy.[3]

Current Medicinal Use

The use of nettle depends on the part of the plant used. Products made from the leaf are primarily used to treat arthritic conditions, such as a gout, and hayfever. A growing amount of scientific research suggests that nettle root, either alone or with other herbal medicines, may be useful in treating benign prostatic hypertrophy (enlargement of the prostate gland).

Relevant Research

Preventative and Therapeutic Effects

CONSTITUENTS

Leaf[1,2,5,7-9]

❖ AMINES: histamine, choline, acetylcholine, serotonin, etc. (especially in stinging hairs).
❖ FLAVONOIDS: including isoquercetin, rutin, kaempferol and quercetin.
❖ MINERALS: including calcium, potassium, iron and silicon.
❖ ACIDS: including silicic acid, malic acid, carbonic acid and formic acid.
❖ MISCELLANEOUS: sitosterol, glycoprotein, high levels of chlorophyll, tannins.

Roots[2,4,10,11]

❖ LECTINS: Urtica dioica agglutinin (separated into 6 isolectins).
❖ STEROLS (AND THEIR GLUCOSIDES): including 3-beta-sitosterol and sitosterol −3-D-glucoside.
❖ MISCELLANEOUS: including lignans, various fatty acids and scopoletin.

COMMON USES

Within the traditional herbal medicine paradigm, nettle leaves are considered very nutritive and consequently they are often used in situations of convalescence and recuperation.[1] They are also used to aid milk production in nursing mothers.[1] In addition, nettle is used for its astringent properties in the treatment of bleeding conditions such as wounds, hemorrhoids and even uterine hemorrhage.[1,12]

GENITOURINARY TRACT EFFECTS

Stinging nettle root has become one the major phytomedicines used in the management of benign prostatic hyperplasia (BPH), especially in Europe.[13,14] It can be taken alone, but is more commonly administered with other phytomedicines used in the management of BPH such as *Serenoa repens* (Bartr.) Small, *Arecaceae/Palmae* (Saw Palmetto) and *Prunus africana* (Hook. F.) Kalkman, Rosaceae (African Pygeum).[15,16] The European Scientific Cooperative on Phytotherapy (ESCOP) lists the symptomatic treatment of micturition disorders (nocturia, pollakisuria, dysuria, urine retention) in benign prostatic hyperplasia as one of the indications for stinging nettle root.[4]

BENIGN PROSTATIC HYPERPLASIA (BPH)

Preparations made primarily from the roots of *Urtica dioica* L. have been shown *in vitro* and *in vivo* to affect many aspects of prostate physiology thought to be implicated in BPH. These include: inhibition of sex hormone-binding globulin (SHBG) to human prostatic tissue; possible suppression of prostate cell metabolism and growth; and weak inhibition of aromatase activity.[4,17] A number of human studies and clinical trials have demonstrated the therapeutic benefit of nettle root in the management of BPH. A more detailed review of these trials, which are primarily published in German, has been published in the ESCOP Urtica radix fascicule. In general, the clinical trials lasted between 9 weeks and 6 months.[4] A randomized, double-blind clinical trial published after that review compared the effects of a fixed combination of extracts of saw palmetto and nettle root (PRO 160/120®) or finasteride. The results of the study indicated that PRO 160/120® was equally as effective as finasteride regardless of prostate volume and that patients tolerated PRO 160/120® better.[18] Since saw palmetto has been found to be as effective as finasteride in other studies,[19] it is unclear how much nettle contributed to the effects noted in this trial. It has been suggested that the inclusion of the relatively inexpensive nettle root with more expensive phytomedicines used in the treatment of BPH may form a very cost effective method of treatment.[20]

MUSCULOSKELETAL CONDITIONS

Oral preparations made from nettle leaf have long been used in the management of various arthritic conditions, including rheumatism and gout.[1,6] It has been suggested that the nettle leaf could have a diuretic effect, resulting in an increased elimination of 'toxins' such as uric acid.[1,6] The localized irritation resulting from topical application of the stinging leaves of this plant is also reputed to be beneficial.[6]

In vitro trials have demonstrated that an hydroalcoholic preparation of the leaves of *Urtica dioica* possesses anti-inflammatory properties. The mechanism of action proposed is that it influences the synthesis of leukotrienes and cyclo-oxygenase derived prostaglandins.[5] It was also reported to decrease the production of a number of inflammatory related cytokines in whole human blood.[21]

An open randomized pilot study of patients (n=40) suffering from acute arthritis compared the effectiveness of stewed *Urtica dioica* L. leaves (50 g daily) plus diclofenac (50 mg daily) to a larger daily dose of diclofenac (200 mg). Both treatments were administered for 14 days. The drug/herb combination was found to be as effective as the higher dose of NSAID in decreasing elevated acute phase protein concentrations and relieving the clinical arthritic symptoms. The authors concluded that the action of diclofenac was potentiated by nettle leaves.[22] Although this may seem promising, it was only a pilot study and some criticism has been made regarding the research design.[23]

Another randomized, placebo-controlled, double-blind crossover trial in 27 patients with osteoarthritic pain at the base of the thumb or index finger investigated the effects of daily topical application of stinging nettle leaf. The placebo used in this trial was white deadnettle leaf. After one week of treatment, score reductions on both the pain visual analogue scale and a disability health assessment questionnaire were significantly greater in the nettle group than in the placebo group.[24]

EFFECT ON HAYFEVER

In a double-blind randomized study, the anti-allergic action of a freeze-dried preparation of *Urtica dioica* was compared to placebo. The study was carried out during the peak season for allergic rhinitis. Volunteers (n=98) were assigned to the treatment (300 mg capsules of freeze-dried *Urtica dioica*) or the placebo group and were advised to take two capsules at the onset of the symptoms of allergic rhinitis. Assessment was made by comparing diary symptoms and global response at a follow-up appointment after one week of therapy. Stinging nettle was rated higher than placebo according to the global assessment and slightly higher according to patient diary ratings.[25]

MISCELLANEOUS EFFFECTS

In vitro trials have demonstrated that nettle leaves have diuretic, hypotensive, hyperglycemic, central nervous system depressant and analgesic action.[2,5] The implication of these findings to clinical practice has not yet been elucidated. In an open study, administration of 15 mL of nettle herb juice was shown to significantly increase the volume of urine excreted by 32 patients suffering from myocardial or chronic venous insufficiency.[5]

ADVERSE EFFECTS

Adverse effects following oral consumption of products containing nettle seem rare. Instances of scanty urination, skin irritation and gastric distress have been noted.[2,4]

CAUTIONS/CONTRAINDICATIONS

No safety details exist regarding the use of this phytomedicine in pregnancy. Significant contraction of pregnant mouse uterine muscle has been reported *in vitro*.[2,5]

DRUG INTERACTIONS

No specific cases of drug interactions could be found. Given the information from *in vitro* and *in vivo* studies, caution is advisable in cases of concomitant administration with conventional anti-hypertensive, diabetes and diuretic medications.[2]

DOSAGE REGIMENS

Aerial Parts [2,26]

❖ DRIED HERB (NORMALLY AS AN INFUSION): 3-6 g three times daily.
❖ LIQUID EXTRACT (1:1 in 25% alcohol): 3-4 mL three times daily.
❖ TINCTURE (1:5 in 45% alcohol): 2-6 mL three times daily.

Root [4]

❖ DRIED ROOT: 4-6 g daily.
❖ FLUID EXTRACT (1:1 in 45% ethanol): 1.5-7.5 mL daily.
❖ TINCTURE (1:5 in 40% ethanol): 5 mL daily.

Passionflower
Passiflora incarnata L.

THUMBNAIL SKETCH

Common Uses
❖ Restlessness, Tension, Insomnia

Active Constituents
❖ Flavonoids
❖ Alkaloids

Adverse Effects
❖ Sedation

Cautions/Contraindications
❖ Pregnancy and Lactation

Drug Interactions
❖ Potential exists for interactions with concomitant administration of centrally acting medications

Doses
❖ *Dried Herb:* 0.25-1.0 g three times daily
❖ *Liquid Extract* (1:1 in 25% alcohol): 0.5-2.0 mL three times daily
❖ *Tincture* (1:8 in 45% alcohol): 2-4 mL three times daily

Introduction

Family
- ❖ Passifloraceae

Synonyms
- ❖ Maypop
- ❖ Maypop passion flower
- ❖ Passiflora
- ❖ Apricot vine
- ❖ Wild passion flower
- ❖ Passion vine
- ❖ Grenadille[1,2]

Medicinal Forms
- ❖ Dried Herb
- ❖ Liquid Extracts

Description

Passionflower is a perennial climbing vine growing up to 9 meters or 30 feet in length, native to the southern United States. The vine has clusters of three leaves, purple-to-red flowers, and oblong fruit. Other members of the genus *Passiflora* are found throughout North, South and Central America.[1] The name arises from the plant's intricate and elaborate flower that blooms only for a maximum of 48 hours.[3] The flower parts are thought to represent the elements of Christ's Passion. For example, the fringe-like crown is said to represent the crown of thorns, while the five anthers represent the five stigmata. 'Passio' means suffering and 'incarnata' means incarnate.[3]

Parts Used

The part used medicinally is the leaf.

Traditional Use

Passionflower was used within many traditional healing models in America. For example, the Aztecs prized it as a sedative.[4] Modern phytotherapy has expanded upon these historical uses. In addition, passionflower has been used for similar indications within the homeopathic tradition.[3] While many species of Passiflora produce edible fruits, the ones commonly available are not from *P. incarnata* but rather *P. edulis* Sims.[3]

Current Medicinal Use

Passionflower products are now used primary to treat conditions associated with nervous tension, restlessness, irritability and insomnia.

Relevant Research

Preventative and Therapeutic Effects

CONSTITUENTS [1,2,4-11]

- ❖ FLAVONOIDS: including vitexin, isovitexin, vitexin-4-O-rhamnoside, rutin, quercetin, kaempferol, apigenin and luteolins (orientin, homoorientin and lucenin).
- ❖ ALKALOIDS: including harman, harmalin, harmalol and harmine (referred to in some texts as harmala alkaloids).
- ❖ MISCELLANEOUS: maltol, fatty acids, sugars and gum.

COMMON USES

Passionflower is reputed to have hypnotic;[4,12,13] sedative;[4,12-14] anodyne (analgesic);[4,12] and anti-spasmodic properties.[4,12] The ESCOP monograph lists therapeutic indications of "tenseness, restlessness and irritability with difficulty in falling asleep."[11] In addition, the French and Swiss herbal pharmacopoeia indicate that it is useful in the management of mild heart conditions.[3] It is thought to be particularly useful in individuals that are weak or exhausted whether from overwork, illness or age.[4] A number of references mention its use in conditions of hysteria and convulsions.[4,12]

MECHANISM OF ACTION

It was initially thought that the harmala alkaloids were the primary active constituents;[3,13] however, it has since been shown that they are present only in trace amounts.[3,4] Another theory is that the medicinal effects may be due at least in part to maltol, which has been shown to have physiological activity in animal models.[15] However, other researchers have argued that maltol may not be present in the original plant, but is formed during the heat extraction processes.[3] While it is likely that no one group of constituents is solely responsible for this plant's medicinal action, it appears that the flavonoid components are the ones of most importance.[3]

CENTRAL NERVOUS SYSTEM EFFECTS

Psychotropic, sedative and anxiolytic properties have been demonstrated following the administration of very large doses of extracts of *P. incarnata* L. in a number of animal models.[3,11,16-18] These actions appear to be influenced by the solvent used in the extraction process.[16] Anxiolytic properties are reported to be evident at lower doses with sedation occurring on administration of larger amounts.[17]

Other studies have reported conflicting findings to those mentioned above.[11] Chrysin, a monoflavonoid found in a related species (*P. caerulea* L.), has been shown to exert an anxiolytic action in mice with no subsequent sedation or muscle relaxation. The authors hypothesize that this could be due to its action as a partial antagonist of the central benzodiazepine receptors.[19] An increase in the nociceptive threshold and reduction in locomotor activity have been noted in rats following administration of an hydroalcoholic extract of *P. incarnata* L (160 mg/kg).[18]

A randomized, double-blind pilot study (n=36) that was designed to compare the efficacy of passion flower (Passiflora® extract 45 drops/day) with oxazepam (30 mg daily) for 4 weeks in the treatment of generalized anxiety disorder reported that both passion flower and oxazepam were effective in treating the patients' symptoms, with no difference between the protocols at the end of the study. Oxazepam appeared to have a more rapid onset of action, but was also associated with significantly more problems relating to impairment of job performance. While the results are promising, a large-scale trial of passionflower is needed before any definitive conclusions can be drawn.[20] Another multi-centered, double-blind study (n=182) demonstrated that a commercial product containing passionflower (Euphytose®), was significantly beneficial when compared to placebo in the management of adjustment disorder with anxious mood. The product was given at a dose of two tablets three times daily for 28 days.[21] The impact of passionflower on this outcome is unknown since Euphytose® contains a number of centrally acting phytomedicines, including valerian (*Valeriana officinalis* L. (Valerianaceae)).

Finally, a randomized, double-blind controlled study compared the effects of clonidine (0.8 mg daily) plus passionflower (60 drops of Passiflora® extract daily) with clonidine plus placebo in the outpatient detoxification of 65 opiates addicts over a 2-week period. Both protocols were found to be equally effective in treating the physical symptoms of withdrawal and the group that received passionflower in addition to clonidine scored significantly better with respect to their mental symptoms.[22] While these results are promising, a larger study is necessary to confirm these findings.

CARDIAC EFFECTS

The evidence supporting the action of passionflower in the treatment of cardiac conditions appears to come from the presence of C-glycosylflavones. These agents (e.g. vitexin, isovitexin) extracted from another plant, hawthorn (*Cratageus monogyna* Jacq., Rosaceae), have been shown to be clinically beneficial in the management of a number of cardiac conditions.[23] Newall makes reference to a randomized, placebo-controlled clinical trial of patients suffering from congestive heart failure (n=42) following administration of a hawthorn/passionflower product (standardized to flavonoid content). While improvement was noted using a number of outcome measures, the importance of the passionflower in the product is not known. Although a hypotensive action from passionflower has been noted *in vivo*,[1] concerns have been raised regarding the lack of clinically relevant information available for this herbal product given its widespread use.[3,24]

ADVERSE EFFECTS

A case of hypersensitivity vasculitis was noted in a 77-year-old man suffering from rheumatoid arthritis following administration of a herbal product in which 'Passiflora extract' was the primary ingredient. The patient had been taking conventional medication (diclofenac and cyclopenthiazide) for a period of 5 years and was applying a placebo gel as part of a clinical trial. The authors conclude that the herbal product was the most likely culprit and make reference to another case reported to the CSM (Committee on Safety of Medicines). No reference is made as to whether the authenticity of the product was confirmed.[25] In addition 'altered consciousness' was reported in five people resulting from the consumption of a commercial product made primarily from the fruit of *P. incarnata* L. (Relaxir®). Once again, no information is available as to whether attempts were made to authenticate the product.[26]

Another case report describes a 34-year-old female who developed severe nausea, vomiting, drowsiness, prolonged QT_c, and episodes of nonsustained ventricular tachycardia following self administration of passionflower (Sedacalm®, 500 mg). Upon cessation of the passionflower product, her symptoms resolved and did not return. A sample of the product ingested was analyzed and found to contain passionflower. The mechanism for the adverse effects experienced by this patient is unclear.[27]

CAUTIONS/CONTRAINDICATIONS

Excessive use should be avoided during pregnancy and lactation.[2] Passionflower may cause sedation and inhibit the ability to drive or use heavy machinery.[11] No reference could be found regarding the influence of alcohol.

Concerns have been raised because harmala alkaloids found in other plants have been shown to act as monoamine oxidase inhibitors (MAOI). Given the small amounts present in *P. incarnata* L., it is unlikely that this will require the restrictions applied to conventional MAOI therapy.[4]

DRUG INTERACTIONS

Passionflower extracts have been shown to increase the sleeping time induced by pentobarbital or hexabarbital in a number of animal models.[15-18] Extracts of passionflower have also be shown to offer protection against convulsions induced by pentylenetetrazole in mice.[15-18] The clinical relevance of these findings is unknown since the evidence comes solely from animal models and the doses and modes of administration are not generally comparable to those seen in clinical practice. Until more is known, it would be prudent to be cautious when administering products containing this herb concurrently with centrally acting conventional medications.

DOSAGE REGIMENS[2,28]

- ❖ DRIED HERB: 0.25-1.0 g (can be taken as an infusion) three times daily.
- ❖ LIQUID EXTRACT (1:1 in 25% alcohol): 0.5 -2.0 mL three times daily.
- ❖ TINCTURE (1:8 in 45% alcohol): 2-4 mL three times daily.
  Note: A number of references note that passionflower is rarely given as a single remedy but rather combined with other phytomedicines determined by the indication.[3,4] Since the constituents responsible for the reputed therapeutic action of passionflower have yet to be conclusively determined, Bergner advises against the use of standardized extracts.[4]

Peppermint
Mentha x piperita L.

THUMBNAIL SKETCH

Common Uses
- ❖ Irritable Bowel Disease
- ❖ Spastic Colon
- ❖ Colonoscopy and Barium Enema Adjunctive Therapy
- ❖ Gastritis
- ❖ Dyspepsia

Active Constituents
- ❖ Menthol (and its derivatives)

Adverse Effects
- ❖ Rare — Heartburn, Esophageal Reflux, Contact Irritation (when used as flavoring agent in oral products)

Cautions/Contraindications
- ❖ Infants and Young Children
- ❖ Achlorhydria

Drug Interactions
- ❖ None known

Doses
- ❖ *Tea:* 1.5 g (1 tablespoonful) of recently dried leaves taken on an empty stomach three to four times daily to relieve upset stomach
- ❖ *Enteric Coated Peppermint Oil Capsules:* 1-3 capsules three times daily away from meals
- ❖ *Tincture* (1:5 in 45% ethanol): 2-3 mL three times daily away from meals

Introduction

Family

❖ Laminaceae (also known as Labiatae)

Synonyms

A number of varieties exist, including:

❖ *M. x piperita* L. var *vulgaris* Sole (Black Mint)

❖ *M. x piperita* L. var *officinalis* Sole (White Mint)[1]

Medicinal Forms

❖ Enteric Coated Tablets (Peppermint Oil)

❖ Dried Herb

❖ Tincture

Description

Peppermint (*Mentha x piperita* L.), once thought to be a unique species, is now considered a hybrid of two other members of the mint family: water mint (*Mentha aquatica* L.) and spearmint (*Mentha spicata* L.).[2,3] Although it is native to Europe, peppermint is now an important aromatic/medicinal crop grown throughout North American temperate zones, especially in the states of Indiana, Wisconsin, Oregon, Washington and Idaho. This perennial grows to a height of approximately 1 meter or 40 inches, spreads by surface runners, and has pink-to-purple flowers.[4] In addition, it has a square stem characteristic of all members of the mint family.[5]

Parts Used

The leaf, as an infusion and as an essential oil, is the part used medicinally.

Traditional Use

Both the peppermint leaf, often taken as a tea, and the essential oil, which is distilled from the leaves, have a long history of medicinal use. Peppermint is considered a carminitive.[6-8] Peppermint leaf tea has been used for indigestion, nausea, diarrhea, colds, headache and cramps.[4,9] The most common use of peppermint oil today is as a flavoring agent in a variety of oral products, including toothpastes, chewing gum and after-dinner mints.[4,6,10] This review will primarily deal with the use of peppermint when taken orally or applied topically and not on its use as an aromatherapy agent.

Current Medicinal Use

Peppermint is now primarily used for its digestive actions in the treatment of such conditions as irritable bowel syndrome and indigestion. It is also used in the management of nausea.

Relevant Research

Preventative and Therapeutic Effects

CONSTITUENTS [4,6,9]

❖ VOLATILE OIL: (-)-menthol and its esters (acetate and isovalerate), (+)- and (-)-menthone, (+)-isomenthone, (+)-neomethone, (+)-menthofuran, eucalyptol, (-)-limonene.

❖ MISCELLANEOUS: flavonoids, phytol, tocopherols, carotenoids, betain, choline, azulenes, rosmarinic acid, tannins.

Note: 1-Menthol makes up 29-48% of the essential oil, but is considered to be a distinctly different agent, not to be confused with the volatile oil of peppermint.[4] Although menthol can be obtained from peppermint oil, the high price of peppermint oil makes this use very uncommon. Today, menthol is usually produced synthetically by the hydrogenation of thymol. Synthetic menthol differs from that produced from peppermint in that it is racemic.

COMMON USES

Peppermint is reputed to have anti-spasmodic, carminative, anti-emetic, diaphoretic, hepatic and anti-septic properties.[1,3,11] As with all carminatives, oral consumption is considered useful in the treatment of many digestive disorders especially nausea, vomiting, bloating, nervous bowel and indigestion.[11,12] It is also commonly used to treat colds and flus.[11]

GASTROINTESTINAL EFFECTS

According to a 1990 study of a variety of over-the-counter (OTC) products conducted by the Food and Drug Administration (FDA) in the United States, there is not sufficient evidence to demonstrate that peppermint oil is effective as a digestive aid. However, this conclusion was based solely on evidence submitted by the manufacturers of the OTC products being reviewed.[13] Tyler heavily criticizes this review.[6] In contrast, the German Commission E's review of the scientific literature has concluded that there is sufficient evidence to demonstrate that peppermint and its volatile oil are effective spasmolytics, and that they promote gastric secretions and the flow of bile.[14]

Several studies have found that in order for peppermint oil to alleviate effectively the symptoms of a variety of bowel conditions, including irritable bowel and spastic colon, the oil must reach the colon in its original state (i.e., unmetabolized state). Thus, most peppermint oil products sold for this purpose in Canada are enteric-coated. Gelatin-coated capsules release the peppermint oil in the stomach where it is metabolized before reaching the colon.[15]

Irritable Bowel Syndrome

Irritable bowel presents with symptoms such as abdominal pain, feelings of distention, and "variations in bowel habits."[4] Several clinical trials have demonstrated the clinical effectiveness of enteric-coated peppermint oil (most often the brand Colpermin®) in relieving these symptoms.[16,17] In one double-blind, placebo-controlled, cross-over trial (n=18), enteric-coated peppermint oil capsules (1-2 caps three times daily depending on severity of symptoms) given between meals significantly decreased patients' symptoms when compared with a placebo (peanut oil).[16]

In another randomized, double-blind, placebo-controlled trial in 42 children (all over 8 years of age) with irritable bowel syndrome, enteric-coated peppermint oil capsules (Colpermin® consisting of 187 mg of peppermint oil per dose) were found to reduce the severity of pain after a two-week treatment period. Patients weighing more that 45 kg received 2 peppermint oil or placebo capsules daily and those weighting between 30 and 45 kg received 1 capsule three times daily.[18]

Anti-Spasmodic

Several in vitro studies have demonstrated peppermint oil's ability to relax smooth muscle via blockade of the calcium channel transport mechanism.[19,20] One research team reported that colon spasms during endoscopy were relieved within 30 seconds when diluted suspension of peppermint oil injected along the biopsy channel of the colonoscope in 20 patients. [21] They called for a prospective clinical trial for this indication, but our literature search found none to date.

Several clinical studies have noted that the addition of peppermint to barium enema suspension decreased the incidence of spasm.[22,23] One double-blind study (n=141) found that peppermint oil (added to barium sulphate suspension) was significantly effective at relieving colonic muscle spasm during double contrast barium enema examination. The authors suggest that this simple, safe and inexpensive technique could decrease the need for intravenous spasmolytic agents during barium enema procedures.[23]

Miscellaneous Gastrointestinal Effects

One double-blind, placebo-controlled, crossover study (n=6) found that peppermint oil decreases colonic motility in humans.[24] Another double-blind, placebo-controlled, multi-center trial (n=45) found that a peppermint oil (90 mg)/Caraway oil (50 mg) combination significantly reduced the symptoms of non-ulcer dyspepsia after four weeks of treatment.[25] Promising results were reported from from another four-week randomized, controlled trial comparing a peppermint oil (90 mg) / Caraway oil (50 mg) combination with cisapride (30 mg daily) in 120 outpatients with functional dyspepsia. In this case, both treatment regimens were found to be equally effective and well tolerated.[26]

ANTI-MICROBIAL ACTIVITY
Anti-Bacterial

In vitro testing indicates that peppermint inhibits the growth of a variety of bacteria including: *S. aureus, B. brevis, B. circulans, Citrobacter sp., E. coli, Klebsiella sp., S. Typhi, S. Typhimurium, S. boydii, S. flexneri,* and *V. cholerae.*[27] In addition, peppermint oil was found to be ineffective against *Pseudomonas aeruginosa.*[28] The clinical significance of these findings is unknown.

Anti-Fungal

Peppermint is reported to inhibit the growth *in vitro* of a variety of fungi, including: *C. albicans, C. neoformans, S. schenkii, A. citrii, A. fumigatus, A. oryzae, F. oxysporum, F. solani, H. compactum, M. phaseolina, S. rolfsii,* and *T. mentagrophytes.*[27] The clinical significance of these findings is unknown.

Anti-Viral

Peppermint is reported to have activity against herpes simplex virus and Newcastle disease *in vitro.*[9] The clinical significance of this is unknown.

MISCELLANEOUS EFFECTS

Peppermint oil has traditionally been used externally for a wide range of indications, including headaches. One double-blind, placebo-controlled, randomized, crossover clinical trial (n=32) reports that a combination of peppermint oil (10 g), eucalyptus oil (5 g) and ethanol (ad 100 g) significantly increased cognitive performance as well as produced mental and pericranial muscle relaxation. In addition, peppermint oil (10 g) in combination with ethanol (*ad* 100 g) produced a significant analgesic effect.[29]

ADVERSE EFFECTS

Regular consumption of peppermint leaf tea is considered safe; however, excessive use of the volatile oil (>0.3 g or 12 drops) may cause problems.[6] Clinical trials of enteric-coated peppermint oil capsules for a variety of gastrointestinal complaints report few side effects. Heartburn and esophageal reflux can occur if the peppermint oil is accidentally released in the stomach.[16] In addition, a burning sensation during defecation (thought to be due to unabsorbed menthol reaching the rectum) has occasionally been observed when peppermint oil is taken in high doses. Reducing the dose reduces this adverse effect.

There have also been several reports of contact-sensitivity to the peppermint in a variety oral products, including toothpaste.[30-33] Symptoms include: burning sensation in the mouth, recurrent oral ulceration, stomatitis, glossitis, gingivitis, and perioral dermatitis.

One case report describes veno-occlusive disease in an 18-month-old boy who had regularly consumed a tea believed to contain peppermint and coltsfoot (*Tussilago farfara* L., Asteraceae) for the previous 12 months. Analysis of the tea revealed that the tea contained

Adenosyles alliariae (Gouan) Kern., Asteraceae, rather than the reported coltsfoot. The peppermint was not thought to play any role in the toxicity of the product.[34]

Cardiac fibrillation has been reported in patients whose condition was controlled with quinidine following the use of mentholated cigarettes or consumption of peppermint candy.[35]

CAUTIONS/CONTRAINDICATIONS

Peppermint should generally be given between meals and it should not be taken by patients with achlorhydria (i.e., patients with no hydrochloric acid in gastric juices).[16] Generally, peppermint (tea and topical application to nostrils) should be avoided in young children or infants because the menthol may cause a choking sensation.[6,33] In addition, oral consumption of peppermint oil should be avoided in situations of glucose-6 phosphate dehydrogenase deficiency since menthol may be implicated in this condition.[33]

DRUG INTERACTIONS

No known drug interactions.

DOSAGE REGIMENS

❖ ENTERIC-COATED PEPPERMINT OIL CAPSULES (0.2 mL peppermint oil/capsule): 1-2 capsules three times daily between meals.[36]

❖ TINCTURE (1:5 in 45% ethanol): 2-3 mL three times daily away from meals.

❖ TEA: Mix 160 mL (⅔ cup) of boiling water with 1.5 g (1 tablespoonful) of recently dried leaves and steep for 5-10 minutes. This amount is taken on an empty stomach three to four times daily to relieve upset stomach.[6]

Red Raspberry

Rubus idaeus L.

THUMBNAIL SKETCH

Common Uses
❖ Pregnancy Aid
❖ Diarrhea

Active Constituents
❖ Tannins

Adverse Effects
❖ None known

Cautions/Contraindications
❖ Pregnancy (concerns given lack of evidence)

Drug Interactions
❖ None known

Doses
❖ *Dried Leaf:* 4-8 grams taken as an infusion three times a day

❖ *Liquid Extract* (1:1 in 25% ethanol): 4-8 mL three times a day

Introduction

Family
* ❖ Rosaceae

Synonyms
* ❖ Raspberry
* ❖ Framboisier
* ❖ Wild raspberry
* ❖ Rubus
* ❖ Hindberry[1]

Medicinal Forms
* ❖ Dried Leaves
* ❖ Liquid Extract

Description

Red raspberry is a deciduous shrub, native to Europe and Asia, but now widespread in North America, growing wild and cultivated primarily for its fruit. The plant grows 5 to 6 feet or 2 meters tall, with prickly woody stems, small green leaves, and red berries.

Parts Used

Many fruit berries are used for their medicinal properties. In this case, rather than the berries, the leaves are the part of the plant used therapeutically.

Traditional Use

The very astringent tannins in the red raspberry leaf have a drying effect and have long been taken as an infusion or tea for a number of reasons. Red raspberry leaf has a long history of use in women's health, most particularly pregnancy.[1,2] It has long been claimed that raspberry leaf tea can be used to "cleanse and purify the blood."[3]

Current Medicinal Use

Red raspberry is an herbal medicine steeped in tradition but with little modern evidence to support its use.[4]

Because of the lack of clear scientific evidence, the German Commission E has suggested that no therapeutic use can be recommended for red raspberry at this time.[3] Nevertheless, under the supervision of an appropriately trained healthcare practitioner, red raspberry is often used to aid pregnancy. The nutritious value of the berries should not be forgotten, being rich in many vitamins and minerals.[1]

Relevant Research

Preventative and Therapeutic Effects

CONSTITUENTS [1,2,5]
* ❖ TANNINS: gallotannins, elagitannins.
* ❖ MISCELLANEOUS: flavonoids (rutin), polypepetides.

COMMON USES

Red raspberry leaf is considered by many herbalists to be particularly useful as a *partus praeparator*, preparing the uterus for childbirth and aiding delivery.[2,6,7] Red raspberry is arguably the most commonly used herbal medicine for childbirth and is recommended by a number of health-care professionals, including midwives, medical herbalists and naturopaths.[8-11]

It is also often recommended in cases of morning sickness and as a general tonic in women's health. Due to the drying effect of the tannins, leaves are also used as a mouthwash in tonsilitis; to treat diarrhea, skin conditions and abrasions, and urinary tract infections.[5,6] Red raspberry leaf is also considered by many to be useful for diabetics.[1]

MEDICINAL ACTION

Extracts of red raspberry leaf have been shown to inhibit the contraction of rat uterus muscle and increase regularity of contractions in human uterine tissue.[12] The actions appeared to be more pronounced in tissue taken from pregnant women rather than women who were not expecting. A published abstract makes mention of one Australian double-blind, randomized, placebo controlled trial. While precise details of the study could not be found, it was suggested that 1.2 g of raspberry leaf herb taken twice a day from 32 weeks of gestation to commencement of labor shortened the second stage of labor and decreased rate of forceps delivery.[13] While these results are promising, more research is needed before a definitive conclusion can be reached.

ADVERSE EFFECTS

Red raspberry leaves appear to be quite safe in most cases.[3] There are been no reported cases of significant adverse effects in the literature.

CAUTIONS/CONTRAINDICATIONS

The main controversy regarding red raspberry leaf is its use in pregnancy. The lack of any scientific studies to show that it is safe, together with the fact that it has been shown to act on uterine tissue, has led many to suggest that red raspberry leaf should not be taken during pregnancy.[5] This goes against the recommendations of many complementary healthcare providers, which are based on historical use of the product. In light of the lack of scientific evidence from clinical trials of both safety and efficacy of red raspberry, many feel that the recommendation of its use by women who are pregnant is inappropriate and may in fact be the biggest risk associated with this particular herbal medicine.[8]

DRUG INTERACTIONS

No drug interactions could be found for red raspberry leaf. Theoretically, the high tannin concentration may decrease the absorption of certain minerals notably calcium and magnesium.[14]

DOSAGE REGIMENS [5]

❖ DRIED LEAF: 4-8 g taken as an infusion three times a day.
❖ LIQUID EXTRACT (1:1 in 25% ethanol): 4-8 mL three times a day.

Saw Palmetto
Serenoa repens (Bartram) Small

Common Uses
❖ BPH (benign prostatic hyperplasia or enlargement of the prostate gland)

Active Constituents
❖ Fatty Acids and Sterols

Adverse Effects
❖ Gastro-Intestinal Upset (rare)

Cautions/Contraindications
❖ Pregnancy and Lactation (safety not established)

Drug Interactions
❖ Hormonal Therapy (theoretical)

Doses
❖ *Dried Berries:* 0.5-1.0 g taken as a tea three times daily
❖ *Liquid Extract:* 0.6 -1.5 mL daily
❖ *Liposterolic Extract:* 160 mg twice daily

Introduction

Family
❖ Arecaceae
   (also known
   as Palmae)

Synonyms
❖ *Serenoa*
   serrulata
   (Michx.) Nichols.

❖ *Sabal serrulata*
   (Michx.) Nutall
   ex. Schultes &
   Schultes

❖ Sabal[1,2]

Medicinal Forms
❖ Dried Fruit
   Berries

❖ Liquid Extract

Description
The only surviving species of *Seronoa* is *Seronoa repens*, which can be found growing along the Atlantic coast of North America.[3] The shrub grows up to 3 meters or 10 feet in height with fan-shaped crowns of palm-like leaves, bearing white flowers and dark-red-to-deep-purple oblong berries.

Parts Used
The dried berries are used medicinally.[4]

Traditional Use
Saw palmetto was used as a food source for early settlers in North America.[5] Historically, the ripe fruit was partially dried and used for a variety of conditions of the bladder, urethra and prostate.[3] It was called the "plant catheter." This herb was considered primarily a "male" remedy and was used to "improve flagging reproductive function" as well as "debility and senility in men."[6]

Current Medicinal Use
Today, saw palmetto is best known for it use as a treatment for benign prostatic hyperplasia (BPH). Several excellent reviews have been written on this topic.[3,7,8]

Relevant Research

Preventative and Therapeutic Effects

CONSTITUENTS [1-4]
❖ FATTY ACIDS: lauric acid, linoleic acid, linolenic acid, capric acid, caproic acid, palmitic acid, oleic acid, caprylic acid, myristic acid, stearic acid.
❖ PHYTOSTEROLS: beta-sitosterol, stigmasterol, campesterol.
❖ ALCOHOLS: docosanol, hexacosanol, octacosanol, triacontanol.
❖ MISCELLANEOUS: carotenes, lipase, tannins.

BENIGN PROSTATIC HYPERPLASIA
Mechanism of Action
Currently, most saw palmetto products are composed of 'liposterolic extracts' (i.e., containing the fatty acids and sterols) of the fruit.[3] There are three primary mechanisms by which these extracts appear to work against BPH:[3]

1. Androgen receptor blockade.[9-13] Dihydrotestosterone (DHT) is an active androgen (more active than testosterone) which has been implicated as a causative factor BPH.[11]

2. 5a-reductase inhibition.[13-18] 5a-reductase catalyzes the metabolism of testosterone to DHT. One recent study does not support this hypothesis; however, the researchers used half the usual dose of saw palmetto (80 mg BID) in their experiments.[19] Several recent *in vitro* studies which support this hypothesis suggest that the inhibition of saw palmetto extract is non-competitive in nature.[15,17]

3. Disruption of the arachidonic cascade. Saw palmetto is reported to inhibit both the cyclooxygenase and lipoxygenase pathways,[20] which is believed to result in an anti-inflammatory effect which will provide added relief for the symptoms of BPH.

In addition, saw palmetto has a phytoestrogenic effect; it appears to compete with endogenous estrogen for receptor sites.[21,22] One research team suggests that this may play a key role in its ability to decrease the symptoms of BPH.[22] It does not appear to affect plasma levels of testosterone, follicle-stimulating hormone (FSH) or luteinizing hormone (LH).[23] One study in rats demonstrated that saw palmetto extract was able to inhibit estradiol/testosterone-induced experimental prostate enlargement.[24]

Clinical Trials

A number of clinical studies have been completed to date, including open trials;[25-30] double-blind, placebo-controlled trials;[31-38] and double-blind trials comparing saw palmetto with other treatments for benign prostatic hyperplasia (BPH).[39-42] The majority of human clinical trials tested 160 mg of a liposterolic extract containing 85-95% fatty acids and sterols twice daily. This is equivalent to approximately 10 g crude berries twice daily.

Three systematic reviews and/or meta-analyses have concluded that saw palmetto use is associated with a significant improvement in peak flow rate and reduction in nocturia in men diagnosed with BPH compared with placebo.[43-45] In addition, compared with finasteride, saw palmetto has been shown to produce similar improvement in urinary tract symptoms and urinary flow and has been associated with fewer adverse effects in clinical trials.[41,45] In a large (n=811) randomized, double-blind comparison study, saw palmetto (Permixon® (320 mg daily) was found to be equivalent to tamsulosin (an alpha-blocker) in the treatment of symptoms of BPH over a 12-month period.[42] Several herbal blends containing saw palmetto have also been reported to be effective in the management of BPH symptoms.[46,47]

MISCELLANEOUS EFFECTS

A randomized, double-blind, placebo-controlled pilot study (n=26) reported that a product containing 200 mg saw palmetto (standardized to 85%-95% liposterolic content) and 50 mg beta-sitosterol that was taken once or twice daily appeared to significantly improve androgenetic alopecia (receding hairline and/or hair loss). The authors argue that these results justify the investigation of this combination product in larger clinical trials.[48] Although no human clinical trials were available for review, saw palmetto has also been reported to be useful in the treatment of hirsutism.[8]

ADVERSE EFFECTS

Clinical trials report that saw palmetto is well-tolerated; however, the FDA in the USA lists saw palmetto as an herb of unknown safety.[1] Gastrointestinal upset is rare, but possible.[34]

CAUTIONS/CONTRAINDICATIONS

Safety has not been established in pregnancy and lactation.[1]

DRUG INTERACTIONS

Theoretically, because of its anti-androgen and estrogenic activity, saw palmetto may interact with existing hormonal therapy, including hormone replacement therapy and contraceptive pills.[1]

DOSAGE REGIMENS

❖ DRIED BERRIES: 0.5-1.0 g taken as a tea three times daily.[1]
❖ LIQUID EXTRACT: 0.6 -1.5 mL daily.[1]
❖ LIPOSTEROLIC EXTRACT: 160 mg twice daily.[29,49]

Scullcap

Scutellaria lateriflora L.i

THUMBNAIL SKETCH

Common Uses
- ❖ Nervous Tension, Exhaustion, Spasms, Hysteria

Active Constituents
- ❖ Flavonoids
- ❖ Volatile Oils
- ❖ Iridoids
- ❖ Tannins

Adverse Effects
- ❖ Drowsiness, Giddiness, Confusion, Convulsions (in large doses)
- ❖ Hepatotoxicity (may be due to adulteration of products with germander)

Cautions/Contraindications
- ❖ Pregnancy and Lactation

Drug Interactions
- ❖ None known but caution is suggested in patients taking other centrally acting drugs

Doses
- ❖ *Dried Herb:* 0.5-2 g up to four times daily
- ❖ *Liquid Extract* (1:1 in 25% alcohol): 0.5-2 mL up to four times daily
- ❖ *Tincture* (1:8 in 25% alcohol): 2-4 mL up to four times daily

Introduction

Family
* Laminaceae also known as Labiatae

Synonyms
* Helmet flower
* Hoodwort
* Quaker bonnet
* Scutellaria
* Mad-dog scullcap
* Skullcap
* European or greater skullcap[1-3]

Medicinal Forms
* Dried Herb
* Liquid Extract
* Tincture

Description
Many different species of the genus *Scutellaria* are used medicinally, although most texts identify *lateriflora* as the most common species.[2] In addition, *Scutellaria baicalensis* Georgi (Baikal Scullcap/Huang-qin) is a major medicinal herb used in Traditional Chinese Medicine.[3] *Scutellaria lateriflora* is native to North America, where it still grows wild, reaching 60 centimeters or two feet, with a straight stem and pink-to-blue flowers. The dried seed husks look like skullcaps. *Scutellaria baicalensis* is a perennial native to China, Japan and Russia, with a fibrous roots and erect stems growing up to 4 feet or 120 centimeters, topped with purple flowers.

Parts Used
In the Western tradition the aerial parts of *Scutellaria lateriflora* are used medicinally, whereas the roots of *Scutellaria baicalensis* (Baikal Scullcap) are used in the Traditional Chinese Medical model.[2,3]

Traditional Use
The native peoples of Native America used *Scutellaria lateriflora* for ailments associated with menstruation and breast pain. In the 19th century, herbalists used it for treating hysteria, epilepsy, convulsions, schizophrenia, and even rabies. In Traditional Chinese Medicine, *Scutellaria baicalensis* was used to treat fevers, colds, coughs, diarrhea and dysentery.[4]

Current Medicinal Use
Based on traditional evidence, scullcap is now primarily used to treat conditions of nervous tension and exhaustion, such as insomnia and anxiety.

Relevant Research

Preventative and Therapeutic Effects

CONSTITUENTS [1,2,5-7]

Since there is a lack of information specifically relating to *Scutellaria lateriflora* L., the information provided here refers to a number of species contained in the *Scutellaria* genus.

* FLAVONOIDS: including apigenin, luteolin, scutellarin (baicalein, wogonin, baicalin are found in S. baicalensis Georgi).
* VOLATILE OILS: primarily monoterpenes and sesquiterpenes.
* IRIDOIDS: catalpol is found in both S. *lateriflora* and S. *galericulata* L.
* MISCELLANEOUS: including tannins and resin.

COMMON USES

Scutellaria lateriflora L. is reputed to have sedative,[1,8] nervine,[1,8] anti-spasmodic,[1,8] and anti-convulsant properties.[1,8] Oral consumption is considered useful in the treatment of conditions related to nervous tension and exhaustion.[8] It is often used in patients with hysteria, spasms or convulsions.[1,8]

MISCELLANEOUS EFFECTS

Little or no clinical information could be found relating to the pharmacology of *Scutellaria lateriflora* L., with most of the available work referring to *Scutellaria baicalensis* Georgi.[2,5] Extracts of *Scutellaria baicalensis* Georgi and its constituents have been shown *in vivo* and *in vitro* to inhibit lipid peroxidation;[9,10] possess antibacterial and antiviral properties;[11] influence arachidonate metabolism;[12] influence lipolysis and lipogenesis;[13] decrease release of histamine from rat mast cells;[6] and decrease serum lipid levels.[14] Given the different species and the fact that the aerial parts rather than the root are used in Western herbalism, it is unknown how applicable the above information is to scullcap products used medicinally in North America.[15]

ADVERSE EFFECTS

Large doses of scullcap can cause giddiness, confusion, drowsiness and convulsions.[16] In addition, herbal products containing scullcap as one of the ingredients have been implicated in a number of cases of hepatotoxicity,[16,17] which has resulted in the removal of a number of herbal scullcap preparations from the market in the United Kingdom.[17] Instances of hepatotoxicity may have been due to adulteration or substitution of scullcap with any of several species of germander (*Teucrium canadense* L., *T. chamaedrys* L., etc.).[18]

There is one case report of a 53-year-old Japanese man with recurrent interstitial pneumonia which appears to have been induced by skullcap (species not specified) contained in a traditional herbal medicine.[19]

CAUTIONS/CONTRAINDICATIONS

Given the lack of information and the cases of possible hepatotoxicity mentioned above, products containing scullcap should not be used in pregnancy or lactation.[2]

DRUG INTERACTIONS

While no clinical examples could be found, given the reputed sedative action of scullcap, it should be used with caution in patients taking conventional centrally acting medications.[20]

DOSAGE REGIMENS

❖ DRIED HERB: 0.5-2 g up to 4 times daily.
❖ LIQUID EXTRACT (1:1 in 25% alcohol): 0.5-2 mL up to 4 times daily.
❖ TINCTURE (1:8 in 25% alcohol): 2-4 mL up to 4 times daily.[21]

Slippery Elm

Ulmus rubra Muhl.

THUMBNAIL SKETCH

Common Uses
Internal

❖ Mucous Membranes Irritations (including gastritis, peptic ulcer disease)

❖ Coughs, Sore Throats

❖ Diarrhea

Topical

❖ Sores, Ulcers and Abscesses

Active Constituents
❖ Mucilage

❖ Tannins

Adverse Effects
❖ None known

Cautions/Contraindications
❖ Bark may be abortifacient (producing abortion)

Drug Interactions
❖ None known

Doses
❖ *Liquid Extract* (1:1 in 60% alcohol): 5 mL three times daily

❖ *Decoction of Powdered Bark* (1:8): 4-16 mL three times daily

❖ *Lozenges:* Many proprietary lozenges containing slippery elm may be found on the North American market.

Introduction

Family
❖ Ulmaceae

Synonyms
❖ *Ulmus fulva* Michx.
❖ Red elm
❖ Moose elm
❖ Indian elm
❖ American elm[1-3]

Medicinal Forms
❖ Liquid Extract
❖ Powdered Bark Decoction
❖ Lozenges

Description
Slippery elm is a deciduous tree standing 15-20 meters or 50-65 feet in height, native to the United States and Canada.[4] The leaves are yellow/olive in color and the fruit produced is winged and round.[1] The bark has a brownish yellow outer surface and an inner yellow white color, with a distinctive 'fenugreek-like odor'.[4] Commercial harvesting of the bark often results in the death of the tree.[5]

Parts Used
The part used medicinally is the inner part of the bark.

Traditional Use
Slippery elm gained favor amongst the First Nations. When the bark is mixed with water, it produces a thick viscid mucilage was used in conditions where the mucous membranes were inflamed and irritated, both externally and internally.[6] It was also applied externally to sores, wounds and abscesses.[1] It is often used as a food during convalescence because it is nutritious and easy to digest.

Current Medicinal Use
Based primarily on traditional evidence, slippery elm is used to treat inflammation of the mucosa membranes, notably gastritis, peptic ulcers and diarrhea. Slippery elm is often available as lozenges to treat sore throats. In addition, the herb may also be used externally to sooth sores, ulcers and abscesses.

Relevant Research

Preventative and Therapeutic Effects

CONSTITUENTS [2,3]
❖ CARBOHYDRATES: complex mucilage containing a number of sugars.
❖ MISCELLANEOUS: tannins, sesquiterpenes and calcium oxalate.

COMMON USES
Slippery elm is reputed to have demulcent,[3-6] nutrient,[3,5] emollient,[3,5] astringent[5] and antitussive[3,5,6] properties. Oral consumption is considered useful in the treatment of any condition presenting with inflamed mucous membranes, including gastritis, peptic ulcer disease, enteritis and colitis.[3,5,7] Due to their astringent action, slippery elm products are also used within the herbal tradition to treat diarrhea and food poisoning.[5,7] In addition, slippery elm is also often taken as a lozenge for the relief of coughs and minor throat irritation.[6] External application, usually as a poultice, is used for ulcers, boils, wounds and abscesses.[5]

No information regarding the pharmacology of slippery elm in particular could be found. Research on other plant species has shown that mucilage has a demulcent action and that tannins have astringent properties.[2,7]

ADVERSE EFFECTS
No adverse effects could be found regarding the use of this medicinal herb.

CAUTIONS/CONTRAINDICATIONS
Products prepared from the whole bark were used as abortifacients. However, it appears that the same caution is not applicable to powdered slippery elm.[2]

DRUG INTERACTIONS
None could be found.

DOSAGE REGIMENS [2]
- ❖ LIQUID EXTRACT (1:1 in 60% alcohol): 5 mL of three times daily.
- ❖ DECOCTION OF POWDERED BARK (1:8): 4-16 mL three times daily. The decoction should be made in the following manner: "Use 1 part of the powdered bark to 8 parts of water. Mix the powder in a little water initially to ensure it will mix. Bring to the boil and simmer gently for 10-15mins. Drink half a cup three times a day."[5]
- ❖ LOZENGES: Many proprietary lozenges containing slippery elm may be found on the North American market.

  Note: Slippery elm is often mixed with other demulcents, notably marshmallow (*Althaea officinalis* L. Malvaceae).

St John's Wort
Hypericum perforatum L.

Common Uses
- Depression (mild to moderate)
- Muscle Aches (topically)

Active Constituents
- Hypericin
- Isohypericin
- Protohypericin
- Flavinoids
- Hyperforin
- Adhyperforin

Adverse Effects
- Photosensitivity
- Gastrointestinal Upset and Dizziness
- Sedation
- Hypomania

Cautions/Contraindications
- Pregnancy and Lactation

Drug Interactions
- Combined oral contraceptives, cyclosporin, digoxin, general anesthesia, inidinivir, nefazadone, paroxetine, phenprocoumon, sertraline, theophylline, trazadone, warfarin, drugs causing photosensitivity

Dose
- *Standardized Extract* (equivalent to 0.4-2.7 mg hypericin daily): 350-1800 mg daily in divided doses
- *Standardized Extract* (0.3% hypericin): 300 mg three times daily
- *Standardized Extract* (5% hypeforin): 300 mg three times daily
- *Dried Herb:* 2-4 g three times per day
- *Infused Oils or Creams:* applied externally as needed

Introduction

Family
❖ Clusiaceae (also known as Guttiferae, sometimes placed in Hypericaceae)

Synonyms
❖ Hypericum

❖ Millepertuis

❖ Amber

❖ Goatweed

❖ Johnswort

❖ Klamath weed

❖ Tipton weed[1,2]

Medicinal Forms
❖ Dried Flowers

❖ Standardized Extracts

❖ Infused Oil

Description

St. John's wort is a shrub-like perennial plant that reaches a height of 60 centimeters or 2 feet. The leaves grow from cylindrical or oval stems in an irregular, oblong shape and produce a red sap when crushed. The underside of the leaves is distinguished by pin-pricks and black spots. The five-petal yellow flowers bloom in the summer months. The plant has a turpentine-like odor and a bitter, acidic flavor. It is indigenous to all of Europe and Asia but now is also found in North America,[1,3,4] where it is listed as a noxious weed in many provinces and states due to its invasion of rangeland and photosensitization of livestock. This makes it necessary to take special precautions when the herb is being cultivated.[5]

Parts Used

The flower tops and petals are used medicinally.

Traditional Use

St. John's wort has been recognized in the West as having medicinal properties since the classical period. The name itself has been associated with a colorful mythology involving Saint John the Baptist, and there are varied customs using the plant as a talisman to ward off misfortune. It was mentioned in the texts of Hippocrates, Pliny, and Galen as helpful for wound healing, pain, and as a diuretic. The use of this herb continued though the Renaissance and Victorian eras,[1,3,6] when it was also used as a treatment for emotional and nervous complaints. Oil infused with St. John's wort can be applied topically and massaged into the tissue for muscle and nerve pain.[4]

Current Medicinal Use

Both traditional and modern scientific evidence support the use of St. John's Wort products in the treatment of mild to moderate depression. Oil infused with St. John's wort is used topically to treat muscle cramps and nerve pain.

Relevant Research

Preventative and Therapeutic Effects

CONSTITUENTS [2,7-9]

❖ ANTHRAQUINONE DERIVATIVES: hypericin, isohypericin, protohypericin, psuedohypericin.

❖ FLAVONOIDS: quercetin, hyperoside, quercitrin, isoquercitrin, rutin, campherol, luteolin, I3-II8-biapigenin.

❖ PRENYLATED PHLOROGLUCINOLS: hyperforin and adhyperforin.

❖ PROCYANIDINES.

❖ PHENOLS.

❖ PHLOROGLUCINOLS.

❖ TANNINS.

❖ VOLATILE OILS.

❖ XANTHONES.

❖ Miscellaneous organic acids, hydrocarbons and alcohols.

MECHANISM OF ACTION

Extracts of St. John's wort contain many constituents that vary depending on the strain.[10] The compounds responsible for the main putative therapeutic effects (anti-retroviral and anti-depressive) have not been identified definitively, however.[7] The red-pigmented hypericins were found to be absorbed in a dose-dependent manner within two hours, to be widely distributed, and to have a plasma half-life of approximately 24 hours, allowing steady-state concentrations to be reached within four days of thrice-daily dosing.[11,12] Approximately 14-21% of the compounds were estimated to be systemically available.[12] *In vitro* experiments localize hypericin primarily in the cytoplasmic membrane and cytoplasm, with smaller amounts in the nucleus.[13]

ANTI-RETROVIRAL EFFECTS

Relatively recent investigations into the potential anti-retroviral activity of St. John's wort have paralleled the search for other effective treatments for HIV infection and AIDS. Anti-bacterial and anti-fungal effects of some constituents have been demonstrated *in vitro*.[9,14] Anti-viral activity against Sindbis, human poliovirus-1, and herpes simplex virus-1 has been found *in vitro*.[15] Murine cytomegalovirus, and human immunodefficiency virus-1 (HIV-1) were also inactivated *in vitro*. Light was found to potentiate the anti-viral effects both on isolated virions and on virally infected cells. No damage to the cultured cells was observed.[16,17] Although the mechanism of the antiviral effects are not known, researchers have found evidence for the ability of the hypericins to inhibit protein kinase C.[18] A more detailed review of the potential mechanisms can be found in Diwu.[19]

The best data on the anti-retroviral activity of hypericins comes from a trio of papers from the Proceedings of the National Academy of Science (PNAS). Meruelo et al. reported *in vitro* and *in vivo* antiretroviral activity with little toxicity.[20] The same group found increased survival in retro-virus infected animals treated with hypericin and pseudohypericin. These compounds were thought to affect retrovirus assembly and to inactivate mature viral particles.[21] Lenard et al. found that both hypericin and Rose Bengal (another pigmented compound) were able to photoinactivate enveloped viruses (human stomatits and HIV) at nanomolecular concentrations. Fusion or hemolysis of cells was inhibited in cells infected by these as well as Sendai and influenza viruses. In cells induced to express the HIV gp120 protein, sycytium formation with CD4⁺ cells was photoinhibited.[22]

ANTI-DEPRESSANT EFFECTS

Although there is considerable evidence that St. John's wort has some anti-depressant effects, clinical recommendations about its use at present must be tempered by the lack of long-term human data and studies in severe depression, uncertainty regarding mechanism of action, interaction with other medications and concerns regarding standardization and regulation of the content of commercial products in North America.[23-25] Extracts of St. John's wort have reported affinities for a variety of neurotransmitter receptors, including: adenosine, $GABA_A$, $GABA_B$, $5HT_1$, central benzodiazepine, forskolin, inositol triphosphate, and the monoamine oxidase A and B enzymes. However, based on the concentrations normally attained after oral administration, only GABA binding appears possible *in vivo*.[26] Non-clinical studies have found evidence for inhibition of serotonin uptake,[27,28] decreased serotonin receptor expression,[29] inhibition of benzodiazepine binding,[30] changes on animal behavioral tests of antidepressant activity,[31] increased excretion of adrenergic metabolites,[32] modulation of cytokine expression,[33] and inhibition of monoamine oxidase.[34-36] Changes in behavioral test outcomes of animal studies caused by St. John's wort extracts are similar to those documented with other anti-depressants.[31,37,38]

Mild to Moderate Depression

In humans, there is clear evidence of efficacy in mild to moderate depression.[24,39-54] The most recent update of the Cochrane Collaboration's review of St. John's wort for depression assessed 27 randomized trials including a total of 2291 patients and concluded that "there is evidence that extracts of hypericum are more effective than placebo for the short-term treatment of mild to moderately severe depressive disorders."[51] This review also noted that further studies are needed comparing St. John's wort with conventional therapies as well as over longer periods of time and comparing different extracts and doses.[51] One study suggests that the efficacy of St. Johns' wort extracts may be related to their hyperforin content (a 5% hyperforin extract was more effective than a 0.5% hyperforin extract).[55,56] Another found no significant difference in the efficacy of extracts that provided total hypericin content of 0.17 mg vs. 0.33 mg vs. 1.0 mg daily.[57] Several reviews have concluded that there is currently insufficient evidence to establish whether or not St. John's wort is as effective as conventional antidepressants.[50,51] Several studies suggest that it may have similar effects in patients with mild to moderate depression.

St. John's wort extracts have been compared directly with several tricyclic anti-depressants[48] and found to be equally as effective as imipramine;[44,53,58] maprotiline;[40] or amitriptyline.[59] However, these studies have been criticized due to the small numbers of patients and the low doses of conventional tricyclic anti-depressants to which the St. John's wort was compared.[47]

A systematic review of studies comparing St. John's wort extracts and fluoxetine in the management of sub-threshold and mild depression concluded that there was no relevant efficacy difference between the two, based on the studies reviewed. However, the authors cautioned that the St. John's wort products tested in the studies differed widely and there was wide methodological variability in the studies reviewed making it impossible to conduct a meta-analysis of the data.[60] Several additional studies have also reported that St. John's wort is as effective as fluoxetine and is associated with fewer adverse effects when used in the treatment of mild to moderate depression.[61-63] A Canadian study published after this review that compared the efficacy of St. John's wort (300 mg standardized to 0.3% hypericum three times daily) and sertraline (50 mg daily) over a 12-week period concluded that there were no important differences between the two treatments and that significantly more adverse effects were reported by individuals taking sertraline.[64] This finding is further supported by another USA comparison trial.[65]

Severe Depression

Several systematic reviews and meta-analyses have concluded that St. John's wort does not appear to be effective in the management of severe depression.[49] A randomized, double-blind, placebo-controlled trial reported that St. John's wort (standardized 900 mg/day for at least 4 weeks; increased to 1200 mg/day if necessary for the second 4 weeks) was not effective (compared to placebo) in treating patients (n=200) diagnosed with severe (defined as Hamilton Depression Scale scores of 20 or greater) major depression.[66] The publication of this study generated significant debate.[67-71]

The findings of this study are supported by another randomized, double-blind, controlled study (n=340) that compared St. John's wort (250 mg twice daily of extract LI160) to placebo and fluoxetine (20 mg daily) in patients with severe depression (defined as Hamilton Depression Scale scores of 20 or greater) over an 8-week period. In this study, neither treatment (St. John's wort nor fluoxetine) was found to be significantly better than placebo on the two primary outcome measures of the trial (change in Hamilton Depression total score and rates of full response).[72] This study also stimulated much discussion.[73-80] For example, there were concerns that the trial had a low assay sensitivity for a number of reasons including that there may have been a relatively large number of treatment-resistant participants; inadequate assessment of the adequacy of blinding; and used an inclusion criteria of 20 or more on the Hamilton Depression scale, which is higher than many earlier trials.

In contrast to the studies described above, a randomized, double-blind trial comparing 1800 mg daily of St John's wort extract LI 160 to 150 mg daily of imipramine in 209 severely depressed patients from 20 psychiatric centers reported that both were equally effective (Hamilton Depression Scales) over the 6 week treatment period.[8]

MISCELLANEOUS EFFECTS

One randomized, double-blind, placebo-controlled, 6-week study (n=151) reported that St. John's wort (600 mg daily of LI 160 extract) was significantly more effective than placebo in treating the symptoms of somatisation disorder independent of depressive symptomatology.[82]

One randomized, double-blind, placebo-controlled, crossover study (n=47) reported that St. John's wort (3 tablets each containing 900 mcg total hypericin daily) over 5 weeks had no effect on pain associated with polyneuropathy.[83]

ADVERSE EFFECTS

In general there are few side effects associated with St. John's wort when used for depression.[41,84,85] St. John's wort is associated with fewer adverse effects than conventional anti-depressants, but they may include: photodermatitis (very rare);[86] gastrointestinal irritation; dizziness; dry mouth; sedation; restlessness; constipation; serotonin syndrome-like symptoms;[87] hair loss;[87] elevation in thyroid-stimulating hormone levels;[88] sexual dysfunction (appears to be very rare);[89] induction of mania or hypomania;[90-94] and hypertensive crisis.[95] Characteristic EEG and sleep changes seen with tricyclic anti-depressants are not observed with St. John's wort,[96] although there is some shortening of evoked potential latencies and enhancement of theta and beta-2 regions in the resting EEG.[97]

CAUTIONS/CONTRAINDICATIONS

Prolonged or intense exposure to sunlight should be avoided by patients ingesting St. John's wort.[2] St. John's wort should by used with caution by pregnant or lactating women due to the lack of research available establishing the safety in these populations.

DRUG INTERACTIONS

Several reviews of drug interactions with St. John's wort exist.[98-101] Cases describing possible drug interactions between St. John's wort and the following drugs have been reported:

- Combined oral contraceptive (resulting in breakthrough bleeding).[102,103]
- Cyclosporin (resulting in decreased cyclosporin levels).[102,104-110]
- Digoxin (resulting in decreased digoxin levels).[111]
- General anesthesia (resulting in delayed emergence).[112]
- Indinivir (resulting in decreased indinivir levels).[113]
- Nefazadone (resulting in symptoms of serotonin syndrome).[114]
- Paroxetine (resulting in symptoms of serotonin syndrome).[115]
- Phenprocoumon.[116]
- Sertraline (resulting in symptoms of serotonin syndrome).[114]
- Theophylline (resulting in decreased theophylline levels).[117]
- Trazadone (resulting in symptoms of serotonin syndrome).[118]
- Warfarin (resulting in decreased warfarin levels).[119]

St. John's wort appears to induce cytochrome P450 enzymes, specifically CYP1A2,[117] CYP3A2[120] and CYP3A4,[121,122] thus enhancing the metabolism of these (and potentially other) medications. St. John's wort has also been reported to reduce the expression of serotonin receptors.[29] A 2-week washout period is recommended between usage of St. John's wort and a selective serotonin reuptake inhibito (SSRI) such as paroxetine or fluoxetine.[98,115] In addition, it probably activates P-glycoprotein, which can further increase the elimination of many drugs.[99-120]

Until more information is available, the following drugs should also be used with caution in combination with St. John's wort:[2,123]

❖ Anti-convulsants: carbamazepine, phenobarbitone and phenytoin.

❖ HIV protease inhibitors: indinivir, nelfinavir, ritonavir, saquinavir.

❖ HIV non-nucleoside reverse transcriptase inhibitors: elfavirenz nevirapine.

❖ Monoamine Oxidase Inhibitors (MAOIs): phenelzine, tranylcypromine, isocarboxazid.

❖ Selective Serotonin Reuptake Inhibitors (SSRIs): fluoxetine.

❖ Sympathomimetics: amphetamines, ephedrine (found in many cold and hay fever remedies), methyldopa, dopamine, levodopa, trytophan.

❖ Triptans: sumatriptan, naratriptan, rizatriptan, zolmitriptan.

Theoretically, St. John's wort may also have an additive effect with other drugs causing photosensitization (e.g., piroxicam, tetracycline and others).[98,123]

DOSAGE REGIMENS

❖ STANDARDIZED EXTRACT (equivalent to 0.4-2.7 mg hypericin daily): 350-1800 mg daily in divided doses.[2]

❖ STANDARDIZED EXTRACT (0.3% hypericin): 300 mg three times daily.[64]

❖ STANDARDIZED EXTRACT (5% hyperforin): 300 mg three times daily.[56]

❖ DRIED HERB: 2-4 g three times per day.[2]

❖ INFUSED OIL OR CREAM: applied externally as needed.[124]

Tea Tree Oil

Melaleuca alternifolia (Maiden & Betche) Cheel

Common Uses
❖ Fungal Infections

Active Constituents
❖ Terpinen-4-ol

Adverse Effects
❖ Skin Irritation

Cautions/Contraindications
❖ Oral Administration

Drug Interactions
❖ None found

Doses
❖ No guidelines could be found but products should contain 30% or more terpinen-4-ol and less than 15% cineole. Preparations used in clinical trials have a tea tree oil concentration range from 5-100%.

Introduction

Family
- ❖ Myrtaceae

Synonyms
- ❖ None found

Medicinal Forms
- ❖ Essential Oil

Description

Tea tree is a member of the myrtle family and is found only in Southeastern Australia. The tree grows to a height of 20 feet or 6 meters, with layered, paper-like bark, narrow pointed leaves and white-to-yellow brush-shaped flowers.

Parts Used

The essential oil produced from steam distillation of the leaves is the part used medicinally.

Traditional Use

The indigenous people of Australia have long prized the aromatic leaves both for religious purposes and for medicinal use as an anti-septic and anti-fungal agent in treating skin, oral, and vaginal infections. Its name comes from the fact that a 'tea' was made from it by the early European settlers.[1] Due to increased popular demand, the commercial production of Australian tea tree oil increased in the early 1990s from 20 tonnes/annum to 140 tonnes/annum. In addition to its medicinal applications, it is now used extensively in the cosmetic and skin-care industry.[2]

Current Medicinal Use

Tea tree oil products are now primarily used as creams and gels in the treatment of fungal infections, such as athletes foot and infections of the nail beds.

Relevant Research

Preventative and Therapeutic Effects

CONSTITUENTS [3,4,5]

- ❖ VOLATILE OIL: contains various terpenes, including: terpinen-4-ol, pinene, terpinene, cymene and cineole.

COMMON USES

The essential oil is considered to be both an anti-septic and anti-microbial. It is reputed to be useful in the management of many conditions, including acne, fungal infections (tinea pedis, onychomycosis, ringworm), vaginal yeast infections, oral thrush and a number of skin conditions.[1,6]

MECHANISM OF ACTION

Tea tree oil has been reported to act against a number of bacteria, fungi and yeasts, most notably *Candida* spp., *Trichophyton rubrum* and *Staphylococcus aureus in vivo.*[1,2,6] It appears that *Staphylococcus aureus* is less susceptible to tea tree oil than *Candida albicans.*[2] A small (n=30) pilot randomized controlled study compared a 4% tea tree oil nasal ointment and 5% tea tree oil body wash with usual care (2% mupirocin nasal ointment and triclosan body wash) for the eradication of methicillin-resistant *Staphylococcus aureus* carriage. The authors report that "the tea tree oil combination appeared to perform better than the standard combination, although the difference was not statistically significant due to the small number of patients."[7] Additional research in this area appears warranted.

ACNE VULGARIS

In a clinical trial of patients (n=124) suffering from acne vulgaris, the effectiveness of a 5% tea tree oil gel was compared to that of a 5% benzoyl peroxide lotion after 3 months. While the tea tree oil product was considered effective, it had a longer onset of action and it was found to be less active on the inflamed lesions than the benzoyl peroxide product. However, the tea tree oil treatment resulted in an appreciably lower incidence of side effects, including skin dryness, pruritis and skin scaling than the benzoyl peroxide.[8]

TOPICAL FUNGAL INFECTIONS

In a randomized, double blind trial of patients (n=104) suffering from tinea pedis, the effectiveness of a tea tree oil cream (10%) was compared to 1% tolnaftate cream or placebo. Outcome measures included culture and clinical symptoms (skin scaling, inflammation, itching and burning). While the tea tree oil was shown to be as effective as tolnaftate and superior to placebo in causing relief of symptoms, it was no better than placebo with respect to the culture samples. The study was carried out over a 5-week period.[9] A second randomized, double-blind, controlled study (n=158) compared the safety and efficacy of 25% and 50% tea tree oil applied twice daily for 4 weeks in the treatment interdigital tinea pedis. The authors concluded that both 25% and 50% tea tree oil were effective, but that 25% tea tree oil was associated with fewer complications and thus should be recommended.[10]

Another randomized, multi-center, controlled trial in patients (n=117) suffering from onychomycosis (a superficial fungal infection that destroys the entire nail) compared the effectiveness of tea tree oil (100%) to a conventional treatment of 1% clotrimazole cream over 6 months. Comparable improvement (cure, clinical assessment and subjective improvement) was seen in both groups. The two preparations were also comparable in cost and shared the same incidence of adverse effects (7%). Another randomized, double-blind, placebo-controlled, 16-week trial of a cream containing 5% tea tree oil and 2% butenafine hydrochloride in 60 outpatients with onychomycosis reported that 80% of those using the cream were cured as compared to no cures in the placebo group.[11]

A randomized, single-blind, placebo-controlled 4-week study in patients with mild to moderate dandruff (n=126) reported that 5% tea tree oil was more effective than placebo and appeared to be well-tolerated. Additional research is needed to confirm these findings.[12]

MISCELLANEOUS EFFECTS

There is one randomized, placebo-controlled, investigator-blinded pilot study (n=20) that investigated tea tree oil gel (6%) for the treatment of recurrent herpes labialis and reported that the tea tree oil gel appeared to have some benefit over placebo with respect to decreased time to re-epitheliazation after treatment and reduction in median duration of culture positivity. None of the differences between the tea tree oil group and the placebo group reached statistical significance, but the authors argue that this is likely due to the small sample size in this pilot study and recommend a larger study to confirm these preliminary findings.[13]

ADVERSE EFFECTS

Tea tree oil is considered 'very mildly irritating' on topical application but 'strongly irritant' following oral administration. It is not considered to result in either sensitization or phototoxicity;[14] however, it is recommended that care should be taken when using very concentrated tea tree oil products in children and fair-skinned individuals.[15]

CAUTIONS/CONTRAINDICATIONS

Given the lack of guidelines available, tea tree oil should not be administered orally.

DRUG INTERACTIONS

No cases of interactions between conventional therapy and tea tree oil could be found.

DOSAGE REGIMENS

No dosage guidelines for tea tree oil could be found. The Australian guidelines for terpinen-4-ol/cineole content should be considered when using a tea tree oil product therapeutically. In 1985, an 'Australian Standard, Oil of Melaleuca' was established, suggesting that the essential oil should contain 30% or more terpinen-4-ol and less than 15% cineole.[1,3] Tyler cautions, "it is important that the commercial product not be derived from other *Melaleuca* species, some of which contain high concentrations of cineole, a skin irritant that also reduces the antiseptic effectiveness of terpinen-4-ol."[5]

Note: Preparations used in clinical trials range from 5-100%; however, in general, the concentrations of tea tree oil used in the clinical trials described are considerably lower than those often seen in clinical practice.[15,16] Many 'tea tree oil products' used in the cosmetic and toiletries industry contain only small amounts of active substance and the medicinal efficacy is often questionable.[2]

Thyme
Thymus vulgaris L.

THUMBNAIL SKETCH

Common Uses
- ❖ Spasmodic Respiratory Conditions
- ❖ Dyspepsia
- ❖ Parasites and Fungal
- ❖ Infections

Active Constituents
- ❖ Volatile Oil (thymol and carvacrol)
- ❖ Flavonoids

Adverse Effects (volatile oil portion)
Oral
- ❖ Nausea, Vomiting, Gastric Distress
- ❖ Headache, Dizziness, Convulsions, Coma
- ❖ Cardiac and Respiratory Collapse

Topical
- ❖ Irritating (moderately)

Cautions/Contraindications
- ❖ Pregnancy

Drug Interactions
- ❖ None known

Doses
Oral
- ❖ *Dried Herb:* 1-4 g (often taken as an infusion)
- ❖ *Tincture* (1:5 in 45% alcohol): 2-6 mL three times daily
- ❖ *Tincture* (1:10 in 70% alcohol): 40 drops up to three times daily

Topical
- ❖ Thyme oil should only be used after diluting with a suitable carrier oil

Introduction

Family
- ❖ Laminaceae (also know as mint or Labiatae)

Synonyms
- ❖ Common thyme
- ❖ French thyme
- ❖ Garden thyme
- ❖ Rubbed thyme[1,2]

Medicinal Forms
- ❖ Dried Herb
- ❖ Liquid Extract
- ❖ Tincture
- ❖ Oil

Description

Thyme is a shrub native to Mediterranean Europe but is also cultivated in the United States. It is an evergreen standing up to 45 centimeters or 18 inches in height, with multiple hairy stems arising from a single woody fibrous root and mauve-to-pink flowers. Like other members of the mint family, it is rich in volatile oils, producing a characteristic aromatic scent.

Parts Used

The aerial parts are used medicinally as dried herb or as an oil, which is extracted from the leaves and flowering tops by steam distillation.[2] Two oils exist, red and white oil. The red oil is made by redistilling the white oil and has often been seen to be adulterated.[2] Many subspecies exist and this can result in differences in medicinal action and composition of the volatile oil, primarily due to differences in the proportion of phenols.[3-5]

Traditional Use

Thyme has been a popular medicinal plant among British herbalists, praised by Nicholas Culpepper and used externally as an antiseptic and internally as tonic, for treating coughs and strengthening the respiratory system. The herb is also used widely for culinary purposes.

Current Medicinal Use

As with its traditional uses, thyme is primarily used now in cough mixtures for irritating spasmodic coughs and as an agent to aid digestion.

Relevant Research

Preventative and Therapeutic Effects

CONSTITUENTS [1,2,5-7]

- ❖ VOLATILE OILS: containing monoterpenoids, predominately the phenols thymol and carvacrol, as well as unsubstituted cymene and terpinene and the alcohols alpha-terpineol, linalool, and thujan-4-ol.
- ❖ PHENYLPROPANOIDS: including eugenol, caffeic acid, and rosmarinic acid.
- ❖ TRITERPENES: including ursolic acid and oleanolic acid,
- ❖ MISCELLANEOUS: including flavonoids, dimethylbiphenyl and tannins.

COMMON USES

Thyme is reputed to have many therapeutic actions, including carminative;[4,8,9] antimicrobial/antiseptic;[8,9] expectorant;[3,4,8,9] anti-tussive;[3,9] and diaphoretic actions.[8] Oral consumption is considered to be useful in the treatment of conditions associated with spasm, including upper respiratory tract conditions (e.g., bronchitis, pertussis and asthma) and digestive upset.[4,8] It is also used both orally and topically for a number of parasitic and fungal infections.[4,8]

MISCELLANEOUS EFFECTS

General anti-spasmodic activity and specific bronchospasmolytic action has been demonstrated *in vitro*.[6,10] The flavonoid and phenolic components are thought to be responsible for this property with a proposed mechanism of action being calcium channel antagonism.[1,11]

The volatile oil has been shown to possess anti-bacterial and anti-fungal activity *in vitro*.[2,12] The anti-bacterial action against *Staphylococcus aureus* was shown to be decreased by agents known to inhibit the action of the phenolic components.[13] An aqueous extract of thyme has been reported to inhibit *Helicobacter pylori in vitro*.[14] In addition, anti-mutagenic properties have been demonstrated *in vitro*.[15]

Thyme oil has been shown to increase respiration and exert a hypotensive action in a number of animal models.[1,2] Rosmarinic acid has also been shown to exert an anti-inflammatory action in both *in vivo* and *in vitro* models.[6,16] Dimethylbiphenyl and a flavonoid, eriodictyol, have been shown to exert profound anti-oxidant action, possibly by inhibiting superoxide generation.[17]

ADVERSE EFFECTS

Thyme oil is considered to be a moderate dermal irritant and strong mucous membrane irritant.[5] Adverse effects of the volatile oil include: nausea, vomiting, digestive distress, headache, dizziness, sweating, convulsions, coma and respiratory/cardiac collapse.[1,2,18] Local irritation has resulted from the use of toothpaste containing thyme extracts.[1] In addition, a case of occupational asthma was noted in an individual in contact with a number of aromatic herbs including thyme. A sensitivity to thyme was confirmed later by skin prick test.[19]

CAUTIONS/CONTRAINDICATIONS

Thyme is reputed to be an emmenagogue and so should be used with caution in pregnancy, especially if given in high doses.[1,4,18] Experimentally cross-sensitivity with other members of the mint (Laminaceae) family has been noted.[20]

DRUG INTERACTIONS

No cases of drug interaction could be found.

DOSAGE REGIMENS

❖ DRIED HERB: **1-4 g** (often taken as an infusion) or 0.5-1.0 g in children under 1 year of age several times a day.[6]

❖ TINCTURE (1:5 in 45% alcohol): 2-6 mL three times daily.[1]

❖ TINCTURE (1:10 in 70% alcohol): 40 drops up to three times daily.[6]

Note: Thyme oil should only be applied topically after it has been diluted with a suitable carrier oil.[1]

Turmeric

Curcuma longa Linn.

THUMBNAIL SKETCH

Common Uses
- ❖ Inflammation (e.g., arthritis)
- ❖ Liver Disorders

Active Constituents
- ❖ Curcumin

Adverse Effects
- ❖ None known

Cautions/Contraindications
- ❖ Bile Duct Blockage and Gallstones
- ❖ Pregnancy and Lactation (safety not yet established)

Drug Interactions
- ❖ None known

Doses
- ❖ *Dried Turmeric Root:* 1.5-3.0 g three times daily
- ❖ *Curcumin:* 250-500 mg three times daily

Introduction

Description
Turmeric is a perennial herb, native to Southern Asia and culti-vated throughout the tropics, including many parts of the Caribbean.[2] A member of the ginger family, this herb grows to 3 feet or 90 centimeters in height and produces large oblong leaves which arise from a tuberous rhizome with a distinctive bright orange-yellow pulp.[2]

Parts Used
The parts used medicinally are the primary and secondary rhizomes, which are usually cured (i.e., boiled, cleaned and sundried) and polished.[3]

Traditional Use
Turmeric has been used historically for both its flavor (e.g., it is a major ingredient in curry powder) and its color (e.g., it is used in the preparation of mustard). Turmeric is used medicinally in both Traditional Chinese and Ayurvedic Medicine for a variety of inflammatory conditions (arthritis and allergies), liver disorders (jaundice), flatulence, menstrual difficulties, bruises and colic.[2]

Current Medicinal Use
Turmeric products are primarily used today in the treatment of joint inflammation, such as arthritis and sports injuries. It is increasingly becoming popular in protecting the liver against environmental toxins.

Relevant Research

Preventative and Therapeutic Effects

CONSTITUENTS [2-4]
* VOLATILE OIL: turmerone, zingiberene, bisabolane, guaiane, curlone curcumin.
* MISCELLANEOUS: sugars: glucose, fructose, arabinose, resins, protein, vitamins and minerals.
  Note: Curcumin is a phenylpropanoid derivative responsible for the characteristic yellow color as well as the main pharmacological activity.[4]

MECHANISM OF ACTION
Curcumin is reported to be a potent anti-inflammatory agent — its action is reported to be comparable to hydrocortisone and phenylbutazone.[3] Several hypotheses have been offered regarding its mechanism of action, including: (1) it has an indirect action via the adrenal cortex;[3] (2) it inhibits cortisone metabolism in the liver, thus increasing the amount of circulating cortisone;[3] (3) it inhibits 5-lipoxygenase;[5-6] and (4) it inhibits lipopolysaccharide (LPS)-induced production of tumor necrosis factor (TNF) and interleukin-1beta (IL-1).[7]

In addition, curcumin has been shown to have a variety of other direct effects, including inhibition of leukotriene formation and platelet aggregation, as well as increasing the breakdown of fibrin and promoting liver function in a variety of ways.[6,8-10] Turmeric has also been reported to increase bile secretion and bile flow.[3,11] It has also been shown to have a significant anti-oxidant activity.[12,13]

ANTI-INFLAMMATORY EFFECTS
Several experimental models have demonstrated the anti-inflammatory activity of the volatile oil component of turmeric,[14-15] as well as curcumin and its analogs.[6,8,9,16]

Rheumatoid Arthritis
Several clinical studies have reported curcumin's effectiveness in the treatment of rheumatoid arthritis.[17,18] One study found that symptoms such as joint swelling, walking speed and morning stiffness were improved to the same degree in patients taking either curcumin (1200 mg daily) or phenylbutazone (300 mg daily).[17] Another used the postoperative inflammation model for evaluating non-steroidal anti-inflammatory drugs (NSAIDs) and found 400 mg of curcumin to be as effective as 100 mg of phenylbutazone.[18]

GASTROINTESTINAL EFFECTS
Turmeric has a long history of use in the management of ulcerative conditions; however, the evidence supporting its use not consistently positive.[19] Despite this, the German Commission E has approved turmeric as an effective cholagogue and digestive aid.[20] Duke reviews a study in which turmeric, given at a dose of 250 mg three times daily, relieved ulcer pain.[21] Yet, another randomized, double-blind, placebo-controlled trial of patients newly diagnosed with duodenal ulcers (n=130) reported no significant difference in the symptom relief of those receiving turmeric (6 g daily in three divided doses) when compared with those taking a placebo after the 8-week study period.[22]

HEPATO-PROTECTIVE EFFECTS
Historically, turmeric was used for a variety of liver conditions. Experimental evidence from animal studies confirms that it appears to increase bile flow and may play a role in protecting the liver from toxins.[8,23] In addition, a related species, *Curcuma xanthorrhiza* Roxb., has been shown in animal experiments to provide protection from hepatotoxin-induced liver damage.[24] However, our literature review did not find any human studies which investigated turmeric's efficacy for these indications.

ANTI-CANCER EFFECTS
Animal studies suggest that curcumin may have an inhibitory effect on a variety of experimentally-induced cancer, including: carcinogen-induced cancers of the duodenum, colon and forestomach in mice;[25,26] Ehrlich ascites tumor in mice;[27] carcinogen-induced skin tumor formation in mice;[28] aflatoxin-induced hepatocarcinogenicity in rats;[29] and carcinogen-induced cancer of the oral mucosa in hamsters.[26] *In vitro* experiments have shown that curcumin may inhibit the growth of estragen-positive human breast MCF-7 cells induced by a variety of carcinogens,[30] and that it is phototoxic to rat basophilic leukemia cells in the presence of oxygen.[31] Researchers hypothesize that these effects are due in part to curcumin's anti-oxidant action (it appears to inhibit superoxide production).[27] The clinical significance of these findings remains unknown.

ANTI-MICROBIAL EFFECTS
Several studies have reported that curcumin has the ability to inhibit the replication of human immunodeficiency virus.[32-34] Researchers suggest that this activity is due in part to its inhibition of HIV-1 integrase.[32] Clinical trials of curcumin in AIDS patients are reportedly scheduled.[32]

Turmeric has been shown to have some nematocidal,[35] anti-fungal activity,[36] and anti-bacterial activity.[37-39]

MISCELLANEOUS EFFECTS

A 12-week, open-label, clinical trial reported that 375 mg curcumin capsules (taken three times daily) alone (n=18) and in combination with anti-tubercular treatment (n=18) were effective in treating chronic anterior uveitis (inflammation of the eye) without any reported adverse effects. The efficacy and ability to prevent recurrences in a 3-year follow-up period were comparable to those reported in trials of corticosteroid therapy, presently the only available standard treatment for this disease. The authors suggest that the lack of adverse effects associated with curcurmin could be a significant advantage over corticosteroid therapy and recommend conducting a randomized, double-blind, clinical trial to confirm these preliminary findings.[40]

Curcumin has been reported to decrease cholesterol and lipid levels in animal studies.[41,42] Anti-oxidant properties have been reported in animal studies.[2]

ADVERSE EFFECTS

Turmeric and curcumin appear to have no adverse effects.[3,43] Prolonged use may occasionally result in gastrointestinal upset.[1]

CAUTIONS/CONTRAINDICATIONS

Individuals with blockage of the common bile duct or gallstones should avoid consuming turmeric due to its reputed ability to increase bile flow.[1] An animal study has demonstrated that the active constituents of turmeric are transferred translactationally.[44] Safety in pregnancy and lactation has not yet been established.

DRUG INTERACTIONS

No known drug interactions.

DOSAGE REGIMENS

❖ DRIED ROOT: 1.5-3 g daily.[1]

   Note: The clinical trials reviewed used 400 mg curcumin three times daily.[17,18]

Uva-Ursi

Arctostaphylos uva-ursi (L.) Spreng.

THUMBNAIL SKETCH

Common Uses
- ❖ Lower Urinary Tract Infections (uncomplicated)

Active Constituents
- ❖ Phenolic Glycosides (arbutin, methylarbutin)

Adverse Effects
- ❖ Nausea and Vomiting
- ❖ Hydroquinone Toxicity Symptoms (large doses)

Cautions/Contraindications
- ❖ Pregnancy and Lactation
- ❖ Kidney Disease

Drug Interactions
- ❖ None known

Doses
- ❖ *Dried Leaves:* 1.5-4.0 g three times a day for a maximum of 2 weeks
- ❖ *Fluid Extract* (1:1 in 25% alcohol): 1.5-4.0 mL three times a day for a maximum of 2 weeks

Introduction

Description
Uva-ursi is a trailing evergreen shrub, growing to 20 inches or 50 centimeters in height, native to many regions of the Northern Hemisphere, including Canada. It produces small shiny, leathery oblong leaves, small pale pink flowers, and glossy red berries.[2] Bears are thought to like the sour red berries, giving rise to the popular name of bearberry.[3] This also gave rise to its Latin binomial name, *Arctostaphylos*, meaning bearberry or bear grape in Greek, and *uva-ursi*, meaning the same in Latin.[4] The leaves have an astringent and bitter taste.[5]

Parts Used
The leaves are used medicinally.

Traditional Use
Uva-ursi has been considered one of the most effective herbal antiseptics for urinary tract infections (bladder and kidney) and cystitis. It has also been used for treating venereal diseases.

Current Medicinal Use
As with its traditional use, uva-ursi is still primarily used for uncomplicated urinary tract infections, such as cystitis.

Relevant Research

Preventative and Therapeutic Effects

CONSTITUENTS [1,2,6-10]
❖ PHENOLIC GLYCOSIDES: arbutin (hydroquinone beta-glucoside), methylarbutin, piceoside and para-methoxyphenol.
❖ FLAVONOIDS: including glycosides of quercetin, kaempferol and myricetin.
❖ IRIDOIDS: monotropein, unedoside (root).
❖ MISCELLANEOUS: including hydrolysable tannins, ursolic acid, terpenoids and allantoin.

COMMON USES
Uva-ursi is used primarily for its action as a urinary anti-septic, often in the management of uncomplicated infections of the lower urinary tract (e.g., cystitis, urethritis and prostatitis).[3,11,12] While it has been reported to be a diuretic,[2,13] other research suggests that this is probably not the case.[11,12,14] As a result of its astringent properties, uva-ursi has also been used in conditions of the lower digestive tract (e.g., diarrhea) and for enuresis.[3,13] It is also reputed to be useful in bronchitis and urinary stones.[2,13,15]

MECHANISM OF ACTION
The phenolic glycosides, especially arbutin, appear to be the primary active agents. However, the therapeutic effectiveness of uva-ursi is dependent on the conversion of these phenolic glycosides to a known anti-microbial agent, hydroquinone. Arbutin appears to be absorbed intact, undergoing hydrolysis in the urine to hydroquinone.[1,16] It has been suggested that

other agents in the whole extract may protect the arbutin from degradation in the gastrointestinal tract.[1]

Other researchers have argued that this conversion occurs in the gastrointestinal tract with the hydroquinone being transported as a conjugate systemically and free hydroquinone being liberated in the urine.[12] Anti-microbial action is noted only when the urine is alkaline with a pH of 8 or greater.[10,12] Since uva-ursi exerts an anti-bacterial action in the genitourinary tract, it has been suggested that the resultant uroepithelial protection may prevent the retention of microcalculi.[17] Anti-microbial properties have been demonstrated *in vitro* for uva-ursi against a number of organisms, including *Staphylococcus aureus*, *Bacillus subtilis*, *Escherichia coli* and *Shigella sp.*[18]

ADVERSE EFFECTS

One randomized, crossover study investigated the urinary excretion of arbutin metabolites after a single dose of uva ursi leaves (dry extract) delivered using either film coated tablets or acqueous extract to 16 healthy volunteers. The total amounts of hydroquinone equivalents excreted in the urine were similar in both groups; however, there was substantial inter-subject variability. No significant differences were found in metabolite patterns detected.[19]

Randomized, blinded, controlled clinical trials are still needed to assess the clinical efficacy of uva ursi for any specific medical condition.

Consumption of large doses of uva-ursi has resulted in nausea and vomiting. In addition, hydroquinone is known to have a toxic potential causing tinnitus, nausea, vomiting, shortness of breath, cyanosis, convulsions, delirium and collapse.[20]

CAUTIONS/CONTRAINDICATIONS

Uva-ursi should be considered contraindicated in kidney disorders,[10,14] pregnancy and lactation.[10,14] Due to the presence of hydroquinone and the large amount of tannins, prolonged use or the consumption of large amounts of uva-ursi should be avoided.[1]

DRUG INTERACTIONS

No cases of interactions with conventional medications could be found. Theoretically, caution should be exercised with drugs known to interact with hydroquinone.

DOSAGE REGIMENS

❖ DRIED LEAVES: 1.5-4.0 g three times daily.[1]
❖ FLUID EXTRACT (1:1 in 25% alcohol): 1.5-4.0 mL three times daily.[1]

Note: The ESCOP monograph recommends "cold water infusions of the crude drug equivalent to 400-800 mg arbutin per day in divided doses."[10] The duration of treatment should be limited to 2 weeks and medical attention sought if there is a worsening of symptoms.[10] Cold water infusions are preferable to hot ones because they contain fewer tannins. Uva-ursi is often given with an alkalinizing agent such as sodium bicarbonate.

Valerian

Valeriana officinalis L. and other species of *Valeriana*

Common Uses
* Sleep Aid
* Anxiety

Active Constituents
* Gamma-aminobutyric Acid (GABA)
* Alkaloids
* Valepotriates
* Volatile Oils

Adverse Effects
* Sedation

Cautions/Contraindications
* Pregnancy and Lactation (contraindicated)
* May impair driving and operation of hazardous machinery

Drug Interactions
* May potentiate the sedative effects of other CNS depressants

Doses
* *Dried Root and Rhizome* (or equivalent dry extracts): 2-3 g three times daily or at bedtime
* *Tincture* (20% concentration by volume in a 70% ethanol solution): 1-3 mL of three times daily or at bedtime

Introduction

Family
❖ Valerianaceae

Synonyms
❖ Belgian valerian
❖ Common valerian
❖ Fragrant valerian
❖ Garden valerian[1-3]

Medicinal Forms:
❖ Dried Root or Rhizome
❖ Tincture

Description
There are over 200 valerian species and variants found in Australia, China, Europe, India, Japan, and North America (including Mexico). This perennial plant grows up to 4 feet or 125 centimeters in height, with pairs of opposing, almond-shaped, serrated-edge leaves arising from a grooved, hollow stem. Small, rose-colored flowers bloom from the top of the stem in the summer months. The root produces an odor variously described as offensive, distinctive, and penetrating.[4,5]

Parts Used
The tuberous root and dried rhizome of three species — *V. officinalis* L., *V. jatamansi* Jones (Indian Valerian) and *V. edulis* Nutt. ex. Torr. & Gray spp. *procera* F.G. Meyer (Mexican Valerian) — are most often used as for medicinal purposes.[2-4,6,7]

Traditional Use
Although not specifically mentioned in classical Greek or Roman medical writings, the use of valerian has been attributed to Hippocrates as early as 425 B.C.[8] Valerian's medicinal use in Asia, Australia, Europe, the Middle East and North America has been documented in Greek, Anglo-Saxon, Medieval and Renaissance texts. It has been used as a sedative and an anti-nauseant, as well as for gastrointestinal and urinary symptoms.[3]

Current Medicinal Use
While valerian is primarily used in the treatment of mild insomnia, it is increasingly being found in herbal products used to treat muscle spasms and pain.

Relevant Research

Preventative and Therapeutic Effects

CONSTITUENTS [1,7,9-12]
❖ AMINO ACIDS: gamma-aminobutyric acid (GABA).
❖ ALKALOIDS: actinidine, chatinine, skyanthine, valerianine, valerine.
❖ IRIDOIDS (VALEPOTRIATES): valerate(s), dihydrovalerate(s), valerosidate.
❖ VOLATILE OILS: monoterpenes, sesquiterpenes (e.g. valerenic acid), valerenyl esters.
❖ PHENYLPROPANOIDS: caffeic and chlorogenic acids.
❖ SESQUITERPENOIDS: valerenolic acid and acetylvalerenolic acid.

COMMON USES
Valerian is most often used as a sedative-hypnotic agent. Due to its reputed muscle relaxing properties it is often used, alone or in combination with other herbs, in the management of musculoskeletal conditions.

MECHANISM OF ACTION

Because of valerian's historical use as a sedative, anti-convulsant, migraine treatment and pain reliever, most basic science research has been directed at the interaction of valerian constituents with the GABA neurotransmitter receptor system. These studies remain inconclusive and all require independent replication. The mechanism of action of valerian in general, and as a mild sedative in particular, remains unknown.

Valerian extracts appear to have some affinity for the $GABA_A$ (benzodiazepine) receptor,[13,14] but this activity does not appear to be mediated by valerenic acid, but rather by the relatively high content of GABA itself.[15,16] The amount of GABA present in aqueous extracts of valerian is sufficient to account for the release of GABA from synaptosomes, and also may inhibit reuptake.[17,18] However, GABA does not cross the blood-brain barrier efficiently at low concentrations, so these *in vitro* results cannot account for the clinical data. Catabolism of GABA may be inhibited by valerenolic acid and acetylvalerenolic acid.[19]

Interactions with the serotonin neurotransmitter system have also been investigated and hydroxypinoresinol was found to have high affinity for the $5\text{-}HT_{1A}$ receptor.[12,20] One paper reports an interaction with the adenosine receptor but not with the benzodiazepine receptor.[21]

Valerian has been reported to decrease gastrointestinal motility.[22] There is also some suggestion of an anti-pyretic or anti-inflammatory effect of valerian extracts.[23-25]

Animal Studies

Behavioral studies on rodents have demonstrated that valerian has some sedative properties. Valerian extracts produce changes in behavioral tests such as rotorod performance, activity and augmentation of barbiturate-induced sleep similar to changes observed with benzodiazepines.[12,26-35] Only weak anticonvulsive effects were found.[36] In contrast, Hiller et al. found no sedative effects in mice but did report some anticonvulsant effects.[37] One study reported that *Valeriana coreana* Briq. methanol extracts were able to decrease immobility in the forced swimming test in mice,[38] and reversed resperpine-induced hypothermia,[32] which suggests potential anti-depressant activity. EEG changes in rats have also been found,[39] but these effects were not confirmed in cats.[40] Cerebral nuclear medicine imaging in rats using radio-labelled glucose showed central nervous system (CNS) depressant effects for a dichloromethane extract of valerian but not for the essential oil, valerenic acid, valeranone, valtrate, didrovaltrate, or homobaldrinal.[12,41,42]

Human Clinical Studies

The human clinical studies of valerian have concentrated on evaluating its use as a sleep aid. As would be expected from the basic science and animal data, valerian appears to have a mild sedative effect making it suitable as a sleep aid.[43] Its precise effects on the components of sleep are not consistent in the small number of studies conducted to date. There are reports that valerian root improves subjective sleep quality and produces a decrease in the latency of sleep onset.[5,44-51] Some objective laboratory sleep observations showed no significant difference between placebo and valerian, including no change in sleep stages, sleep latency, awakening, subjective sleep quality or EEG patterns;[52] while others noted increased rapid eye movement sleep,[53] increased slow wave sleep,[50,52] decreased stage I sleep,[50,52,53] increased density of K-complexes,[52] and decrease in wake time after sleep onset.[51]

A randomized, double-blind, placebo-controlled study (n=37) assessing the use of valerian (100mg Valmane® three times daily) on benzodiazepine withdrawal reported subjective sleep quality improvement after two weeks of treatment of insomniacs that had withdrawn from benzodiazepines. The sleep study also reported an objective decrease in wake time after sleep onset in those treated with valerian, but those taking valerian also took longer to get to sleep compared with the placebo control group. Overall, the authors concluded that valerian had a positive effect on withdrawal from benzodiazepine use.[51]

One randomized, double-blind, controlled pilot study (n=36) found no significant differences in total Hamilton Anxiety scores between individuals diagnosed with generalized anxiety disorder that took valerian (81.3 mg valepotriates daily), compared with diazepam (mean daily dose 6.5 mg) and placebo. Given the small number of participants in this pilot study, the authors indicate that their results must be viewed as preliminary and recommended additional studies.[54]

Another randomized, placebo-controlled trail assessed the effect of valerian on five children with varying intellectual deficits and different primary sleep problems over 8 weeks. The results indicate that compared to baseline and placebo, valerian treatment was associated with "significant reduction in sleep latencies and nocturnal time awake, lengthened total sleep time and improved sleep quality" that was particularly apparent in children with hyperactivity problems.[55] While promising, these findings must be seen as preliminary with further research warranted.

ADVERSE EFFECTS

Clinical trials report very few adverse effects associated with valerian.[50,53-56] Data on the toxicity associated with valerian preparations are sparse, but there is some evidence of cytotoxicity.[4] Braun et al. found no *in vivo* toxicity of valerian derivatives on hematopoietic precursor cells in contrast to *in vitro* data.[57,58,59] Hepatotoxicity has been reported with herbal sleep remedies but these contained other ingredients in combination with valerian.[60,61] Bounthanh et al. report that valpotriates significantly inhibit both DNA and protein synthesis.[62] Potential teratogenicity has been investigated in rats with no adverse effects identified.[63] However, this single study does not establish that valerian is safe to use in pregnancy, and therefore its use should be avoided until further data are available even though some authors have suggested that valerian is safe to use in pregnancy.[64,65] Large doses (400mg/kg) of valerenic acid were found to be fatal in mice.[32]

A randomized, double-blind, placebo-controlled trial (n=102) reported that valerian (600 mg of LI156 extract) did not have a relevant negative impact on reaction time, alertness or concentration the morning after intake of a single dose nor after two weeks of evening administration.[56]

CAUTIONS/CONTRAINDICATIONS

Valerian should be used with caution in children under 3 years of age; and pregnant or lactating women. Individuals taking valerian should be cautious when operating a motor vehicle or hazardous machinery.[9]

DRUG INTERACTIONS

Little data on specific drug interactions exist at present. However, given the evidence of hypnotic-sedative effects, the use of valerian preparations in conjunction with other CNS depressants should be avoided or approached with caution. Valerian may potentiate the effects of other CNS depressants, including ethanol.[23,28,32,66]

DOSAGE REGIMENS

❖ DRIED ROOT OR RHIZOME (or equivalent dry extracts) ❖ 2-3 g three times daily or at bedtime.
❖ TINCTURE (20% concentration by volume in a 70% ethanol solution) ❖ 1-3 mL of three times daily or at bedtime.[9]

Wild Yam

Dioscorea villosa L.

THUMBNAIL SKETCH

Common Uses
- ❖ Abdominal Colic, Diverticulitis, Irritable Bowel Syndrome
- ❖ Arthritis and Rheumatism
- ❖ Gynecological Problems (dysmennorhoea and ovarian pains)

Active Constituents
- ❖ Steroidal Glycosides (based on the sapogenin diosgenin)

Adverse Effects
- ❖ None could be found for the plant itself but consumption of the sapogenins may result in bruising

Cautions/Contraindications
- ❖ Pregnancy

Drug Interactions
- ❖ None could be found

Doses
- ❖ *Tincture:* 2-4 mL three times daily

Introduction

Family
❖ Dioscoreaceae

Synonyms
❖ Colic root
❖ Rheumatism root[1]

Medicinal Forms
❖ Tincture
❖ Creams

Description

Many different species of the genus Dioscorea exist but within the complementary medical model, *Dioscorea villosa* is the one most often used. Wild yam (*Dioscorea villosa*) is distinct from the vegetable often referred to as yam (*Ipomoea batatas* (L.) Lam., Convolvulaceae).[5] *Dioscorea villosa* is a perennial vine, growing to 6 meters or 20 feet, with small green flowers, heart-shaped leaves, and a large fibrous root stock. The plant is native to the Eastern United States and Central America.[2] It has a characteristic taste often described as insipid.[3,4]

Parts Used

The tuberous roots are the part used medicinally. The therapeutic actions disappear on storage and it is best harvested annually.[4]

Traditional Use

The Aztecs, Mayans, and other native peoples of North and Central America used wild yam for treating painful menstruation and labor. The plant was also known as colic root and rheumatism root. This herb was used extensively by eclectic physicians in the United States during the mid to latter part of the 19th century.[5] Diosgenin, a steroid-like substance found in wild yam, was used in the development of modern contraceptives.

Current Medicinal Use

Unprocessed wild yam products are primarily used to treat digestive disorders such as colic, diverticulitis and irritable bowel syndrome. Semi-synthetic products containing hormones made from diosgenin are used in treating a number of gynecological conditions, although more research is needed to confirm this use.

Relevant Research

Preventative and Therapeutic Effects

CONSTITUENTS [1,3]

Steroidal saponins (based on the sapogenin diosgenin) including dioscin and dioscorin. Dioscorein is not an actual constituent but refers to a dried solid extract.[5]

COMMON USES

Wild yam is reputed to have anti-spasmodic,[2,4,6] anti-inflammatory,[2,6] diuretic,[2] hepatic,[2,6] and anti-rheumatic properties.[2,6] Oral consumption is considered useful in the treatment of digestive conditions such as intestinal colic, diverticulitis, irritable bowel syndrome and bilious indigestion.[2,6] As a traditional 'anti-rheumatic' it is used in situations of arthritis and joint inflammation.[2,5,6] It is also considered a 'relaxing remedy' and is used to treat a number of gynecological problems such as ovarian pain, painful menstruation and in labor.[2,5,6]

MISCELLANEOUS EFFECTS

No details regarding the mode of action of *Dioscorea villosa* itself could be found for this monograph.

Diosgenin, isolated from Mexican yam, was originally considered of prime importance in the pharmaceutical manufacture of steroidal substances, including early oral contraceptives.[2,3] Confusion has arisen because of claims made that diosgenin can be converted into steroidal substances, including dehydroepiandrosterone (DHEA) and progesterone, following oral or topical administration. Some products have been marketed as 'hormonal precursors'. No evidence could be found to substantiate these claims. Araghiniknam et al. demonstrated that oral administration of a compound containing 90% 'wild yam extract' did not increase serum dehydroepiandrosterone sulfate (DHEA-S) levels in a group of elderly patients (over 65 years of age, n=7).[7] The results of this study were supported by a similar investigation in which saliva specimens were analyzed in a group of women taking products containing Mexican yam.[8]

Concerns have been expressed regarding the use and marketing of 'wild yam' extracts as 'hormonal precursors'. There appears to be no evidence to support this claim. This confusion seems to be particularly important regarding the use of natural progesterone products.[5]

ADVERSE EFFECTS

No situations of adverse reactions could be found for the plant itself. Cases of 'hormonal effects' (early menopause symptoms, masculinization of females and hypertension) have been attributed to one commercial product.[9] No details were given with respect to the exact composition of this product and therefore the clinical relevance to the use of *Dioscorea villosa* in general cannot really be ascertained.

CAUTIONS/CONTRAINDICATIONS

Concerns have been raised regarding the safety of products referred to as 'Mexican Wild Yam' for individuals diagnosed with conditions with a strong hormonal element such as breast and prostate cancer.[9] A case of occupational allergy caused by frequent exposure to Sanyak / Chinese yam (*Dioscorea oppositifolia* L.) has been reported in a 25-year-old male who worked in a herbal pharmacy.[10] Given the lack of information and the fact that the herb acts as on smooth muscle, wild yam should be avoided in pregnancy.

DRUG INTERACTIONS

No cases of drug interaction could be found.

DOSAGE REGIMENS

❖ TINCTURE: 2-4 mL three times daily.[6]

Willow

Salix spp

Common Uses
- ❖ Arthritic Conditions
- ❖ Analgesic

Active Constituents
- ❖ Phenolic Glycosides (including salicin and salicortin)

Adverse Effects
- ❖ Rare — Nausea, Headache, Digestive Upset

Cautions/Contraindications
- ❖ Classic ones applicable to salicylates (e.g., aspirin)

Drug Interactions
- ❖ Classic ones applicable to salicylates (e.g., aspirin)

Doses
- ❖ *Raw Herb:* 5-10 g three times daily
- ❖ *Willow Preparations* (dried, hydroalcoholic or aqueous extracts, tinctures or fluid extracts): equivalent to 60-120 mg (up to 240 mg) of salicin daily
- ❖ *Salicin:* 20-40 mg three times daily (maximum of 240 mg of salicin daily)
- ❖ *Liquid Extract* (1:1 in 25% ethanol): 1-2 mL three times daily
- ❖ *Hydroalcoholic Tincture* (1:5 in 25% ethanol): 5-8 mL three times daily

Introduction

Description
Members of the this genus of trees, native to Europe, Asia and North America, range in height from 30 to 70 feet or 10 meters to 25 meters, with soft green, 'willowy' leaves and a soft bark that is easily separated or peeled from the young branches. While in North America white willow and black willow are most often used,[3,4] pharmacologically these may not be the most active since other members of the genus (e.g., *S. fragilis* L., *S. purpurea* and *S. daphnoides* Villars) are richer in the medicinally active phenolic glycosides.[4]

Parts Used
The bark of young branches is the part most commonly used medicinally. However, it has been shown that the leaves of some species may contain as much, and maybe more, of the phenolic glycosides than the bark. Accordingly, it has been argued that there is no reason why these parts cannot be used therapeutically.[5]

Traditional Use
Willow has a long history in many different healing traditions. It was especially popular in the treatment of rheumatism and ague (e.g., fever, chills).[3]

Current Medicinal Use
Willow products are considered to be 'natural painkillers' and are typically used in the treatment of joint pains, notably from arthritis, and in low back pain. Since willow does not contain aspirin (acetylsalicylic acid), it should not used as an aspirin substitute in thinning the blood.

Relevant Research

Preventative and Therapeutic Effects

CONSTITUENTS [1,5-8]

❖ PHENOLIC GLYCOSIDES: including salicin, salicortin, tremulacin and salireposide.

❖ MISCELLANEOUS: including condensed tannins, flavonoids and catechins.

Note: There is great variability among species of the salix genus; of particular importance are the phenolic glycoside components. While *Salix purpurea* L. can contain up to 8% salicin and *Salix fragilis* L. up to 10%,[4,7], *S. alba* L. often has less than 1% salicin.[4]

COMMON USES

Preparations of white willow bark have been used in the treatment of feverish conditions, rheumatism and as mild pain-killers in such conditions as headache.[7,9] Given the relatively low amount of phenolic glycosides (notably salicin) when compared to conventional salicylate medications, it has been argued that, in pharmacological terms, it is unlikely that any willow preparation will be effective in the management of these conditions.[4]

MECHANISM OF ACTION

The pharmacological action of willow appears to be determined not only by salicin content. The other phenolic glycosides also have therapeutic properties.[4] It is hypothesized that the phenolic glycosides do not act directly but rather act as pro-drugs. They are converted in multiple stages, primarily in the liver and intestines, to the active moieties (most notably salicylic acid).[7] The action is therefore slower in onset than conventional salicylic acid but has a longer duration of action.[4] It should be noted that salicin does not irreversibly inhibit platelet aggregation, as is the case with acetylsalicylic acid.[7]

Limited *in vivo* studies demonstrate that a number of the phenolic glycosides have anti-inflammatory properties.[7] Little research has been conducted on the salicylates and salicylic acid obtained from plant sources such as willow.

LOW BACK PAIN

One randomized, double-blind, placebo-controlled, 4-week trial reported that willow bark extract (120 mg or 240 mg of salicin) was more effective (dose-dependent effects were noted) than placebo in treating patients (n=210) with exacerbations of chronic low pack pain.[10] While promising, more research is necessary to confirm these findings.

OSTEOARTHRITIS

A randomized, double-blind, placebo-controlled 2 week trial (n=78) reported that willow (extract containing 240 mg salicin daily) significantly decreased pain (as assessed by the WOMAC osteoarthritis index, patient diary and visual analogue scores) associated with osteoarthritis.[11] As with the results for back pain, additional studies are needed to confirm these findings.

ADVERSE EFFECTS

Side-effects seem to be rare and mild, limited to nausea, digestive upset and headache.[7] A case of hemorrhage in a 64-year-old women with glucose-6-phosphate dehydrogenase (G6PD) deficiency has been documented following the consumption of an ayurvedic product containing *Salix caprea* L. No information is given in the case report with regards to other ingredients present in the preparation.[12] A clinical trial (n=35) confirms that willow extract (with 240 mg salicin in a daily dose) reduces arachidonic acid-induced platelet aggregation compared to placebo, but does not reduce it as much as 100 mg of acetylsalicylate. The authors suggest that further research is necessary to determine if these effects are of clinical relevance for patients with impaired thrombocyte function.[13]

One participant in a clinical trial who was randomized to the willow bark group experienced a severe allergic reaction (swollen eyes and pruritis) whose symptoms resolved 2 days after discontinuing willow (containing 120 mg of salicin).[10]

CAUTIONS/CONTRAINDICATIONS
The contraindications applicable to the use of conventional salicylate preparations are believed to be applicable to the consumption of willow products. Consequently, use should be avoided in individuals with conditions such as asthma, diabetes, gout, haemophilia, hyperthrombinaemia, hepatic/renal disease, active peptic ulcer disease, glucose-6-phosphate dehydrogenase (G6PD) deficiency and individuals sensitive to aspirin.[1] Until more detailed information is available, preparations containing willow should not be administered during pregnancy or lactation. No information could be found regarding the use of willow products in children given that salicylate-containing products are normally restricted to individuals over 12 years of age.

DRUG INTERACTIONS
No cases could be found but drug interactions common to conventional salicylates appear applicable.[1]

DOSAGE REGIMENS
- ❖ RAW HERB: 5-10 g three times daily.
- ❖ WILLOW PREPARATIONS (dried, hydroalcoholic or aqueous extracts, tinctures or fluid extracts): equivalent to 60-120 mg (up to 240 mg) of salicin daily.[7]
- ❖ SALICIN: 20-40 mg three times daily.
- ❖ LIQUID EXTRACT (1:1 in 25% ethanol) ❖ 1-2 mL three times daily.
- ❖ HYDROALCOHOLIC TINCTURE (1:5 in 25% ethanol) ❖ 5-8 mL three times daily.[14]

References

Foreword

1. Northcott H, Bachynsky J. Concurrent Use of Chiropractic, Prescription Medicines, Nonprescription Medicines and Alternative Health Care. Social Science and Medicine. 1993; 37(3):431-35.

2. Canada Health Monitor. Highlights Report. Survey #9. March 1993. Toronto: Price Waterhouse, Suite 3300, Box 190, 1 First Canadian Place, Toronto, Ontario, M5X 1H7; 1993.

3. Eisenberg DM, Kessler RC, Foster C, Norlock FE, Calkins DR, Delbanco TL. Unconventional medicine in the United States: Prevalence, costs and patterns of use. The New England Journal of Medicine. 1993; 328 (4):246-52.

4. Clarke K. Herbs, homeopathy rising stars. Pharmacy Post. 1996; November 17.

5. Health Management Institute. Plant derived pharmaceuticals — A renewed direction. Reference HMI 960201 White Paper. Fredericton, New Brunswick: Health Management Institute (HMI):1996.

6. Anonymous. Pharmacy Trends. Pharmacy Practice. 1997; 13(6): 48-50.

7. Dundass H. The Herbal Niche. The Canadian Pharmaceutical Journal. 1993; 125(6):292-95.

8. Howden KM, Sheard LM, Christensen IP, et al. Counter prescribing of herbal remedies: A comparative study of pharmacies and health food shops. The Pharmaceutical Journal. 1989; Sepember 30:R28.

Introduction

1. Drugs Directorate (Canada). Drugs Directorate Guideline. Traditional Herbal Medicines (Revised). Ottawa: Health Protection Branch, Health Canada;October 1995.

2. Drugs Directorate. Good Manufacturing Guidelines for the Manufacture of Herbal Medicinal Products. Final Version. Ottawa: Drugs Directorate;October 1996.

3. Transition Team of the Office of Natural Health Products. A Fresh Start: Final Report of the ONHP Transition Team. Ottawa: Office of Natural Health Products;March 31, 2000.

4. Her Majesty the Queen in Right of Canada. Natural Health Products Regulations. Canada Gazette Part I 2001;135(51):4912-71.

5. Her Majesty the Queen in Right of Canada. Natural Health Products Regulations. Canada Gazette Part II 2003;137(13).

6. Blumenthal M, Brusse WR, Goldberg A, Gruenwald J, Hall T, Riggins CW, et al., ed. The Complete German Comission E Monographs. Austin, TX: American Botanical Council; 1998.

7. US Food and Drug Administration. Dietary Supplement Health and Education Act of 1994 http://www.cfsan.fda.gov/~dms/dietsupp.html; 1995.

8. Mills S. The Essential Book of Herbal Medicine. London: Penguin; 1991:677.

9. Bone K. Dosage considerations in herbal medicine. The British Journal of Phytotherapy. 1993-4; 3(3):128-37.

10. Werback M, Murray M. Botanical Influences on Illness. Tarzana, CA: Third Line Press; 1994:344.

11. Chevalier A. The Encyclopedia of Medicinal Plants. London: Readers Digest: 1996:336.

12. O'Neill A. Danger and safety in medicines. Social Science and Medicine. 1994;38(4): 497-507.

13. Mills S. Safety awareness in complementary medicine. Complementary Therapies in Medicine. 1996; 4:48-51.

14. Coremans P, Lambrecht G, Schepens P et al. Anti-cholinergic intoxication with commercially available thornapple tea. Journal of Toxicology: Clinical Toxicology. 1994; 32: 589-92.

15. Tennekoon K, Jeevathayaparan S, Angunawala P et al. Effect of *Momordica charantia* on key hepatic enzymes. Journal of Ethnopharmacology. 1994;44:93-97.

16. D'Arcy P. Adverse reactions and interactions and herbal medicine. Part 1 Adverse reactions. Adverse Drug React. Toxicol. Rev. 1991;10(4):189-208.

17. Smith A, Feddersen R, Gardner K et al. Cystic renal cell carcinoma and acquired renal cystic disease associated with consumption of chaparral tea: A case report. Journal of Urology. 1994; 152:2089-91.

18. Atherton D. Towards the safer use of traditional remedies. British Medical Journal. 1994; 308:673-74.

19. Itami N, et al. Herbal medicine can induce hypertension. Nephron. 1991; 59:339-40.

20. Hogan R. Hemorrhagic diathesis caused by drinking an herbal tea. Journal of the American Medical Association. 1983; 249(19):2679-80.

21. Perharic L, Shaw D, Colbridge M et al. Toxicological problems resulting from exposure to traditional remedies and food supplements. Drug Safety. 1994;11(4):284-94.

22. Vanhaelen M, Vanhaelen-Fastre R, But P et al. Identification of aristocholic acid in Chinese herbs. Lancet. 1994:174.

23. Bryson P, Watanabe A, Rumack B et al. Burdock root tea poisoning. Journal of the American Medical Association. 1978;239(20):2157.

24. Raman A, Jamal J. 'Herbal' hayfever remedy found to contain conventional drugs. The Pharmaceutical Journal.1997;258:105-06.

25. Hughes J, Higguis E, Pembroke A et al. Oral dexamethasone masquerading as a Chinese herbal remedy. British Journal of Dermatology. 1994;130:261.

26. Markowitz S, Nuuez C, Klitzman S et al. Lead poisoning due to hai ge fen. Journal of the American Medical Association. 1994; 271:932-34.

27. Stricht B. Remedies may contain cocktail of active drugs. British Medical Journal. 1994; 308:1162.

28. Mcrae S. Elevated serum digoxin levels in a patient taking digozin and Siberian ginseng. Canadian Medical Association Journal. 1996;155(3):293-95.

29. Jones, B, Runikis A. Interaction of ginseng with phenelzine. Journal of Clinical Psychopharmacology. 1987;7(3):201-02.

30. Lepik K. Safety of herbal medicines in pregnancy. Canadian Pharmaceutical Journal. 1997; May:29-33.

31. Jonas W. Safety in complementary medicine. In: Ernst E, ed. Complementary Medicine, An Objective Appraisal. Oxford: Butterworth-Heinermann; 1996:127-49.

Alfalfa

1. Briggs C. Alfalfa. Canadian Pharmaceutical Journal. 1994;March:84-86.

2. Leung AY, Foster S. Encyclopedia of Common Natural Ingredients Used in Food, Drugs, and Cosmetics. 2nd ed. New York: John Wiley and Sons Inc; 1996:649.

3. Chevallier A. The Encyclopedia of Medicinal Plants. London: Readers Digest; 1996:336.

4. Natelson S. Canavanine to arginine ratio in alfalfa (*Medicago sativa*), clover (*Trifolium*), and the jack bean (*Canavalia ensiformis*). Journal of Agriculture and Food Chemistry. 1985;33:413-419.

5. Natelson S. Canavanine in alfalfa (*Medicago sativa*). Experentia. 1985;41:257-59.

6. Polachek I, Zehavi V, Naim M, et al. Activity of compound G2 isolated from alfalfa roots against medically important yeasts. Antimicrobial Agents and Chemotherapy. 1986;30:290-94.

7. Berrang B, Davis KHJ, Wall ME, Hanson CH, Pedersen ME. Saponins of two alfalfa cultivars. Phytochemistry. 1974;13:2253-60.

8. Newall CA, Anderson LA, Phillipson JD. Herbal Medicines: A Guide for Health Care Professionals. London: The Pharmaceutical Press; 1996:296.

9. Malinow MR, McLaughlin P, Kohler GO, Livingston AL. Prevention of elevated cholesterolemia in monkeys by alfalfa saponins. Steroids. 1977;29:105-110.

10. Malinow MR, McLaughlin P, Papworth L, et al. Effect of alfalfa saponins on intestinal cholesterol absorption in rats. American Journal of Clinical Nutrition. 1977;30(12):2061-67.

11. Cookson FB, Altschul R, Federoff S. The effects of alfalfa on serum cholesterol and in modifying or preventing cholesterol induced atherosclerosis in rabbits. Journal of Atherosclerosis Research. 1967;7:69.

12. Cookson FB, Fedoroff, S. Quantitative relationships between administered cholesterol and alfalfa required to prevent hypercholesterolaemia in rabbits. British Journal of Experimental Pathology. 1968;49:348.

13. Kritchevsky D, Tepper SA, Story JA. Isocaloric, isogravic diets in rats, Part 3 (Effect of non-nutritive fibre (alfalfa or cellulose) on cholesterol metabolism). Nutrition Reports International. 1974;9:301.

14. Yanaura S, Sakamoto M. Influence of alfalfa meal on experimental hyperlipidemia. Nippon Yakurigaku Zasshi – Folia Pharmacologica Japonica. 1975;71:387.

15. Malinow MR, McLaughlin P, Stafford C, Livingstone AL, Kohler GO. Alfalfa saponins and alfalfa seeds: Dietary effects on cholesterol-fed rabbits. Atherosclerosis. 1980;37:433-38.

16. Malinow MR, Connor WE, Mclaughlin P, et al. Cholesterol and bile acid balance in *Macaca fascicularis*: Effects of alfalfa saponins. Journal of Clinical Investigation. 1981;67:156-62.

17. Malinow MR, McLaughlin P, Naito HK, et al. Effect of alfalfa meal on shrinkage (regression) of atherosclerotic plaques during cholesterol feeding in monkeys. Atherosclerosis. 1978;30(1):27-43.

18. Malinow MR, McNulty, WP, Houghton, DC, et al. Lack of toxicity of alfalfa saponins on cynomolgus macaques. Journal of Medical Primatology. 1982;11:106-18.

19. Malinow MR, McLaughlin P, Stafford C. Alfalfa seeds: Effects on cholesterol metabolism. Experimentia. 1980;36:562-63.

20. Molgaard J, von Schenck H, Olsson AG. Alfalfa seeds lower low density lipoprotein cholesterol and apolipoprotein B concentrations in patients with type II hyperlipoproteinemia. Atherosclerosis. 1987; 65:173-79.

21. Malinow MR, McLaughlin P, Stafford C, et al. Comparative effects of alfalfa saponins and alfalfa fiber on cholesterol absorption in rats. American Journal of Clinical Nutrition. 1979; 32(9):1810-12.

22. Barichello AW, Federoff S. Effect of ileal bypass and alfalfa on hypercholesterolemia. British Journal of Experimental Pathology. 1971;52:81.

23. Hornick B, Cookson FB, Federoff S. Effect of alfalfa feeding on the excretion of fecal neutral sterols in the rabbit. Circulation. 1967;36 (Suppl. II):II-18.

24. Story JA, LePage SL, Petro MS, et al. Interactions of alfalfa plant and sprout saponins with cholesterol *in vitro* and in cholesterol-fed rats. American Journal of Clinical Nutrition. 1984; 39:917-29.

25. Zhao WS, Zhang YQ, Ren LJ, Zhang L, Yang J. Immunopotentiating effects of polysaccharides isolated from *Medicago sativa* L. (Chinese; English abstract). Acta Pharmacologica Sinica. 1993; 14(3):273-76.

26. De Smet PA, et al. Adverse Effects of Herbal Drugs. 2nd ed. Verlag: Springer; 1992.

27. Malinow MR, McNulty WP, McLaughlin P, et al. The toxicity of alfalfa saponins in rats. Food and Cosmetics Toxicology. 1981;19:443-45.

28. Anderson JO. Effect of alfalfa saponin on the performance of chicks and laying hens. Poultry Science. 1957;36:873-76.

29. Reshef G, Gestetner B, Birk Y. Effect of alfalfa saponins on the growth and some aspects of lipid metabolism of mice and quails. Journal of the Science of Food and Agriculture. 1976;27:63-72.

30. Wilcox EB, Galloway LS. Serum and liver cholesterol, total lipids and lipid phosphorus levels of rats under various dietary regimes. American Journal of Clinical Nutrition. 1961;9:236-43.

31. White RD, Kauperman PH, Cheeke PR, Buhler DR. An evaluation of acetone extracts from six plants in the Ames mutagenicity test. Toxicology Letters. 1983;15:25-31.

32. Malinow MR, Bardana EJ, Goodnight SH. Pancytopenia during ingestion of alfalfa seeds. Lancet. 1981:i:615.

33. Malinow MR, Bardana EJ, Pirofsky B, et al. Systemic lupus erythematosus-like syndrome in monkeys fed alfalfa sprouts: Role of a non-protein amino acid. Science. 1982;216:415-17.

34. Roberts JL, Hayashi JA. Exacerbation of SLE associated with alfalfa ingestion. [Letter]. New England Journal of Medicine. 1983;308(22):1361.

35. Rosenthal GA. The biological effects and mode of action of L-canavanine, a structural analogue of L-arginine. Quarterly Review of Biology. 1977;52:155-78.

36. Alcocer-Varela J, Iglesias A, llorente L, Alarcon-Segovia D. Effects of L-canavanine on T cells may explain the induction of systemic lupus erythematosus by alfalfa. Arthritis and Rheumatology. 1985;28(1):52-57.

37. Oakenfull D. Saponins in food. Food Chemistry. 1980;6:19-40.

38. Marles RJ, Associate Professor, Department of Botany, Brandon University, Brandon, Manitoba. Review of Medicinal Plant Modules for CCNM; 1997.

Aloe Vera

1. Marles RJ, Associate Professor, Department of Botany, Brandon University, Brandon, Manitoba. Review of Medicinal Plant Modules for CCNM; 1997.

2. Tyler VE. Herbs of Choice. The Therapeutic Use of Phytomedicinals. Binghamton, NY: Pharmaceutical Products Press; 1994.

3. Klein SD, Penneys NS. Aloe vera. Journal of the American Academy of Dermatol. 1988;18:714-19.

4. Harding TBC. Aloes of the world: A checklist, index and code. Excelsa. 1979;9:57-94.

5. Budavari SE. An Encyclopedia of Chemicals, Drugs, and Biologicals. Rahway, NJ: Merck and Co.; 1989.

6. Grindlay D, Reynolds T. The Aloe vera leaf phenomena: A review of the properties and modern use of the leaf parenchyma gel. Journal of Ethnopharmacology. 1986;16:117-51.

7. Mapp RK, McCarthy TJ. The assessment of purgative principles in Aloes. Planta Medica. 1970;18:361-5.

8. Cole HN, Chen KK. Aloe vera in oriental dermatology. Archives of Dermatology and Syphilology. 1943;47:250.

9. Morton JF. Atlas of Medicinal plants of Middle America: Bahamas to Yucatan. Springfield, IL: Charles C. Thomas; 1981.

10. Shelton RW. Aloe vera, its chemical and therapeutic properties. International Journal of Dermatology 1991;30(10):679-683.

11. Coats BC, Ahola R. Aloe vera the Silent Healer. A Modern Study of Aloe vera. Dallas,TX: Bill C. Coats; 1979.

12. Gunther RT. The Greek Herbal of Dioscorides. Oxford: Oxford University Press; 1934.

13. Chopra RN, Nayar SL. Glossary of Indian Medicinal Plants. New Delhi, India: Council of Scientific and Industrial Research; 1956.

14. Dastur JF. Aloe barbadensis Mill. In: Medicinal Plants of India and Pakistan. Bombay: D.B.: Taraporevala Sons and Co. Private Ltd.; 1962:16-17.

15. Morton JF. Aloe. In: Major Medicinal Plants — Botany, Culture and Uses. Springfield, IL: Charles C. Thomas; 1977:46-50.

16. Canigueal S, Vila R. Aloe. British Journal of Phytotherapy. 1994;3(2):67-75.

17. Rowe TD, Parks LM. A phytochemical study of aloe vera leaf. Journal of the American Pharmaceutical Association. 1941;30:262-65.

18. Tyler VE, Brady LR, Roberts JE. Pharmacognosy. Philadelphia, PA: Lea and Febiger; 1976.

19. Robson MC, Heggers JP, Hagstrom WJ. Myth, magic, witchcraft or fact? Aloe vera revisited. Journal of Burn Care and Rehabilitation. 1982;3:157-62.

20. Bruce WGG. Medicinal properties in the Aloe. Excelsa. 1975;5:57-68.

21. Suga T, Hirata T. The efficacy of the Aloe plant chemical constituents and biological activities. Cosmetics and Toiletries. 1983;98:105-8.

22. Reynolds T. The compounds in Aloe leaf exudates: a review. Botanical Journal of the Linnean Society. 1985;90:157-77.

23. Sabeh F, Wright T, Norton SJ. Purification and characterization of a glutathione peroxidase from the Aloe vera plant. Enzyme Protein. 1993;47:92-98.

24. Yamaguchi I, Mega N, Sanada H. Components of the gel of Aloe vera (L.) Burm. f. Biosci. Biotech. Biochem. 1993;57(8):1350-52.

25. Afzal M, Ali M, Hassan RAH, Sweedan N, Dhami MSI. Identification of some prostanoids in Aloe vera extracts. Planta medica. 1991;57:38-40.

26. Fujita K, Shasike I, Teradaira R, et al. Properties of a carboxypeptidase from aloe. Biochem Pharmacol. 1979;28:1261-62.

27. Collins CE, Collins C. Roentgen dermatitis treated with fresh whole leaf of Aloe vera. Am J Roentgenol. 1935;33:396.

28. Wright CS. Aloe vera in treatment of roentgen ulcers and telangiectasis. Journal of the American Medical Association. 1936;106:1363-64.

29. Loveman AB. Leaf of aloe vera in treatment of roentgen ray ulcers. Arch Dermatol Syphilol. 1937;36:838-43.

30. Crewe JE. The external use of aloes. Minn Med. 1937;20:670-73.

31. Barnes TC. The healing action of extracts of Aloe vera leaf on abrasions of human skin. Am J Bot. 1947;34:597.

32. Crewe JE. Aloes in the treatment of burns and scalds. Minn. Med. 1939;2:538-39.

33. Tchou MT. Aloe vera (jelly leeks). Arch Dermatol Syphilol. 1943;47:249.

34. Bunyapraphatsara N, Jirakulchaiwong S, Thirawarapan S, Manonukul J. The efficacy of Aloe vera cream in the treatment of first, second and third degree burns in mice. Phytomedicine. 1996;2(3):247-51.

35. Kaufman T, Kalderon N, Ullman Y, et al. Aloe vera gel hindered wound healing of experimental second-degree burns: A quantitative controlled study. Journal of Burn and Care Rehabilitation. 1988;9:156.

36. Ashley FL, O'Loughlin BJ, Peterson BJ, Fernandez R, Fernandez L, Stein H, et al. The use of Aloe vera in the treatment of thermal and irradiation burns in laboratory animals and humans. Plastic and Reconstructive Surgery. 1957;20:383-96.

37. Watcher MA, Wheeland RG. The role of topical agents in the healing of full-thickness wounds. Journal of Dermatologic Surgery and Oncolology. 1989;15:1188-95.

38. Schmidt JM, Greenspoon JS. *Aloe vera* dermal wound gel is associated with a delay in healing. Obstetrics and Gynecology. 1991;78(1):115-17.

39. Fulton JE. The stimulation of post dermabrasion wound healing with stabilized *Aloe vera* gel-polyethylene oxide dressing. Journal of Dermatologic Surgery and Oncolology. 1990;16:460-67.

40. West DP, Zhu YF. Evaluation of *Aloe vera* gel gloves in the treatment of dry skin associated with occupational exposure. American Journal of Infections Control. 2003;31(1):40-2.

41. Blitz J, Smith JW, Gerard JR. *Aloe vera* gel in peptic ulcer therapy: Preliminary report. Journal of the American Osteopathic Association. 1963;63:731-35.

42. Ship AG. Is topical *Aloe vera* plant mucus helpful in burn treatment? Journal of the American Medical Association. 1977;238:1770.

43. Sjostrom B, Weatherly-White RCA, Paton BC. Experimental studies in cold injury. Journal of Surgical Research. 1964;4:12-16.

44. Raine TJ, London MD, Golouch K, et al. Antiprostaglandins and antithromboxanes for treatment of frostbite. Surgery Forum. 1980;31:557-59.

45. McCauley RL, Hing DN, Robson MC, et al. Frostbite injuries: A rational approach based on pathophysiology. Journal of Trauma. 1983;23:143-47.

46. Rodriguez-Bigas M, Cruz NI, Suarez A. Comparative evaluation of *Aloe vera* in the management of burn wounds in guinea pigs. Plastic Reconstruction Surgery. 1988;81:386-89.

47. Zawacki BE. Reversal of capillary stasis and prevention of burns. Annals of Surgery. 1974;180:98-102.

48. El Zawahry M, Hegazy MR, Helal M. Use of aloe in treating leg ulcers and dermatoses. International Journal of Dermatology. 1973;12:68-73.

49. Womble D, Helderman JH. Enhancement of allo-responsiveness of human lymphocytes by acemannan (Carrisyn). International Journal of Immunopharmacology. 1988;10(8):967-74.

50. Shida T, et.al. Effect of aloe extract on peripheral phagocytosis in adult bronchial asthma. Planta Med. 1985;51:273-75.

51. McDaniel HR, et al.. An increase in circulating monocyte/macrophages (MM) is induced by oral acemannan (ACE-M) in HIV-1 patients. American Journal of Clinical Pathology. 1990;94:516-17.

52. Egger SF, Brown GS, Kelsey LS, Yates KM, Rosenberg LJ, Talmadge JE. Studies on optimal dose and administration schedule of a hematopietic stimulatory b-(1,4)-linked mannan. International Journal of Immunopharmacology. 1996;18(2):113-26.

53. Marshall GD, Gibbons AS, Parnell LS. Human cytokines induces by acemannan. Journal of Allergy and Clin. Immunology. 1991;91:295.

54. Ramamoorthy L, Kemp MC, Tizard IR. Effects of acemannan on the production of cytokine in a macrophage cell line RAW264.7. In: Joint Meeting of the European Tissue Repair Society and Wound Healing Society 1993. Amsterdam, The Netherlands; 1993.

55. Zhang L, Tizard IR. Activation of a mouse macrophage cell line by acemannan: The major carbohydrate fraction from Aloe vera gel. Immunopharmacology. 1996;35:119-28.

56. Karaca K, Sharma JM, Nordgren R. Nitric oxide production by chicken macrophages activated by acemannan, a complex carbohydrate extracted form *Aloe vera*. International Journal of immunopharmacology. 1995;17(3):183-88.

57. Chinnah AD, Baig M, Tizard IR, Kemp MC. Antigen dependent adjuvant activity of a polydispersed B-(1-4)-linked acetylated mannan (acemannan). Vaccine. 1992;10:551-57.

58. Ritchie BW, Niagro FD, Latimer KS, Pritchard N, Greenlacre C, Campagnoli RP, et al. Antibody response and local reactions to adjuvant avian polyomavirus vaccines in psittacine birds. J. Assoc. Avian. Vet. 1994;8:21-26.

59. Kahlon JB, et.al. *In vitro* evaluation of the synergistic anti-viral effects of acemannan in combination with azidothymidine and acyclovir. Molecular Biotherapy. 1991;3:214-23.

60. Kahlon JB, Kemp MC, Carpenter RH, McAnalley BH, McDaniel HR, Shannon W. Inhibition of AIDS virus replication by acemannan *in vitro*. Molecular Biotherapy. 1991;3:127-35.

61. Fogelman RW, Chapdelaine JM, Carpenter RH, McAnalley BH. Toxicologic evaluation of injectible acemannan in the mouse, rat, and dog. Veterinary and Human Toxicology. 1992;34:201-05.

62. Benigni R. Substances with antibiotic action contained in anthraquinonic drugs. Chemical Abstracts. 1950;44:11036.

63. Gottshall RY, Jennings JC, Weller LE, et al. Antibacterial substances in seed plants active against tubercle bacilli. Am Rev Tuberc. 1950;62:475-80.

64. Bruce WG. Investigations of antibacterial activity in the aloe. South African Medical Journal. 1967;51:984.

65. Lorenzetti LJ, Salisbury R, Beal JL, et al. Bacteriostatic property of *Aloe vera*. Journal of Pharmaceutical Sciences. 1964;53:1287.

66. Heggers JP, Pineless GR, Robson MC. Dermaide/*Aloe vera* gel comparison of the antimicrobial effects. 1979;41:293-94.

67. Fly LB, Kiem I. Test of *Aloe vera* for antibiotic activity. Economic Botany. 1963;17:46-49.

68. Hanley DC, Solomon WAB, Saffran B, et al. The evaluation of natural substances in the treatment of adjuvant arthritis. Journal of the American Podiatric Medical Association. 1982;72:275-84.

69. Fujita K, Teradaira R. Bradykininase activity of aloe extract. Biochem Pharmacol. 1976;25:205.

70. Rubel BL. Possible mechanisms of the healing actions of Aloe gel. Cosmetics and Toiletries. 1983;98:109-14.

71. Davis RH, Leitner MG, Russo JM, et al. Antiinflammatory activity of aloe vera against a spectrum of irritants. Journal of the American Podiatric Medical Association. 1989;79:263-76.

72. Parish LC, Witkoski JA, Millikan LE. *Aloe vera*: its chemical and therapeutic properties.

International Journal of Dermatology. 1991;30:679.

73. Davis RH, Leitner MG, Russo, et al. Wound healing: oral and topical activity of *Aloe vera*. Journal of the American Podiatric Medical Association. 1989;79:559.

74. Davis RH, DiDonato JJ, Johnson RWS, Stewart CB. *Aloe vera*, hydrocortisone, and sterol influence on wound tensile strength and anti-inflammation. Journal of the American Podiatric Medical Association. 1994;84(12):614-21.

75. Davis RH, Di Donato JJ, Hartman GM, Haas RC. Anti-inflammatory and wound healing activity of a growth substance in *Aloe vera*. Journal of the American Podiatric Medical Association. 1994;84(2):77-81.

76. Davis RH, Parker WL, Murdoch DP. Aloe vera as a biological active vehicle for hydrocortisone acetate. Journal of the American Podiatric Medical Association. 1991;81:1.

77. Hart LA, Nibbering PH, van den Barselaar MT, van Dijk H, Van den Berg AJJ, Labadie RP. Effects of low molecular constituents from aloe vera gel on oxidative metabolism and cytotoxic and bactericidal activities of human neutraphils. International Journal of Immunopharmacology. 1990;12(4):427-34.

78. Cera LM, Heggers JP, Robson MC, Hagstrom WJ. The therapeutic efficacy of *Aloe vera* cream (dermaide aloe) in thermal injuries: Two case reports. Journal of the American Animal Hospital Association. 1980;16:768-72.

79. Yagi A, Harada N, Yamada H, Iwadare S, Nishioka I. Antibradykinin active material in Aloe saponaria. Journal of Pharmaceutical Sciences. 1982;71:1172-74.

80. Cera LM, Heggers JP, Hagstrom WJ, et al. Therapeutic protocol for thermally injured animals and its successful use in an extensively burned rhesus monkey. J Am Anim Hosp Assoc. 1982;18:633-38.

81. Penneys NS. Inhibition of arachidonic acid oxidation *in vitro* by vehicle components. Acta Derm Venereol. 1982;62:59-61.

82. Davis RH, Kabbani JM, Marno NP. Wound healing and antiinflammatory activity of *Aloe vera*. Proc Pa Acad Sci. 1986;60:79.

83. Davis RH, Agnew PS, Shapiro E. Antiarthritic activity of anthaquinones found in aloe for podiatric medicine. Journal of the American Podiatric Medical Association. 1986;76:61-62.

84. Mandeville FB. Aloe vera in the treatment of radiation ulcers of mucous membranes. Radiology. 1939;32:598-99.

85. Rowe TD, Lovell BK, Parks LM. Further observations on the use of *Aloe vera* leaf in the treatment of third degree x-ray reactions. Journal of the American Pharmaceutical Association. 1941;30:265-69.

86. Lushbaugh CC, Hale DB. Experimental acute radiodermatitis following beta irradiation: V. Histopathological study of the mode of action of therapy with *Aloe vera*. Cancer. 1953;6:690-97.

87. Rowe TD. Effect of fresh *Aloe vera* jell in the treatment of third-degree Roentgen reactions on white rats. Journal of the American Pharmaceutical Association. 1940;30:262-66.

88. Williams MS, Burk M, Loprinzi CL, Hill M, Schomberg PJ, Nearhood K, et al. Phase III double-blind evaluation of an *Aloe vera* gel as a prophylactic agent for radiation-induced skin toxicity. International Journal of Radiation Oncology, Biology and Physiology. 1996;36(2):345-49.

89. Heggie S, Bryant GP, Tripcony L, Keller J, Rose P, Glendenning M, et al. A Phase III study on the efficacy of topical *Aloe vera* gel on irradiated breast tissue. Cancer Nursing. 2002;25(6):442-51.

90. Davis RH, et al. *Aloe vera*, a natural approach for treating wounds, edema, and pain in diabetes. Journal of the American Podiatric Medical Association. 1988;78:60-68.

91. Peng SY, Norman J, Curtin G, et al. Decreased mortality of Norman murine sarcoma in mice treated with the immunomodulator, acemannan. Molecular Biotherapy. 1991;3(2):79-87.

92. Harris C, Pierce K, King G, et al. Efficacy of acemannan in treatment of canine and feline spontaneous neoplasms. Molecular Biotherapy. 1991;3(4):207-13.

93. King GK, Yates KM, Greenlee PG, Pierce KR, Ford CR, McAnalley BH, et al. The effect of Acemannan immunostimulant, surgery and radiation on spontaneous canine and feline fibrosarcoma. Journal of the American Animal Hospital Association. 1995;31:439-47.

94. Manna S, McAnalley BH. Determination of the position of the O-acetyl group is a B-(1,4)-mannan (acemannan) from *Aloe barbadensis* Miller. Carbo. Res. 1993;241:317-19.

95. Desai KN. The preventive and therapeutic potential of the squalene-containing compound, Roidex, on tumour promotion and regression. Cancer Letters. 1996;101(1):93-96.

96. Gribel NV, Pashinskii VG. Protivometastaticheskie svoistva soka aloe. Voprosy Onkolojii. 1986;32:38-40.

97. McDaniel HR, McNalley BH, White A. *In vitro* studies on acemannan (Carrisyn™) for antiviral effect. ASCP/CAP. 1987;69:(abstract).

98. McDaniel HR, Perkins S, McAnalley BH. A clinical pilot study using acemannan (Carrisyn™) in the treatment of acquired immunodeficiency syndrome (AIDS). ASCP/CAP. 1987;68:(abstract).

99. McDaniel HR, Rosenberg LJ, McAnalley BH. CD4 and CD8 lymphocyte levels in acemannan (ACM)-treated HIV-1 infected long-term survivors. International Conference on AIDS. 1993;9(1):498: abstract no. PO B29-2179.

100. McDaniel HR, et al. Extended survival and prognostic criteria for acemannan (ACE-M) treated HIV-1 patients. Antiviral Research. 1990;13 (Supp.1):117.

101. Syed TA, Ahmed SA, Holt AH, Ahmed SA, Ahmed SH, Afzal M. Management of psoriasis with *Aloe vera* extract in a hydrophillic cream: A placebo-controlled, double-blind study. Tropical Medicine and International Health. 1996;1(4):505-09.

102. Bovik EG. *Aloe vera*. Panacea of old wives' tale? Texas Dental Journal. 1966;84:13-16.

103. Payne JM. Tissue Response to *Aloe vera* gel following peridontal surgery. Dentistry. Baylor University; 1970.

104. Northway RB. Experimental use of *Aloe vera* extract in clinical practice. Veterinary Medicine/Small Animal Clinician. 1975;70:89.

105. Anderson BC. *Aloe vera* juice: A veterinary medicament? The Compendium on Continuing Education for Practising Veterinarian. 1983;5:S364-68.

106. Leung AY. *Aloe vera* in cosmetics. Drugs and Cosmetic Industry. 1977;120:34-5; 154-55.

107. Madis Laboratories. *Aloe vera* L. and its products, applications and nomenclature. Cosmetics and Toiletries. 1983;98:99-104.

108. Madis Laboratories. *Aloe Vera* Gel. The Ageless Beauty Ingredient. 9th ed. South Hackensack, NJ: Madis Laboratories Inc; 1984.

109. Hattori M, Kanda T, Shu YZ, Akao T, Kobashi K, Namba T. Chemical and Pharmaceutical Bulletin. (Tokyo). 1988;36:4462-66.

110. Che QM, Akao T, Hattori M, Kobashi K, Namba T. Isolation of human intestinal bacterium capable of transforming barbaloin to aloe-emodin anthrone. Planta Medica. 1991;57:15-19.

111. Ishii Y, Tanizawa H, Takino Y. Studies on Aloe. III Mechanism of cathartic effect. Chem. Pharm. Bull. (Tokyo). 1990;38:197-200.

112. Ghannam N. The antidiabetic effect of aloes: Preliminary clinical and experimental observations. Hormone Research. 1986;24:288-94.

113. Ajabnoor MA. Effect of aloes on blood glucose levels in normal and alloxan diabetic mice. Journal of Ethnopharmacology. 1990;28:215-20.

114. Sydiskis RJ, Owen DG, Lohr JL, Rosler KH, Blomster RN. Inactivation of enveloped viruses by anthraquinones extracted from plants. Antimicrobial Agents Chemother. 1991;35:2463-66.

115. Shoji A. Contact dermatitis to *Aloe arborescens*. Contact Dermatitis. 1982;8:164-67.

116. Nakamura T, Kotajima S. Contact dermatitis from *Aloe arborescens*. Contact Dermatitis. 1984;11:51.

117. Hunter D, Frumkin A. Adverse reactions to vitamin E and *Aloe vera* preparations after dermabrasion and chemical peel. Cutis. 1991;47:193-96.

118. Dominguez-Soto L. Photodermatitis to aloe vera. International Journal of Dermatology. 1992;31:372.

119. Ernst E. Adverse effects of herbal drugs in dermatology. British Journal of Dermatology. 2000;143(5):923-29.

120. Hogan DJ. Widespread dermatitis after topical treatment of chronic leg ulcers and stasis dermatitis. Canadian Medical Association Journal. 1988;138:336-38.

121. Morrow DM, Rappaport MJ, Strick RA. Hypersensitivity to aloe. Arch Dermatol. 1980;116:1064-65.

122. Newall CA, Anderson LA, Phillipson JD. Herbal Medicines. A Guide for Health Care Professionals. London: The Pharmaceutical Press; 1996.

123. Gottlieb K. *Aloe vera* Heals: The Scientific Facts. Denver, CO: Royal Publications; 1980.

124. Murray MT. Natural Alternatives to Over-the-Counter and Prescription Drugs. New York, NY: William Morrow and Company, Inc; 1994.

Astragalus

1. Scalzo R. Botanical materia medica for sinusitis. The Protocol Journal of Botanical Medicine. 1997;2(2):147-62.

2. Foster S, Chongxi Y. Herbal Emissaries. Bringing Chinese Herbs to the West. Rochester, VT: Healing Arts Press; 1992:356.

3. Sun Y, Chang YH, Yu GQ, et al. Effect of Fu-zheng therapy in the management of malignant diseases. Chinese Medical Journal.1981;61:97-101.

4. Sun Y, et al. Preliminary observations on the effects of the Chinese medicinal herbs *Astragalus membranaceus* and *Ligustrum lucidum* on lymphocyte blastogenic responses. Journal of Biological Response Modifiers. 1983;2:227-237.

5. Zhao KS, Mancini C, Doria G. Enhancement of the immune response in mice by *Astragalus membranaceus* extracts. Immunopharmacology. 1990;20(3):225-33.

6. Marles RJ, Associate Professor, Department of Botany, Brandon University, Brandon, Manitoba. Review of Medicinal Plant Modules for CCNM; 1997.

7. Leung AY, Foster S. Encyclopedia of Common Natural Ingredients Used in Food, Drugs, and Cosmetics. 2nd ed. Toronto, ON /New York, NY: John Wiley and Sons Inc; 1996:649.

8. Chevallier A. The Encyclopedia of Medicinal Plants. London: Readers Digest; 1996:336.

9. Zhao KW, Kong HY. Effect of Astragalan on secretion of tumour necrosis factor in human peripheral blood mononuclear cells. Chung-Kuo Chung Hsi i Chieh, Ho Tsa Chih. 1993;13(5):263-65.

10. Luo HM, Dai RH, Li Y. Nuclear cardiology study on effective ingredients of *Astragalus membranaceus* in treating heart failure. Chung-Kuo Chung Hsi i Chieh, Ho Tsa Chih. 1995;15(12):709.

11. Hirotani M, Zhou Y, Rui H, Furuya T. Cycloartane triterpene glycosides from the hairy root cultures of *Astragalus membranaceus*. Phytochemistry. 1994;37(5):1403-07.

12. Weng XS. Treatment of leucopenia with pure astragalus preparation — an analysis of 115 leucopenic cases [Chinese]. Chung-Kuo Chung Hsi i Chieh, Ho Tsa Chih. 1995;15(8):462-64.

13. Chu DT, et al. Immunotherapy with Chinese medicinal herbs. II. Reversal of cyclophosphamide-induced immune suppression by administration of fractionated *Astragalus membranaceus in vivo*. Journal of Clinical Laboratory Immunology. 1988;25:125-29.

14. Chen YC. Experimental studies on the effects of danggui buxue decoction on IL-2 production of blood-deficient mice [Chinese]. Chung-Kuo Chung Hsi i Chieh. 1994;19(12):739-41, 763.

15. Liang H, Zhang Y, Geng B. The effect of astragalus polysaccharides (APS) on cell mediated immunity (CMI) in burned mice. Chung-Hua Cheng Hsing Shao Shang Wai Ko Tsa Chih. 1994;10(2):138-41.

16. Jin R, Wan LL, Mitsuishi T. Effects of shi-ka-ron and Chinese herbs in mice treated with anti-tumor agent mito mycin C [Chinese]. Chung-Kuo Chung Hsi i Chieh, Ho Tsa Chih. 1995;15(2):101-03.

17. Sugiura H, Nishida H, Indaba R, Iwata H. Effects of exercise in the growing stage in mice and of *Astragalus membranaceus* on immune functions [Japanese]. Nippon Eiseigaku Zasshi — Japanese Journal of Hygiene. 1993;47(6):1021-31.

18. Yang YZ, Jin PY, Guo Q, et al. Effect of *Astragalus membranaceus* on natural killer cell activity and induction of a- and g- interferon in patients with coxsackie B viral myocarditis. Chinese Medical Journal. 1990;103(4):304-07.

19. Hou YD, Ma GL, Wu SH, Li HT. Effect of radix Astrageli seu Hedysari on the interferon system. Chinese Medical Journal. 1981;94:35-40.

20. Khoo KS, Ang PT. Extract of *Astragalus membranaceus* and *Ligustrum lucidum* does not prevent cyclophosphamide-induced myelosuppression. Singapore Medical Journal. 1995;36(4):387-90.

21. Rui T, Yang Y, Zhou T, et al. Effect of *Astragalus membranaceus* on electrophysiological activities of acute experimental Coxsackie B-3 viral myocarditis in mice. Chinese Medical Sciences Journal. 1993;8(4):203-06.

22. Huang Z, Qin NP, Ye W. Effect *of Astragalus membranaceus* on T-lymphocyte subsets in patients with viral myocarditis [Chinese]. Chung-Kuo Chung Hsi i Chieh, Ho Tsa Chih. 1995;15(6):328-30.

23. Peng T, Yang Y, Riesemann H, Kandolf R. The inhibitory effect of *Astragalus membranaceus* on coxsackie B-3 virus RNA replication. Chinese Medical Sciences Journal. 1995;10(3):146-50.

24. Guo Q, Peng TQ, Yang YZ. Effect of *Astragalus membranaceus* on Ca2+ influx and coxsackie virus B3 RNA replication in cultured neonatal rat heart cells [Chinese]. Chung-Kuo Chung Hsi i Chieh, Ho Tsa Chih. 1995;15(8):483-85.

25. Shi HM, Dai RH, Fan WH. Intervention of lidocaine and *Astragalus membranaceus* on ventricular late potentials [Chinese]. Chung-Kuo Chung Hsi i Chieh, Ho Tsa Chih. 1994;14(10):598-600.

26. Li SQ, Yuan RX, Gao H. Clinical observation of the treatment of ischemic heart disease with *Astragalus membranaceus* [Chinese]. Chung-Kuo Chung Hsi i Chieh, Ho Tsa Chih. 1995;15(2):77-80.

27. Lei ZY, Qin H, Liao JZ. Action of *Astragalus membranaceus* on left ventricular function of angina pectoris [Chinese]. Chung-Kuo Chung Hsi i Chieh, Ho Tsa Chih. 1994;14(4):199-202.

28. Chen LK, Liao JZ, Guo WQ. Effects of *Astragalus membranaceus* on left ventricular function and oxygen free radical in acute myocardial infarction patients and mechanism of its cardiotonic action [Chinese]. Chung-Kuo Chung hsi i Chieh, Ho Tsa Chih. 1995;15(3):141-43.

29. Yang YZ, Guo Q, Jin PY, et al. Effect of *Astragalus membranaceus* injecta on Coxsackie B-2 virus infected rat beating heart cell culture. Chinese Medical Journal. 1987;100:595.

30. Hou YD. Study on the biological active ingredients of *Astragalus membranaceus*. Chung His i Chieh Ho Tsa Chih. 1984;4:420.

31. Zhang XQ, et al. Studies of *Astragalus membranaceus* on antiinfluenza virus activity, interferon induction and immunostiluation in mice. Chinese Journal of Microbiology and Immunology. 1984;4:92.

32. Research Group of Common Cold and Bronchitis. Investigation into *Astragalus membranaceus*. II. A research on some of its mechanism of reinforcing the Qi (vital energy). Journal of Traditional Chinese Medicine. 1980;3:67.

33. Cha RJ, Zeng DW, Chang QS. Non-surgical treatment of small cell lung cancer with chemo-radio-immunotherapy and traditional Chinese medicine [Chinese]. Chung-Hua Nei Ko Tsa Chih — Chinese Journal of Internal Medicine. 1994;33(7):462-66.

34. Lau BH, Ruckle HC, Botolazzo T, Lui PD. Chinese medicinal herbs inhibit growth of murine renal cell carcinoma. Cancer Biotherapy. 1994;9(2):153-61.

35. Chu DT, Lin JR, Wong W. The *in vitro* potentiation of LAK cell cytotoxicity in cancer and AIDS patients indiced by F3 — a fractionated extract of *Astragalus membranaceus* [Chinese]. Chung-Hua Chung Liu Tsa Chih — Chinese Journal of Onocology. 1994;16(3):167-71.

36. Xuan W, Dong M, Dong M. Effects of compound injection of *Pyrola rotunifolia* L. and *Astragalus membranaceus* BGE on experimental guinea pigs' gentamicin ototoxicity. Annals of Otology Rhinology and Laryngology. 1996;194:374-80.

37. Hong C, Ku J, et al. *Astragalus membranaceus* stimulates human sperm motility in vitro. American Journal of Chinese Medicine. 1992;20:289-94.

38. Xiangzhe J. A Clinical Investigation on 30 Cases of Senile Benign Renal Arteriolosclerosis Treated by Huang Qi Gu Jing Yin. J Trad Chin Med. 2001;21(3):177-80.

39. Murray MT. The Healing Power of Herbs. Rocklin, CA: Prima Publishing; 1992:246.

40. Teegarden R. Chinese Tonic Herbs. New York, NY: Japan Publishing Inc; 1985:197.

Black Cohosh

1. Brinker F. A comparative review of eclectic female regulators. British Journal of Phytotherapy.1997;4(3):123-42.

2. Beuscher N. *Cimicifuga racemosa* L.-Black Cohosh. Zeitschrift fur Phytotherapie. 1995;16:301-10. (English translation in Quarterly Review of Natural Medicine).

3. Chevallier A. The Encyclopedia of Medicinal Plants. London: Reader's Digest; 1996:336.

4. Marie Snow J. *Cimicifuga racemosa* (L) Nutt. (Ranunculaceae). The Protocol Journal of Botanical Medicine. 1996;1(4):17-19.

5. Leung A, Foster S. Encyclopedia of Common Natural Ingredient Used in Food, Drugs and Cosmetics. 2nd ed. New York, NY: John Wiley and Sons; 1996:649.

6. Jarry H, Harnischfeger G. Untersuchungen zur endokrinen wirksamkeit von inhaltsstoffen aus *Cimicifuga racemosa*. Einfluss auf die serumspiegel von hypophysenhormonen ovariektomieter ratten. Planta Medica. 1985;51:46-49.

7. Jarry H, Harnischfeger G, Duker E. Untersuchungen zur endokrinen wirksamkeit von inhaltsstoffen aus *Cimicifuga racemosa*. In vitro-bindung von inhaltsstoffen an ostrogenrezeptoren ratten. Planta Medica. 1985;51:316-19.

8. Linde H. Die inhaltsstoffe von *Cimicifuga racemosa*. Mitt: zur struktur des acteins. Archiv der Pharmazie. 1967;300:885-92.

9. Linde H. Die inhaltsstoffe von *Cimifuga racemosa*. Mitt: uber die konstitution der ringe A,B, und C des acteins. Archiv der Pharmazie. 1967;300:982-92.

10. Linde H. Die inhaltsstoffe von *Cimicifuga racemosa*. Mitt: actein: der ring D und seitenkette. Archiv der Pharmazie.1968;301:120-38.

11. Linde H. Die inhaltsstoffe von *Cimicifuga racemosa*. Mitt: 27-desoxyacetylacteol. Archiv der Pharmazie. 1968;301:335-41.

12. Newall C, Anderson L, David Phillipson J. Herbal Medicines: A Guide for Health Care Professionals. London: The Pharmaceutical Press; 1996:296.

13. Duker E-M, Kopanski L, Jarry H, Wuttke W. Effects of extracts from *Cimicifuga racemosa* on gonadotropin release in menopausal women and ovariectomized rats. Plant Medica. 1991;57:420-24.

14. Einer-Jensen N, Zhao J, Andersen K, Kristoffersen K. Cimicifuga and Melbrosia lack estrogenic effects in mice and rats. Maturitas. 1996;25(2):149-53.

15. Warnecke G. Beeinflussung klimakterisch Beschwerden durch ein Phytotherapeutikum. Die Medizinische Welt. 1985;36:871-74.

16. Stoll W. Phytotherapeutikum beeinflust atrophisches Vaginalepithel. Therapeutikon. 1987;1:23-31.

17. Lehmann-Willenbrock E, Riedel H. Klinische und endokrinologischen untersuchungen zur therapie ovarieller aus fallserscheinungen nach hysterekomie unter belassung der adnexe. Zentralblatt fur Gynakologie. 1988;110:611-18.

18. Jacobson JS, Troxel AB, Evans J, Klaus L, Vahdat L, Kinne D, et al. Randomized trial of black cohosh for the treatment of hot flashes among women with a history of breast cancer. Journal of Clinical Oncology. 2001;19(10):2739-45.

19. Borelli F, Ernst E. *Cimicifuga racemosa*: A systematic review of its clinical efficacy. European Jouranl of Clinical Pharmacology. 2002:58:235-41.

20. Daiber W. Menopause symptoms: Success without hormones. Arztliche Praxis. 1983;35:1946-47.

21. Vorberg G. Treatment of menopause symptoms. Zeitschrift Fuer Alternsforshung. 1984;60:626-29.

22. Petho A. Menopause symptoms: is it possible to switch from hormone treatment to a botanical gynecologicum? Arztliche Praxis. 1987;47:1551-53.

23. Linde K, Ramirez G, Mulrow C, et al. St John's Wort for depression — an overview and meta-analysis of randomized clinical trials. British Medical Journal. 1996;313:253-58.

24. Burke BE, Olson RD, Cusack BJ. Randomized, contolled trail of phytoestrogen in the prophylactic treatment of menstrual migraine. Biomed Pharmacolther. 2002;56(6):283-88.

25. Blumenthal M, Brusse WR, Goldberg A, et al. The Complete Commission E Monographs. Austin, TX: American Botanical Council; 1998: 685.

26. Genazzani E, Sorrentino L. Vascular action of acteina: active constituents of *Actea racemosa* L. Nature. 1962;194:544-45.

27. Resing K, Fitzgerald A. Crystal data for 15-o-acetylacerinol and two related triterpenes isolated from Japanese Cimicifuga plants. J.Appl.Cryst. 1978;11:58.

28. Moskalenko S. Preliminary screening of Far-Eastern ethnomedicinal plants for antibacterial activity. Journal of Ethnopharmacology. 1986;15:231-59.

29. Bradley P. British Herbal Compendium. Bournemouth: BHMA; 1992:239.

Burdock

1. Wren R. Potter's New Encyclopedia of Botanical Drugs and Preparations. Saffron Walden: C.W. Daniel Company; 1988:362.

2. Mills S. The Essential Book of Herbal Medicine. 2nd ed. London: Penguin; 1991:677.

3. Chandler F, Osborne F. Burdock. Canadian Pharmaceutical Journal. 1997;130(5):46-49.

4. Leung A, Foster S. Encyclopedia of Common Natural Ingredient Used in Food, Drugs and Cosmetics. 2nd ed. New York, NY: John Wiley and Sons; 1996:649.

5. Newall C, Anderson L, David Phillipson J. Herbal Medicines: A Guide for Health Care Professionals. London: The Pharmaceutical Press; 1996:296.

6. Bever B, Zahnd G. Plants with oral hypoglyceamic action. Quarterly Journal of Crude Drug Research. 1979;17:139-96.

7. Bradley P. British Herbal Compendium. Bournemouth: BHMA; 1992:239.

8. Chevallier A. The Encyclopedia of Medicinal Plants. London: Reader's Digest; 1996:336.

9. Weiss R. Herbal Medicine. Beaconsfield: Beaconsfield Publishers;1988:362.

10. Moskalenko S. Preliminary screening of Far-Eastern ethnomedicinal plants for antibacterial activity. Journal of Ethnopharmacology. 1986;15:231-59.

11. Cappalletti E, Trevisan R, Caniato R. External antirheumatic and antineuralgic herbal remedies in the traditional medicine of North-eastern Italy. Journal of Ethnopharmacology. 1982;6:161-90.

12. Tsujita J, Takeda H, Ebihara K, Kiriyama S. Comparison of protective activity of dietary fiber against the toxicities of various food colours in rats. Nutrition Reports International. 1979;20:635-42.

13. Morita K, Kada T, Namiki M. Desmutagenic factor isolated from burdock (Arctium Lappa L.). Mutation Research. 1986;129:25-31.

14. Bryson P, Watanabe A, Rumack B, Murphy R. Burdock root tea poisoning. Journal of the American Medical Association. 1978;239(20):2157.

15. Bryson P. Burdock root tea poisoning. Journal of the American Medical Association. 1978;240:1586.

16. Tyler V. The Honest Herbal. 3rd ed. Binghamton, NY: Pharmaceutical Products Press; 1993:375.

17. Rhoads P, Tong T, Banner W, Anderson R. Anticholinergic poisonings associated with commercial burdock root tea.

Journal of Toxicology-Clinical Toxicology. 1985;22(6):581-84.

18. Rodriguez P, Blanco S, Juste S, et al. Allergic contact dermatitis due to burdock (*Arctium lappa*). Contact Dermatitis. 1995;33:134-35.

19. Marles RJ, Associate Professor, Department of Botany, Brandon University, Brandon, Manitoba. Review of Medicinal Plant Modules for CCNM; 1997.

20. Hirono I, Mori H, Kato K, Ushimaru Y. Safety examination of some edible plants. Part 2. Journal of Environmental Pathology Toxicology and Oncology. 1977;1:72-74.

21. Farnsworth N, Bingel A, Cordell G, et al. Potential value of plants as sources of new antifertility agents I. Journal of Pharmaceutical Sciences. 1975;64(4):535-98.

Calendula

1. Aldstat E. Calendula off. Eclectic Dispensatory of Botanical Therapeutics. Portland, OR: Eclectic Medical Publishers; 1989.

2. Newall C, Anderson L, David Phillipson J. Herbal Medicine: A Guide for Health Care Professionals. London: The Pharmaceutical Press; 1996:296.

3. Wren R. Potter's New Encyclopedia of Botanical Drugs and Preparations. Saffron Walden: C.W. Daniel Company; 1988:362.

4. Leung A, Foster S. Encyclopedia of Common Natural Ingredient Used in Food, Drugs and Cosmetics. 2nd ed. New York, NY: John Wiley and Sons; 1996:649.

5. Fleischener A. Plant extracts: to accelerate healing and reduce inflammation. Cosmetics and Toiletries. 1985; 100(10): 45-58.

6. Mills S. The Essential Book of Herbal Medicine. 2nd ed. London: Penguin; 1991:677.

7. Chevallier A. The Encyclopedia of Medicinal Plants. London: Reader's Digest; 1996:336.

8. Akihisa T, Yasukawa K, Oinuma H, et al. Triterpene Alcohols from the Flowers of Compositae and their Anti-inflammatory effects. Phytochemistry. 1996; 43(6):1255-60.

9. Willuhn G, Westhaus R. Loliolide (Calendin) from *Calendula officinalis*. Planta Medica. 1987; 53: 304.

10. Vidal-Olivier E, Elias R, Faure F, et al. Flavonol Glycosides from *Calendula officinalis* flowers. Planta Medica. 1989;55(73-74).

11. Mascolo N, et al. Biological screening of Italian medicinal plants for anti-inflammatory activity. Phytotherapy Research. 1987;1(28).

12. Della Loggia R, Tubaro A, Becker H, et al. The role of Triterpenoids in the topical anti-inflammatory activity of *Calendula officinalis* flowers. Planta Medica. 1994;60:516-20.

13. Bezakova L, Masterova I, Paulikova I, Psenak M. Inhibitory activity of isorhamnetin glycosides from *Calendula officinalis* L. on the activity of lipoxygenase. Pharmazie. 1996;51(2):126-27.

14. Boucaud-Maitre Y, Algernon O, Raynaud J. Cytotoxic and antihumoral activity of *Calendula officinalis* extracts. Pharmazie. 1988; 43:221-22.

15. Wagner H. The immune stimulating polysaccharides and heteroglycans of higher plants. A preliminary communication. Arzneimittelforschung. 1984;34(6):659-61.

16. Dumenil G, Chemli R, Balansard G, Guirand H, Lallemand M. Evaluation of antibacterial properties of marigold flowers and homeopathic mother tincture of *Calendula off.* Annales Pharmaceutiques Francaises. 1980;36(6):493-99.

17. Rawi S, El-Gindy H, Abd El Kader A. New possible molluscicides from *Calendula micrantha officinalis* and *Ammi majus*. Ecotoxicology and Environmental Safety. 1996;35:261-67.

18. Hammouda O, Borbely G. Alterations in protein synthesis in the *Cyanobacetrium synechococcus* sp. Strain PCC 6301 in response to *Calendula micrantha* extract with molluscicidal activity. Ecotoxicology and Environmental Safety. 1995;31:201-04.

19. Rawi S, El-Gindy H, Abd El Kader A. New possible molluscides from *Calendula micantra offininalis Ammi majus*. Ecotoxicology and Environmental Safety. 1996;35:262-67.

20. Tyler V. Herbs of Choice. The Therapeutic Use of Phytomedicinals. Binghamton, NY: Pharmaceutical Products Press; 1994:209.

21. Hoffman D. Holistic Herbal. Rockport, MA: Element Books; 1996:256.

22. Weiss R. Herbal Medicine. Beaconsfield: Beaconsfield Publishers;1988:362.

23. Casley-Smith J, Casley -Smith J. The effect of 'Unguentum Lymphaticum' on acute experimental lymphedema and other high-protein edemas. Lymphology. 1983;16:150-56.

24. Reider N, Komericki P, Hausen BM, Fritsch P, Aberer W. The seamy side of natural medicines: contact sensitization to arnica (*Arnica Montana* L.) and marigold (*Calendula officinalis* L.). Contact Dermatitis. 2001;45(5): 269-72.

25. Paulsen E. Contact sensitization from Compositae-containing herbal remedies and cosmetics. Contact Dermatitis. 2002:47(4):189-98.

Capsicum

1. Tyler VE. Herbs of Choice. The Therapeutic Use of Phytomedicinals. Binghamton, NY: Pharmaceutical Products Press; 1994.

2. Leung AY, Foster S. Encyclopedia of Common Natural Ingredients Used in Food, Drugs, and Cosmetics. 2nd ed. Toronto,ON/New York,NY: John Wiley and Sons Inc; 1996.

3. Newall CA, Anderson LA, Phillipson JD. Herbal Medicines. A Guide for Health Care Professionals. London: The Pharmaceutical Press; 1996.

4. Pickersgill B. The domestication of chilli peppers. In: B.J. U, Dimbleby GW, ed. The Domestication and Exploitation of Plants and Animals. London: Gerald Duckworth; 1969.

5. Marles RJ, Associate Professor, Department of Botany, Brandon University, Brandon, Manitoba. Review of Medicinal Plant Modules for CCNM; 1997.

6. Cordell GA, Araujo OE. Capsaicin: Identification, nomenclature, and pharmacology. Annals of Pharmacotherapy. 1993;27:330-36.

7. Mills S. The Essential Book of Herbal Medicine. 2nd ed. London: Penguin Publ; 1991.

8. Chevalier A. The Encyclopedia of Medicinal Plants. London: Reader's Digest; 1996.

9. Govindarajan VS. Capsicum — production, technology, chemistry, and quality. I. History, botany, cultivation and primary processing. CRC Critical Review of Food Science Nutrition. 1985;22:109-76.

10. Govindarajan VS. Capsicum — production, technology, chemistry, and quality. II. Processed products, standards, world production, and trade. CRC Critical review of Food Science Nutrition. 1986;23:207-88.

11. Govindarajan VS. Capsicum — production, technology, chemistry, and quality. III. Chemistry of the color, aroma and pungency stimuli. CRC Critical Review of Food Science Nutrition. 1986;24:245-355.

12. Govindarajan VS, Rajalakshmi D, Chand N. Capsicum — production, technology, chemistry, and quality. IV. Evaluation of quality. CRC Critical Review of Food Science Nutrition. 1987;25:185-283.

13. Govindarajan VS, Sathyanarayana MN. Capsicum — production, technology, chemistry, and quality. V. Impact on physiology, pharmacology, nutrition, and metabolism; structure, pungency, pain and desentization sequences. CRC Critical Review of Food Science Nutrition. 1991;29:435-73.

14. Bennett DJ, Kirby GW. Constitution and biosynthesis of capsaicin. Journal Chem Soc C. 1968:442-46.

15. Jentzsch K, Pock H, Kubelka W. Isolation of dihydrocapsaicin and homodihydrocapsaicin form Capsicum fruits. Monatsch Chem. 1968;99:661-63.

16. Kosuge S, Furata M. Studies on the pungent principles of Capsicum XIV. Chemical constitution of the pungent principles. Agric Biol Chem. 1970;34:248-56.

17. Muller-Stock A, Joshi RK, Buchi J. Components of capsaicinoids: quantitative gas chromatographic determination of individual homologs and analogs of capsaicin in mixtures from a natural source and of vanillylpelargonic amide as an adulteration. Journal of Chromatography. 1971;63:281-87.

18. Muller-Stock A, Joshi RK, Buchi J. Thin-layer and column chromatographic separation of capsaicinoids: Study of the constituents of capsicum. Journal of Chromatography 1973;79:229-41.

19. Todd P, Bensinger M, Biftu T. TLC screening techniques for the qualitative determination of natural and synthetic capsaicinoids. Journal Chromatography Science. 1975;13:577-79.

20. Jurenitsch J, Kubelka W, Jentzsch K. Gas chromatographic determination of the content of individual and total capsaicinoids in Capsicum fruits after thin-layer chromatographic separation. Sci Pharm. 1978;46:307-18.

21. Heresch F, Jurenitsch J. Off-line mass spectrometric monitoring of HPLC effluents — an improved identification and quantitation method for mixtures of similar compounds. Natural Capsaicinoids. Chromatographia. 1979;12:647-50.

22. Jurenitsch J, Leinmuller R. Quantification of nonylic acid vanillylamide and other capsaicinoids in the pungent principle of Capsicum fruits and preparation by gas-liquid chromatography on glass capillary columns. J. Chromatogr. 1980;189:389-97.

23. Ross DR, Varipapa RJ. Treatment of painful diabetic neuropathy with topical capsaicin (Letter). New England Journal of Medicine. 1989;321(7):474-75.

24. Donofrio PD, Walker F, Hunt V, Tandan R, Fries T, Lewis G, et al. Treatment of painful diabetic neuropathy with topical capsaicin: a multicentre, double-blind, vehicle-controlled study. Archives of Internal Medicine. 1991;151:2225-29.

25. Tandan R, Lewis GA, Krusinski PB, Badger GB, Fries TJ. Topical capsaicin in painful diabetic neuropathy. Controlled study with long term follow-up. Diabetes Care 1992;15(1):8-14.

26. Dailey GE. Effect of treatment with capsaicin on daily activities of patients with diabetic neuropathy. Diabetes Care. 1992;15(2):159-65.

27. Scheffler NM, et.al. Treatment of painful diabetic neuropathy with capsaicin 0.075%. Journal of the American Podiatr Med Association. 1991;81(6):288-93.

28. Basha KM, Whitehouse FW. Capsaicin: a therapeutic option for painful diabetic neuropathy. Henry Ford Hospital Medical Journal. 1991;39(2):138-40.

29. Pfeifer MA, et al. A highly successful and novel model for treatment of chronic painful diabetic peripheral neuropathy. Diabetes Care. 1993;16(8):1103-15.

30. Chad D, Ross D, Molitch M, Schipper HM, Stall G, Dyess E, et al. Treatment of painful diabetic neuropathy with topical capsaicin — a double-blind multicentre investigation. Pain. 1990;42:387-88.

31. Chad DA, Aronin N, Lundstrom R, McKeon P, Ross D, Molitch M, et al. Does capsaicin relieve the pain of diabetic neuoropathy? Pain 1990;42:387-88.

32. Watson CP, et.al. Post-herpetic neuralgia and topical capsaicin. Pain. 1988;35:289-97.

33. Watson CPN, et al. Post-herpetic neuralgia: 208 cases. Pain. 1988;35:289-97.

34. Bernstein JE, Korman NJ, Bickers DR, Dahl MV, Millikan LE. Topical capsaicin treatment of chronic postherpetic neuralgia. Journal of the American Academy of Dermatology. 1989;21(2, Pt.1):265-70.

35. Bernstein JE, Bickers DR, Dahl MV, Roshal JY. Treatment of chronic postherpetic neuralgia with topical capsaicin. A preliminary study. Journal of the American Academy of Dermatology. 1987;17(1):93-96.

36. Bernstein JE. Capsaicin in the treatment of dermatologic disease. Cutis. 1987;39:352-53.

37. Peikert A, et al. Topical 0.025% capsaicin in chronic post-herpetic neuralgia: efficacy, predictors of response and long-term course. Journal of Neurology. 1991;238(8):452-56.

38. Bjerring P, et al. Argon laser induced cutaneous sensory and pain thresholds in post-herpetic neuraligia. Quantitative modulation by topical capsaicin. Acta Derm Venereol (Stockholm). 1990;70(2):121-25.

39. Hawk RJ, Millikan LE. Treatment of oral postherpetic neuralgia with topical capsaicin. International Journal of Dermatology. 1988;27(5):336.

40. Watson CPN, Evans RJ, Watt VR. The post-mastectomy pain syndrome and the effect of topical capsaicin. Pain. 1989;38:177-86.

41. Watson CP, Evans RJ. The postmastectomy pain syndrome and topical capsaicin: a randomized trial. Pain. 1992;51(3):375-79.

42. Deal CL, et al. Treatment of arthritis with topical capsaicin: A double-blind trial. Clinical Therapapy. 1991;13(3):383-95.

43. McCarthy G, McCarty D. Effect of topical capsaicin on asteoarthritis of the hands. Journal of Rheumatology. 1992;19:604-07.

44. Sicuteri F, Fusco BM, Marabini S, Campagndo V, Maggia CA, Geppetti P, et al. Beneficial effect of capsaicin application to the nasal mucosa in cluster headache. Clin J Pain. 1989;5:49-53.

45. Marks DR, et al. A double-blind, placebo-controlled trial of intranasal capsaicin for cluster headache. Cephalalgia 1993;13(2):114-16.

46. Chesire WP, Snyder CR. Treatment of reflex sympathetic dystrophy with topcial capsaicin. Pain. 1990;42:307-11.

47. Rayner HC, et al. Relief of local stump pain by capsaicin cream (Letter). Lancet. 1989;ii:1276-77.

48. Fusco BM, Alessandri M. Analgesic effect of capsaicin in idiopathic trigeminal neuralgia. Anesthesia and Analgesia. 1992;74(3):375-77.

49. Heal the burn: Pepper and lasers in cancer pain therapy. Journal of the National Cancer. Institute 1994;86(18):1381.

50. Morgenlander JC, et al. Capsaicin for the treatment of pain in the Guillain-Barré syndrome (Letter). Annals of Neurology. 1990;28(2):199.

51. Bernstein JE, et al. Effects of topically applied capsaicin on moderate and severe psoriasis vulgaris. Journal of the American Academy of Dermatolog. 1986;15(3):504-507.

52. Keitel W, Frerick H, Kuhn U, Schmidt U, Kuhlmann M, Bredehorst A. Capsicum pain plaster in chronic non-specific low back pain. Arzneimittelforschung. 2001;51(11):896-903.

53. Kim KS, Koo MS, Jeon JW, Park HS, Seung IS. Capsicum plaster at the korean hand acupuncture point reduces postoperative nausea and vomiting after abdominal hysterectomy. Anesth Analg. 2002;95(4):1103-7, table of contents.

54. Locock RA. Capsicum. Canadian Pharmaceutical Journal. 1985;118:517-19.

55. Skofitsch G, Donnerer J, et al. Comparison of Nonivamide and Capsaicin with regard to their pharmacokinetics and effects on sensory neurons. Arzneimittel forsch. 1984;34:154-56.

56. Szolesanyi J. Capsaicin, irritation, and desensitization. In: Green BG, Mason JR, Kare MR, editors. Chemical Senses. New York, NY: Marcel Dekker; 1990.

57. Lynn B. Capsaicin: Actions on nociceptive C-fibres and therapeutic potential (review article). Pain. 1990;41:61-69.

58. Nagy JI, Emson PC, et al. A re-evaluation of the neurochemical and antinociceptive effects of intrathecal capsaicin in the rat. Brain Research. 1981;211:497-502.

59. Fitzgerald M. Capsaicin and sensory neurones — a review. Pain. 1983;15:109-30.

60. Nagy JI. Capsaicin's action on the nervous system. Trends in Neurosciences. 1982;5:362-65.

61. Nagy JI. A chemical probe for sensory neuron mechanism. In: Iversen LL, Iverson SD, Snyder SH, ed.. Handbook of Psychopharmacology. New York, NY: Plenum; 1982:185.

62. Buck SH, Burks TF. Capsaicin: Hot new pharmacological tool. Trends in Pharmacological Sciences. 1983;4:84-87.

63. Virus RM, Gebhart GF. Pharmacological action of capsaicin: Apparent involvement of substance P and serotonin. Life Science. 1979;25:1273-84.

64. Lembeck F, Gamse R, Juan H. Substance P and sensory nerve endings. In: von Euler US, Pernow B, editors. Substance P. New York, NY: Raven Press; 1977:169.

65. Jancso G, Kiraly E, Such G, Joo F, Nagy A. Neurotoxic effect of capsaicin in mammals. Acta Physiol Hung. 1987;69:295-313.

66. Baranowski R, Lynn B, Pini A. The effects of locally applied capsaicin on conduction in cutaneous nerves in four mammalian species. British Journal of Pharmacology. 1986;80:267-76.

67. Gamse R, Petsche V, Lembeck F, Jansco G. Capsaicin applied to peripheral nerve inhibits axonal transport of substance P and somatostatin. Brain Research. 1982;239:447-62.

68. Kenins P. Responses of single nerve fibers to capsaicin applied to the skin. Neuroscience Letters. 1982;29:83-88.

69. Jessel TM, Iverson LL, Cuello AC. Capsaicin-induced depletion of substance P from primary sensory neurons. Brain Research. 1978;152:183-88.

70. Sambaiah K, Satyanarayana MN. Hypocholesterolemic effect of red pepper and capsaicin. Indian Journal of Experimental Biology. 1980;18:898-99.

71. Kawada T, al. e. Effects of capsaicin on lipid metabolism in rats fed a high fat diet. Journal of Nutrition. 1986;116:1272-78.

72. Bortolotti M, Coccia G, Grossi G, Miglioli M. The treatment of functional dyspepsia with red pepper. Aliment Pharmacol Ther. 2002;16(6):1075-82.

73. Futrell JM, Rietschel RL. Spice allergy evaluated by results of patch tests. Cutis. 1993;52:288-90.

74. Niinimaki A, Hannuksela M, Makinen-Kiljunen S. Skin prick tests and in vitro immunoassays with native spices and spice extracts. Annals of Allergy, Asthman, & Immunology. 1995;75:280-86.

75. Chan TC, Vilke GM, Clausen J, Clark RF, Schmidt P, Snowden T, et al. The effect of oleoresin capsicum "pepper" spray inhalation on respiratory function. Journal of Forensic Science. 2002;47(2):299-304.

76. Zollman TM, Bragg RM, Harrison DA. Clinical effects of oleoresin capsicum (pepper spray) on the human cornea and conjunctiva. Ophthalmology. 2000;107(12):2186-89.

77. Agrawal RC, Sarode AV, Lalitha VS, Bhide SV. Chili extract treatment and induction of eye lesions in hamsters. Toxicology Letters. 1985;28:1-7.

78. Visudhiphan S, Poolsuppasit S, Piboonnukarintr O, Tumliang S. The relationship between high fibrinolytic activity and daily capsicum ingestion in Thais. The American Journal of Clinical Nutrition. 1982;35:1452-58.

79. Smith JG, Crounse RG, et al. The effects of capsaicin on human skin, liver and epidermal lysomes. J Invest Dermatol. 1970;54:170-73.

80. Carpenter SE, Lynn B. Vascular and sensory responses of human skin to mild injury after topical treatment with capsaicin. British Journal of Pharmacology. 1981;73:755-58.

81. Tandan R, Lewis G, Fries T. Safety of topical capsaicin in diabetic neuropathy. Neurology. 1990;40 (Supplement):160.

82. McMahon SB, Lewin G, Bloom S. The consequences of long-term topical capsaicin application in the rat. Pain. 1991;44:301-10.

83. Desai HG, Venugoplan K, et al. Effect of red chilli powder on DNA content of gastric aspirates. Gut. 1973;14:974-76.

84. Pimparker BND, Donde UM, et al. Effects of commonly used spices on human gastric secretion. Journal of the Association of Physicians India. 1972;20:910.

85. Dugani A, Glavin GB. Capsaicin effects on stress pathology and gastric acid secretion in rats. Life Science. 1985;39:1519-31.

86. Wang JP, Hsu MF, Teng CM. Antiplatelet effect of capsaicin. Thrombosis Research. 1984;36:497-507.

87. Surh YJ, Lee SS. Capsaicin in hot chili pepper: Carcinogen, co-carciogen or anticarcinogen? Food Chem Toxic. 1996;34:313-16.

88. Farnsworth NR. Potential value of plants as sources of new antifertility agents I [Review]. Journal of Pharm Science. 1975;64(4):535-98.

Cat's Claw

1. Duke J. Una de Gato. The Business of Herbs. 1994;May/June:12-13.

2. Jones K. Cats Claw. Herbs for Health. 1996;Sep/Oct:42-46.

3. Chandler F, ed. Herbs: Everyday Reference for Health Professionals. 1st ed. Ottawa: Canadian Pharmacists' Association; 2000.

4. Barnes J, Anderson L, David Phillipson J. Herbal Medicines. 2nd ed. London: Pharmaceutical Press; 2002.

5. Syrimis A. *Uncaria Tomentosa*; A Review. British Journal of Phytotherapy. 1998;5(1):3;29.

6. Foster S. Cat's Claw. Health Foods Business. 1995;June:24-25.

7. Jones K. Cat's Claw: Healing Vine of Peru. Seattle: Sylvan Press; 1995.152

8. Reinhard K. *Uncaria tomentosa* (Willd.) D.C.: Cat's Claw, Una de Gato, or Saventaro. Journal of Alternative and Complementary Medicine. 1999;5(2):143-51.

9. Laus G, Keplinger D. Separation of sterioisomeric oxindole alkaloids from *Uncaria tomentosa* by high performance liquid chromatography. Journal of Chromatography. 1994:243-49.

10. Stuppner H, Sturm S, Geisen G, Zillian U, Konwalinka G. A differential sensitivity of oxindole alkaloids to normal and leukemic cell lines. Planta Medica. 1993;59(Supplement issue):A583.

11. Aquino R, De Simone F, Pizza C. Plant metabolites, structure and *in vitro* antiviral activity of quinovic acid glycosides from *uncaria tomentosa* and *guettarda platypoda*. Journal of Natural Products. 1989;52(4):679-85.

12. Hemingway S, Phillipson J. Alkaloids from South American species of *Uncaria* (Rubiaceae). Journal of Pharmacy and Pharmacology. 1974;26(Supp.):113P.

13. de Matta S, Monache F, Ferrari F, Marini-Bettolo G. Alkaloids and procyanidins of an *Uncaria* sp. from Peru. Farmaco. 1976;31(7):527-35.

14. Steinberg P. Cat's Claw Update (Uncaria tomentosa). That wondrous herb from the Peruvian rain forest. Townsend Letter for Doctors and Patients. 1995;Aug/Sep:70-71.

15. Wagner H, Kreutzkamp B, Jurcic K. The alkaloids of *Uncaria tomentosa* and their phagocytosis-stimulating action. Planta Medica. 1985;5:419-23.

16. Rizzi R, Re F, Bianchi A, De Feo V, de Simone F, Bianchi L, et al. Mutagenic and antimutagenic activities of *Uncaria tomentosa* and its extracts. Journal of Ethnopharmacology. 1993;38(1):63-77.

17. Keplinger K. *Uncaria tomentosa* (Willd.) DC. — Ethnomedicinal use and new pharmacological, toxicological and botanical results. Journal of Ethnopharmacology. 1999;64:23-34.

18. Lamm S, Sheng Y, Pero R. Persistent response to pneumococcal vaccine in individuals supplemented with a novel water soluble extract of *Uncaria tomentosa*, C-Med-100. Phytomedicine. 2001;8(4):267-74.

19. Aguilar J, Rojas P, Marcelo A, Plaza A, Bauer R, Reininger E, et al. Anti-inflammatory activity of two different extracts of *Uncaria Tomentosa* (Rubiaceae). Journal of Ethnopharmacology. 2002;81(2):271-76.

20. Piscoya J, Rodrigeuez Z, Bustamante S, Okuhuma N, Miller M, Sandoval M. Efficacy and safety of freeze dried cat's claw in osteoarthritis of the knee: mechanisms of action of the species *Uncaria guainensis*. Inflammation Research. 2001;50(9):442-48.

21. Mur E, Hartig F, Eibl G, Schirmer M. Randomized double blind clinical trial of an extract from the pentacyclic alkaloid-chemotype of *Uncaria tomentosa* for the treatment of rheumatoid arthritis. Journal of Rheumatology. 2002;29(4):678-81.

22. Santa Maria A, Lopez A, Diaz M. Evaluation of the toxicity of *Uncaria tormentosa* by bioassays in vitro. Journal of Ethnopharmacology. 1997;57:183-87.

23. Hilepo J, Belluci A, Mossey R. Acute renal failure caused by cat's claw herbal remedy in a patient with systemic lupus erythematosus. Nephron. 1997;77:361.

24. Reichert R. Acute renal failure and cat's claw. Quarterly Review of Natural Medicine. 1998;4.

25. Marles RJ, Associate Professor, Department of Botany, Brandon University, Brandon, Manitoba. Review of Medicinal Plant Modules for CCNM; 1997.

26. Anon. Is cat's claw the cat's meow of herbs. Environmental Nutrition. 1998;21(7):1:8.

Chamomile (German)

1. Bradley P. British Herbal Compendium. Bournemouth: BHMA; 1992:239.

2. Wren R. Potter's New Encyclopedia of Botanical Drugs and Preparations. Saffron Walden: C.W. Daniel Company; 1988:362.

3. Newall C, Anderson L, David Phillipson J. Herbal Medicines: A Guide for Health Care Professionals. London: The Pharmaceutical Press; 1996:296.

4. Leung A, S F. Encyclopedia of Common Natural Ingredient Used in Food, Drugs and Cosmetics. 2nd ed. New York, NY: John Wiley and Sons; 1996:649.

5. Berry M. The Chamomiles. The Pharmaceutical Journal. 1995;254:191-93.

6. Tyler V. The Honest Herbal. 3rd ed. Binghampton, NY: Pharmaceutical Products Press; 1993:375.

7. Mann C, Staba EJ. The Chemistry, Pharmacology, and Commercial Formulations of Chamomile. In: Herbs, Spices and Medicinal Plants. Ed. LE Craker and JE Simons. Phoenix, AR: Dryx Press, 1986:235-80.

8. Brown D. Anxiolytic effects of chamomile modulated through central benzodiazepine receptors. Quarterly Review of Natural Medicine. 1996;4(2):87-88.

9. Brown D. Herbal Prescriptions for Better Health. Rocklin, CA: Prima Publishing; 1995:349.

10. Tyler V. The Honest Herbal. 3rd ed. Binghamton, NY: Pharmaceutical Products Press; 1993:375.

11. Isaac O. Pharmakologische Untersuchungen von Kamillen-Inhaltsstoffen.1.Zur Pharmakologie des (-)-alpha Bisabolols under der Bisabololoxide (Ubersicht)/Pharmacological investigations with Compounds of Chamomile 1. On the Pharmacology of (-)-a-Bisabolol and Bisabolol oxides (Review). Planta Medica. 1979;35:118-23.

12. Achterrath-Tuckermann U, Kunde R, Flaskamp E, et al. Pharmacological investigations with compounds of Chamomile V. Investigations on the spasmolytic effect of compounds of chamomile and kamillosan on he isolated guinea gig ileum. Planta Medica. 1980;39:38-50.

13. Della Loggia R, Carle R, Sosa S, Tubaro A. Evaluation of the anti-inflammatory activity of chamomile preparations. Planta Medica. 1990;56:657-58.

14. Jakovlev V, Isaac O, Thiemer K, Kunde R. Pharmacological investigations with compounds of chamomile II. New investigations on the antiphlogistic effects of (-) - alpha bisabolol and bisabolol oxides. Planta Medica. 1979;35:125-40.

15. Szelenyi I, Isaac O, Thiemer K. Pharmacological experiments with compounds of chamomile III. Experimental studies of the ulceroprotective effect of chamomile. Planta Medica. 1979;35:218-27.

16. Jakovlev V, Isaac O, Flakamp E. Pharmacological investigations with compounds of chamomile VI. Investigations on the antiphlogistic effects of chamazulene and matricine. Planta Medica. 1983;49:67-73.

17. Safayhi H, Sabieraj J, Sailer E, Ammon H. Chamazulene: An antioxidant-type inhibitor of leukotriene B4 formation. Planta Medica. 1994;60(5):410-3.

18. Rekka E, Kourounakis A, Kourounakis P. Investigation of the effect of chamazulene on lipid peroxidation and free radical processes. Research Communications in Molecular Pathology and Pharmacology. 1996;92(3):361-64.

19. Holzl J, Ghassemi N, Hahn B. Preparation of 14C-spiro ethers by chamomile and their use by an investigation of absorption. Planta Medica. 1986;52:533.

20. Viola H, Wasowski C, Levi de Stein M, et al. Apigenin, a component of *Matricaria recutita* flowers, is a central benzodiazepine receptors-ligand with anxiolyic effects. Planta Medica. 1995;61:213-216.

21. Miller T, Wittstock U, Lindequist U, Teuscher E. Effects of some components of the essential oil of chamomile, *Chamomila recutita* on histamine release from rat mast cells. Planta Medica. 1996;62:60-61.

22. Wagner H. The immune stimulating polysaccharides and heteroglycans of higher plants. A preliminary communication. Arzneimittelforschung. 1984;34(6):659-61.

23. Mills S. The Essential Book of Herbal Medicine. 2nd ed. London: Penguin; 1991:677.

24. Von Grochulski A, Borkowski B. Influence of chamomile oil on experimental glomerulonephritis in rabbits. Planta Medica. 1972;21:289-92.

25. Ikram M. Medicinal Plants as hypocholesterlemic agents. Journal of the Pakistan Medical Association. 1980;30:278-82.

26. Suganda A, Amoros M, Fauconnier B. Effets inhibiteurs de quelques extraits bruts et semi purifies de plantes indigenes Francaises sur la multiplication de l'herpes virus humain 1 et du poliovirus humain 2 en culture cellulaire. Journal of Natural Products. 1983;46(5):626-32.

27. Blumenthal M, Brusse WR, Goldberg A, et al. The Complete German Commission E Monographs. Austin, TX: American Botanical Council; 1998:685.

28. Carl W, Emrich L. Management of oral mucositis during local radiation and systemic chemotherapy:A study of 98 patients. Journal of Prosthetic Dentistry. 1991;66:361-69.

29. Fidler P, Loprinzi C, O'Fallon J, et al. Prospective evaluation of a chamomile mouthwash for prevention of 5 FU induced oral mucositis. Cancer. 1996;77(3):522-25.

30. Tubaro A, Zilli C, Redaelli C, Della Loggia R. Evaluation of anti-inflammatory activity of a chamomile extract after topical application. Planta Medica. 1984;51:359.

31. Korting H, Schafer-Korting M, Hart H, et al. Anti-inflammatory activity of hamamelis distillate applied topically to the skin. European Journal of Clinical Pharmacology. 1993;44:315-18.

32. Merfort I, Heilmann J, Hagedorn-Leweke U, Lippold B. In vivo skin penetration studies of chamomile flavones. Pharmazie. 1994;49:509-11.

33. Paulsen E, Andersen K, Hausen B. Compositae dermatitis in a Danish dermatology department in one year. Contact Dermatitis. 1993;29:6-10.

34. Hausen B. The sensitizing capacity of Compositae plants III. Test results and cross reactions in Compositae-sensitive patients. Dermatologica. 1979;159:1-11.

35. Hausen B, Busker E, Carle R. The sensitizing capacity of Compositae plants. VII. Experimental investigations with extracts of *Chamomila recutita* (L.) Rauschert and *Anthemis cotula* L. Planta Medica. 1984;50:229-234.

36. Habersing S, Leuschner F, Isaac O, Theimer K. Pharmacological studies with compounds of Chamomile IV. Studies on toxicity of (-) alpha bisabolol. Planta Medica. 1979;37:115-23.

37. Benner M, Lee H. Anaphylactic reaction to chamomile tea. Journal of Allergy and Clinical Immunology. 1973;52:307-308.

38. Van Ketel W. Allergy to *Matricaria chamomila*. Contact Dermatitis. 1987;16:50-51.

39. Casterline C. Allergy to chamomile tea. Journal of the American Medical Association. 1980;4:330-31.

40. Hausen B. A 6-year experience with Compositae mix. American Journal of Contact Dermatitis. 1996;7(2):94-99.

41. Mitchell J, Dupuis G. Allergic contact dermatitis from sesquiterpenoids of the Compositae family of plants. British Journal of Dermatology. 1971;84:139-50.

42. Harris B, Lewis R. Advances in aromatherapy — Chamomile Part 1. International Journal of Alternative and Complementary Medicine. 1994; September:12.

43. Opdyke D. Chamomile oil — German. Food and Cosmetics Toxicology. 1974;12:851-52.

44. Grieves M. A Modern Herbal. London: Pen-Johnson; 1931:912.

Chaste Tree

1. Newall C, Anderson L, David Phillipson J. Herbal Medicines: A Guide for Health Care Professionals. London: The Pharmaceutical Press; 1996:296.

2. Du Mee C. *Vitex agnus castus*. Australian Journal of Medical Herbalism. 1993;5(3):63-65.

3. Brown D. *Vitex agnus castus* Clinical Monograph. Quarterly Review of Natural Medicine. 1994;2(2):111-21.

4. Houghton P. *Agnus castus*. The Pharmaceutical Journal. 1994;253:720-21.

5. Mills S. The Essential Book of Herbal Medicine. 2nd ed. London: Penguin ; 1991:677.

6. Belic I, et al. Constituents of *Vitex agnus castus* seeds. Part 1. Journal of the Chemical Society. 1961:2523-25.

7. Gomaa C, El-Moghazy M, Halim F, El-Sayyad A. Flavonoids and iridoids from *Vitex agnus castus*. Planta Medica. 1978;33:227.

8. Wollenweber E, Mann K. Flavonols from fruits of *Vitex agnus castus*. Planta Medica. 1983;48:126-127.

9. Rimpler H. Iridoids and Ecdysones from Vitex species. Phytochemistry. 1972;11:2653-54.

10. Kustrak D, Kuftinec J, Blazevic N. The composition of the essential oil of *Vitex agnus castus*. Planta Medica. 1992;58(Supp.1):A681.

11. Zwavig J, Bos R. Composition of the essential fruit oil of *Vitex agnus castus*. Pharmacy World and Science. 1993;15(6): Supp H15.

12. Schellenberg R. Treatment for the premenstrual syndrome with agnus castus fruit extract: prospective, randomised, placebo controlled study. Bmj. 2001;322(7279):134-37.

13. Berger D, Schaffner W, Schrader E, Meier B, Brattstrom A. Efficacy of *Vitex agnus castus* L. extract Ze 440 in patients with pre- menstrual syndrome (PMS). Arch Gynecol Obstet. 2000;264(3):150-53.

14. Coeugniet E, Elek E, Kuhnast R. Premenstrual syndrome (PMS) and its treatment. Arztezitchr Naturheilverf. 1986;27(9):619-22.

15. Dittmar F, Bohnert K, Peeters M. Premenstrual syndrome: Treatment with a phytopharmaceutical. Therapiewoche Gynakol. 1992;5(1):60-68.

16. Loch E, Bohnert K, Peeters M. The treatment of menstrual disorders with *Vitex agnus castus* tincture. Der Frauenarzt. 1991;32(8):867-70.

17. Marie-Snow J. *Vitex agnus-castus* L. The Protocol Journal of Botanical Medicine. 1996;1(4):20-23.

18. Halaska M, Beles P, Gorkow C, Sieder C. Treatment of cyclical mastalgia with a solution containing *Vitex agnus castus* extract: results of a placebo-controlled double-blind study. The Breast. 1999;8:175-81.

19. Kubista E, Muller G, Spona J. Treatment of mastopathy with cyclic mastodynia. Clinical results and hormone profiles. Gynakologische Rundschav. 1986;26:65-79.

20. Bleier W. Therapie von Zyklus und Blutungsstorungen und weiteren endokrin bedingten Erkrankungen der Frau mit pflanzlichen Wirkstoffen. Zentralblatt Fur Gynakologie. 1959;81(18):701-09.

21. Propping D, Katzorke T, Belkein I. Diagnosis and therapy of corpus luteum defiociency in general practice. Therapiewoche. 1988;38:2992-3001.

22. Bruckner C. In mitteleuropa genutze heilpflanzen mit milchsekretionsfordernder wirkung (galactagoga). Gleditschia. 1989;17:189-210.

23. Milewicz A, Gejdel E, Sworen H, et al. *Vitex agnus-castus* extract in the treatment of luteal phase defects due to latent hyperprolactinemia: Results of a randomised placebo-controlled double-blind study. Arzneimittelforschung. 1993;43(7):752-66.

24. Bohnert K. The Use of *Vitex agnus castus* for hyperprolactinemia. Quarterly Review of Natural Medicine. 1997;5(1):19-21.

25. Weiss R. Herbal Medicine. Beaconsfield: Beaconsfield Publishers; 1988:362.

26. Jarry H, Leonhardt S, Gorkow C, Wuttke W. *In vitro* prolactin but not LSH and FSH release is inhibited by compounds in extracts of Agnus Castus: direct evidence for a dopaminergic principle by the dopamine receptor assay. Experimental and Clinical Endocrinology. 1994;102:448-54.

27. Muhlenstedt D, Bohnet H, Hanker J, Schneider H. Short luteal phase and prolactin. International Journal of Fertility. 1978;23(3):213-18.

28. Carroll B, Steiner M. The psychobiology of premenstrual dyphoria: The role of prolactin. Psychoneuroendocrinology. 1978;3:171-80.

29. Halbreich U, Assael M, Ben-David M, Bornstein R. Serum Prolactin in women with premenstrual syndrome. Lancet. 1976:654-56.

30. Sliutz G, Speiser P, Schultz A, Spona J, Zellinger R. Agnus castus extracts inhibit prolactin secretion of rat pituitary cells. Hormone and Metabolic Research. 1993;25:253-55.

31. Jarry H, Leonhardt S, Wuttke W. Agnus castus as dopaminergous effective principle in Mastodynon N. Zeitschrift Phytother. 1991;12:77-82.

32. Wuttke W. Dopaminergic Action of extracts of Agnus castus. [Abstract]. Forschende Komplementarmedizen. 1996;3(6):329-30.

33. Merz P, Gorkow C, Schroder A, et al. The effects of a special Agnus castus extract

(BP1095e1) on prolactin secretion in healthy male subjects. Endocrinology and Diabetes. 1996;104:447-53.

34. Bleier W. Phytotherapy in irregular menstrual cycles or bleeding periods and other gynecological disorders of endocrine origin. Zentralblatt fur Gynakologie. 1959;81(18):709-10.

35. Milewicz A, Gejdel E, et.al. *Vitex agnus-castus* in the treatment of luteal phase defects due to hyperprolactinemia: Results of a randomized placebo-controlled double-blind study. Arzneim-Forsch Drug Research. 1993;43:752-56.

36. Propping D, Katzorke T. Treatment of corpus luteum insufficiency. Zeits Allgemeinmedizin. 1987;63:932-33.

37. Gerhard II, Patek A, Monga B, Blank A, Gorkow C. Mastodynon(R) bei weiblicher Sterilitat [Mastodynon(R)] for female infertility randomized, placebo-controlled, clinical double-blind study. Forsch Komplementarmed. 1998;5(6):272-78.

38. Amann W. Akne vulgaris und agnus castus (Agnolyt). Zeits Allgemeinmedizin. 1975;14:1645-48.

39. Cahill D, Fox R, Wardle P, Harlow C. Multiple follicular development associated with herbal medicine. Human Reproduction. 1994;9(8)(Aug):1469-70.

40. Propping D. Multiple follicular development associated with a herbal medicine. Human Reproduction. 1995;10(8):2175.

41. Brown D. Vitex and multiple follicular development. Quarterly Review of Natural Medicine. 1995;3(2):105-06.

42. Cahill D. Comment. Human Reproduction. 1995;10(8):2175-76.

Cranberry

1. Marles RJ, Associate Professor, Department of Botany, Brandon University, Brandon, Manitoba. Review of Medicinal Plant Modules for CCNM; 1997.

2. Leung AY, Foster S. Encyclopedia of Common Natural Ingredients Used in Food, Drugs, and Cosmetics. 2nd ed. New York, NY: John Wiley and Sons Inc; 1996:649.

3. Papas PN, Brusch CA, Ceresia GC. Cranberry juice in the treatment of urinary tract infections. Southwestern Medicine. 1966; 47(1):17-20.

4. Zinsser HH. Newer antibacterial drugs in urological infections. Medical Clinics of North America.1964; 48:293-304.

5. Bodel PT, Cotran R, Kass E. Cranberry juice and the antibacterial activity of hippuric acid. Journal of Laboratory and Clinical Medicine. 1959;64:881.

6. Kahn DH, Panariello V, Saeli J, et al. Effect of cranberry juice on urine. Journal of the American Diet Association. 1967; 51:251.

7. Gibson L, Pike L, Kilbourn JP. Effectiveness of cranberry juice in preventing urinary tract infections in long-termcare facility patients. The Journal of Naturopathic Medicine. 1991; 2(1):45-47.

8. Avorn J, Manone M, Gurwitz JH, Glynn RJ, Choodnovskiy I, Lipsitz LA. Reduction of bacteriuria and pyuria after ingestion of cranberry juice. Journal of the American Medical Association. 1994; 271:751-54.

9. Kilbourne JP. Cranberry juice appears to prevent urinary tract infections. CCML Newsletter. 1986; January.

10. Katz LM. Reduction of bacteriuria and pyuria using cranberry juice [Letter]. Journal of the American Medical Association. 1994; 272(8):589.

11. Hamilton-Miller JMT. Reduction of bacteriuria and pyuria using cranberry juice [Letter]. Journal of the American Medical Association. 1994; 272(8):588.

12. Goodfriend R. Reduction of bacteriuria and pyuria using cranberry juice [Letter]. Journal of the American Medical Association. 1994;272(8):588.

13. Hopkins W, J., Heisey D, M., Jonler M, Uehling DT. Reduction of bacteriuria and pyuria using cranberry juice (Letter). Journal of the American Medical Association. 1994;272(8):588-89.

14. Avorn J, Maonone M, Gurwitz JH, Glynn RJ, Choodnosky I, Lipsitz LA. Reduction of bacteruria and pyuria using cranberry juice [Reply to letters]. Journal of the American Medical Association.1994;272(8):589.

15. Haverkorn MJ, Mandigers J. Reduction of bacteriuria and pyuria using cranberry juice. Journal of the American Medical Association. 1994;272(8):590.

16. Kontiokari T, Sundqvist K, Nuutinen M, Pokka T, Koskela M, Uhari M. Randomised trial of cranberry-lingonberry juice and Lactobacillus GG drink for the prevention of urinary tract infections in women. British Medical Journal. 2001;322(7302):1571.

17. Schlager TA, Anderson S, Trudell J, Hendley JO. Effect of cranberry juice on bacteriuria in children with neurogenic bladder receiving intermittent catheterization. Journal of Pediatrics. 1999;135(6):698-702.

18. Schultz AS. Efficacy of cranberry juice on urinary pH. Journal of Community Health Nursing. 1984;1:155-169.

19. Moen DV. Observations on the effectiveness of cranberry juice in urinary infections. Wisconsin Medical Journal. 1962; 61:282-83.

20. Kinney AB, Blount M. Effect of cranberry juice on urinary pH. Nursing Research. 1979;28:287-90.

21. Fellers CR, Redmon BC, Parrott EM. The effect of cranberries on urinary acidity and blood alkali reserve. Journal of Nutrition. 1933;6:455-63.

22. Nickey NE. Urine pH: effect of prescribed regimens of cranberry juice and ascorbic acid. Archives of Physical Medicine and Rehabilitation. 1975;55:556.

23. McLeod DC, Nahata MC. Methenamine therapy and urine acidification with ascorbic acid cranberry juice. American Journal of Hospital Pharmacology. 1978;35:654.

24. Sobota AE. Inhibition of bacterial adherence by cranberry juice: Potential use for the treatment of urinary tract infection. Journal of Urology. 1984;131:1013-16.

25. Zafriri D, Ofek I, Adar R, et al. Inhibitory activity of cranberry juice on adherence of type I and type P fimbriated *Escherichia coli* to eukaryotic cells. Antimicrobial Agents and Chemotherapy. 1989;33(1):92-98.

26. Schmidt D, Sobota A. An examination of the anti-adherence activity of cranberry juice on urinary and nonurinary bacterial isolates. Microbios. 1988;55:173-81.

27. Ofek I, Goldhar J, Zafriri D, Lis H, et al. Anti-*Escherichia coli* adhesion activity of cranberry and blueberry juices [Letter]. New England Journal of Medicine. 1991;324:1599.

28. Bomser J, Madhavi DL, Singletary K, Smith MAL. *In vitro* anticancer activity of fruit extracts from Vaccinium species. Planta Medica. 1996;62:212-16.

29. Brown D. Herbal Prescriptions for Better Health. Rocklin, CA: Prima Publishing; 1996:349.

Dandelion

1. Cordatos E. *Taraxacum officinale*. Textbook of Natural Medicine. Seattle, WA: Bastyr University; 1992.

2. Mills S. The Essential Book of Herbal Medicine. 2nd ed. London: Penguin; 1991:677.

3. Blanchert K. Dandelion: Leaves are rich source of vitamins and minerals. Alternative and Complementary Therapies. 1995;1(2):115-117.

4. Leung A, Foster S. Encyclopedia of Common Natural Ingredients Used in Food, Drugs and Cosmetics. 2nd ed. New York, NY: John Wiley and Sons; 1996:649.

5. Hobbs C. *Taraxacum officinale*: A monograph and literature review. Eclectic Dispensatory. Portland: Eclectic Medical Publication; 1989.

6. Newall C, Anderson L, David Phillipson J. Herbal Medicines: A Guide for Health Care Professionals. London: The Pharmaceutical Press; 1996:296.

7. Clifford M, Shutler S, Thomas G, Ohiokepehai O. The chlorogenic acids content of coffee substitutes. Food Chemistry. 1987;24:99-107.

8. Williams C, Goldstone F, Greenham J. Flavonoids, Cinnamic acids and coumarins from the different tissues and medicinal preparations of *Taraxacum officinale*. Phytochemistry. 1996;42(1):121-27.

9. Marles RJ, Associate Professor, Department of Botany, Brandon University, Brandon, Manitoba. Review of Medicinal Plant Modules for CCNM; 1997.

10. Stelling K. Restoring the Liver. Canadian Journal of Herbalism. 1991;12(11):7-10.

11. Faber K. The dandelion — *Taraxacum officinale* Weber. Pharmazie. 1958;13(7):423-35.

12. Sankaran J. Livr-Doks in viral hepatitis. The Antiseptic. 1977;74:621-26.

13. Stelling K, Salama, S, Salib M. Phytotherapy an adjunct in cancer treatment. Canadian Journal of Herbalism. 1995(Winter):34-36.

14. Racz-Kotilla E, Racz G, Solomon A. The action of *Taraxacum officinale* extracts on the body weight and diuresis of laboratory animals. Planta Medica. 1974;26:212-17.

15. Houghton P. Bearberry, dandelion and celery. The Pharmaceutical Journal. 1995;255:272-273.

16. Hoffman D. Holistic Herbal. Rockport, MA: Element Books; 1996:256.

17. Chevallier A. The Encyclopedia of Medicinal Plants. London: Reader's Digest; 1996:336.

18. Akhtar MS, Khan Q, Khaliz T. Effects of *Portulaca oleracae* (kulfa) and *Taraxacum officinale* (dhudhal) in non moglycaemic and alloxan-treated hyperglycaemic rabbits. Journal of the Pakistan Medical Association. 1985;35:207-10.

19. Grases F, Melero G, Costa-Bauza A, et al. Urolithiasis and phytotherapy. International Urology and Nephrology. 1994;26(5):507-11.

20. Lovell C, Rowan M. Dandelion dermatitis. Contact Dermatitis. 1991;25:185-188.

21. Dawe R, Green C, MacLeod T, Ferguson J. Daisy, dandelion and thistle contact allergy in the photosensitive dermatitis and actinic reticuloid syndrome. Contact Dermatitis. 1996;35:109-10.

22. Hirono I, Mori H, Kato K, Ushimaru Y. Safety examination of some edible plants. Part 2. Journal of Environmental Pathology Toxicology and Oncology. 1977;1:72-74.

23. Bradley P. British Herbal Compendium. Bournemouth: BHMA; 1992:239.

24. Fernandez C, Martin-Esteban M, Fiandor A, et al. Analysis of cross-reactivity between sunflower pollen and other pollens of the compositae family. Journal of Allergy and Clinical Immunology. 1993;92(5):660-67.

25. Cook C, Sgardelis S, Pantis J, Lanaras T. concentrations of Pb, Zn and Cu in Taraxacum spp. in relation to urban pollution. Bulletin of Environmental Contamination and Toxicology. 1994;53:204-10.

Devil's Claw

1. Newall CA, Anderson LA, Phillipson JD. Herbal Medicines. A Guide for Health Care Professionals. London: The Pharmaceutical Press; 1996.

2. Weiss RF. Herbal Medicine. Gothenburg, Sweden: Ab Arcanum; 1988.

3. Leung AY, Foster S. Encyclopedia of Common Natural Ingredients Used in Food, Drugs, and Cosmetics. 2nd ed. Toronto, ON/New York, NY: John Wiley and Sons Inc; 1996.

4. Grahame R, Robinson B. Devil's Claw (*Harpagophytum procumbens*): pharmacological and clinical studies. Annals of Rheumatic Disease. 1981;40:632.

5. Wren R. Potter's New Encyclopedia of Botanical Drugs and Preparations. Saffron Walden: C.W. Daniel Company; 1988.

6. Ziller K, Franz G. Analysis of the water-soluble fraction from the roots of Harpogophytum procumbens. Planta Medical. 1979;37:340-348.

7. Kikuchi T, Matsuda S, Kubo Y, Namba T. New iridoid glucosides from *Harpagophytum procumbens* DC. Chem Pharm Bulletin. 1983;31:2296-2301.

8. Burger J, Vincent Brandt E, Ferreira D. Iridoid and phenolic glycosides from Harpogophytum. Phytochemistry. 1987;26:1453-57.

9. Bradley P. British Herbal Compendium. Bournemouth, UK: The British Herbal Medical Association; 1992.

10. Czygan F, Krueger A. Pharmaceutical biological studies of the genus harpagophytum. Part 3 Distribution of the iridoid glycoside harpagoside in the different organs of *Harpagophytum procumbens* and *Harpagophytum zeyheri*. Planta Medica. 1977;31:305-307.

11. Weiss R. Herbal Medicine. Beaconsfield: Beaconsfield Publishers Ltd; 1988.

12. Chevallier A. The Encyclopedia of Medicinal Plants. London: Reader's Digest; 1996.

13. Hoffman D. Holistic Herbal. Rockport,MA: Element Books; 1996.

14. Soulimani R, Younos C, Mortier F, Derrieu D. The role of stomachal digestion on the pharmacological activity of plant extracts, using as an example of *Harpagophytum procumbens*. Canadian Journal of Physiology and Pharmacology. 1994;72(12):1532-36.

15. Lanhers M, Fleurentin J, Mortier F, Vinche A, Younos C. Anti-inflammatory and analgesic effects of an aqueous extract of *Harpagophytum procumbens*. Planta Medica. 1992;58:117-23.

16. Erdos A, Fontaine R, Friehe H, Durand R, Poppinghaus T. Beitrag zur pharmakologie und toxokologie verschieder extrakte, sowie des harpagoside aus *Harpagophytum procumbens* DC. Planta Medica. 1978;34:97-108.

17. Whitehouse L, Znamirowska M, Paul C. Devil's Claw (*Harpagophytum procumbens*): No evidence for anti-inflammatory activity in the treatment of arthritic disease. Canadian Medical Association Journal. 1983;129:249-51.

18. Mcleod D, Revell P, Robinson D. Investigations of *Harpagophytum procumbens* (Devil's Claw) in the treatment of experimental inflammation and arthritis in the rat. British Journal of Pharmacology. 1979;66:140-41.

19. Moussard C, Alber D, Toubin M, Thevenon N, Henry J. A drug used in traditional medicine, *Harpagophytum procumbens*: No evidence for NSAID-like effect on whole blood eicosanoid production in human. Prostaglandins Leukotrienes and Essential Fatty Acids. 1992;46:283-86.

20. Pinget M, Lecomte A. The effects of Harpagophytum capsules (Arkocaps) in degenerative rheumatology. Médecine Actuelle. 1985;12(4):65-67.

21. Chantre P, Cappelaere A, Leblan D, Guedon D, Vandermander J, Fournie B. Efficacy and tolerance of *Harpagophytum procumbens* versus diacerhein in treatment of osteoarthritis. Phytomedicine. 2000;7(3):177-83.

22. Leblan D, Chantre P, Fournie B. *Harpagophytum procumbens* in the treatment of knee and hip osteoarthritis. Four-month results of a prospective, multicenter, double-blind trial versus diacerhein. Joint Bone Spine. 2000;67(5):462-67.

23. Laudahn D, Walper A. Efficacy and tolerance of Harpagophytum extract LI 174 in patients with chronic non-radicular back pain. Phytotherapy Research. 2001;15(7):621-24.

24. Chrubasik S, Junck H, Conradt C, Zappe H, Chrubasik J. Effectiveness of oral harpagophytum extract WS 1531 in treating low back pain. Arthr Rheum. 1998;41(Suppl 9):S261.

25. Chrubasik S, Zimpfer C, Schutt U, Ziegler R. Effectiveness of *Harpagophytum procumbens* in treatment of acute back pain. Phytomedicine. 1996;3(1):1-10.

26. Barnes J. *Harpagophytum procumbens* extract for acute low back pain requires further investigation. Focus on Alternative and Complementary Therapies. 1996;1(1):6-7.

27. Occhiuto F, Circosta C, Ragusa S, Ficarra P, Costa De Pasquale R. A drug used in traditional medicine: *Harpagophytum procumbens* DC.IV. Effects on some isolated muscle preparations. Journal of Ethnopharmacology. 1985;13:201-08.

28. Circosta C, et al. A drug used in traditional medicine: *Harpagophytum procumbens* DC.II. Cardiovascular activity. Journal of Ethnopharmacology. 1984;11:259-74.

29. Costa De Pasquale R, Busa G, Circosta C, Iauk L, Ragusa S, Ficarra P, et al. A drug used in traditional medicine: Harpagohytum procumbens DC.III. Effects on hyperkinetic ventricular arrythmias by reperfusion. Journal of Ethnopharmacology. 1985;13:193-99.

30. Guerin J, Revelliere H. Activite antifongique d'extraits vegetaux a usage therapeutique.II.Etude de 40 extraits sur 9 souches fongiques. Ann. Pharmaceutiques francaises. 1985;43:77-81.

31. Tyler V. The Honest Herbal. 3rd ed. Binghamton, N.Y.: Pharmaceutical Products Press; 1993.

Dong Quai

1. Noe J. *Angelica Sinensis*: A Monograph. Journal of Naturopathic Medicine. 1997;7(1):66-72.

2. Foster S, Chongxi Y. Herbal Emissaries. Bringing Chinese Herbs to the West. Rochester, VT: Healing Arts Press; 1992.

3. Bensky D, Gamble A. Chinese Herbal Medicine Materia Medica. Seattle, WA: Eastland Press; 1986.

4. Marles RJ, Associate Professor, Department of Botany, Brandon University, Brandon, Manitoba. Review of Medicinal Plant Modules for CCNM; 1997.

5. Upton R, ed. Dang Gui Root (*Angelica Sinensis* (Oliv.) Diels Standards of Analysis, Quality Control and Therapeutics. Scotts Valley, CA: American Herbal Pharmacopoeia; 2003.

6. Zhu D. Dong Quai. American Journal of Chinese Medicine. 1987;15:117-25.

7. Bensky D, Gamble A. Chinese Herbal Materia Medica. Seattle: Eastland Press; 1986.

8. Mills S. The Essential Book of Herbal Medicine. 2nd ed. London: Penguin Publ; 1991.

9. Chang H-M, But PP-H, editors. Pharmacology and Applications of Chinese Materia Medica. Philadelphia, PA: World Scientific; 1986.

10. Chevalier A. The Encyclopedia of Medicinal Plants. London: Reader's Digest; 1996.

11. Belford-Courtney R. Comparison of Chinese and Western uses of *Angelica Sinensis*. Australian Jouranl of Medical Herbalism. 1993;5(4):87-91.

12. Mei Q-b, Yi T-J, Cui B. Advances in the pharmacological studies of radix *Angelica Sinensis* (Oliv) Diels (Chinese Danggui). Chinese Medical Journal. 1991;104(9):776-81.

13. Yoshiro K. The physiological action of Tang Kuei and Cnidium. Bull. Oriental Healing Arts Institute of U.S.A. 1985;10(7):269-78.

14. Ko F, Wu T, Liou M, Huang T, Teng C. Inhibition of platelet thromboxane formation and phosphoinostides breakdown by osthole from Angelica pubescens. Thrombosis Haemostasis. 1989;62(3):996-99.

15. Hudson T. Balancing the Female Hormonal System. Gaia Symposium Proceedings; 1993 May 29-31,1993; Ashland, MA: Gaia Herbal Research Institute; 1993:119.

16. Hudson T, Standish L, Breed C, Bettenberg R, Dalen C, Noe J, et al. Clinical and endocrinological effects of a menopausal botanical formula. Journal of Naturopathic Medicine. 1997;7(1):73-84.

17. Burke BE, Olson RD, Cusack BJ. Randomized, controlled trial of phytoestrogen in the prophylactic treatment of menstrual migraine. Biomedicine Pharmacotherapeutics. 2002;56(6):283-88.

18. Reichert R. Phyto-estrogens. Quarterly Review of Natural Medicine. 1994;2(1):27-33.

19. Tyler V. The Honest Herbal. 3rd ed. Binghamton, N.Y.: Pharmaceutical Products Press; 1993.

20. Goh S, Loh K. Gynaecomastia and the herbal tonic "Dong Quai". Singapore Medical Journal. 2001;42(3):115-16.

21. Newall CA, Anderson LA, Phillipson JD. Herbal Medicines. A Guide for Health Care Professionals. London: The Pharmaceutical Press; 1996.

22. Page RL, 2nd, Lawrence JD. Potentiation of warfarin by dong quai. Pharmacotherapy. 1999;19(7):870-76.

23. Teegarden R. Chinese Tonic Herbs. New York: Japan Publishing Inc; 1985.

Echinacea

1. Awang DVC, Kindack DG. Echinacea. Canadian Pharmaceutical Journal. 1991;124:512-16.

2. Hobbs C. Echinacea - a literature review. Herbalgram. 1994;30:33-47.

3. Murray M. The Healing Power of Herbs. Rocklin, CA: Prima Publishing; 1992.

4. Foster S. Echinacea: The cold and flu remedy. Alternative and Complementary Therapies. 1995;1(4):254-57.

5. Bauer R. Echinacea drugs — effects and active ingredients [German]. Zeitschrift fur Arztliche Fortbildung. 1996;90(2):111-15.

6. Shemluck M. Medicinal and other uses of the Compositae by Indians in the United States and Canada. Journal of Ethnopharmacology. 1982;5:303-58.

7. Vogel V. American Indian Medicine. Norman: University of Oklahoma Press; 1970.

8. Hobbs C. Echinacea: diminished immune stimulation over time? Medical Herbalism. 1994;6(2):3-5.

9. Bauer R, Wagner H. Echinacea species as potential immunostimulatory drugs. Economic and Medical Plant Research. 1991;5:253-321.

10. Editorial. Echinacea. Journal of the American Medical Association. 1909;53:1836.

11. Brown DJ. Echinacea: Phytotherapy review and commentary. Townsend Letter for Doctors and Patients. 1995;January:134-35.

12. Hobbs C. The Echinacea Handbook. Portland, Oregon: Eclectic Medical Publications; 1989.

13. Bauer R, Wagner H. Ein Handbuch für Ärzte, Apotheker und andere Naturwissenschaftler. Stuttgart: Wissenschaftliche Verlagsgesellschaft; 1990.

14. Foster S. Echinacea: Nature's immune enhancer. Rochester, VT: Healing Arts Press; 1991.

15. Hobbs C. The chemistry and pharmacology of Echinacea species. Herbal Gram (Supplement). 1994;30:1-7.

16. Luettig B, Steinmüller C, Gifford GE, Wagner H, Lohmann-Matthes M-L. Macrophage activation by the polysaccharide arabinogalactan isolated from plant cell cultures of Echinacea purpurea. Journal of the National Cancer Institute. 1989;81(9):669-75.

17. Steinmuller C, Roesler J, Grottrup E, Franklin G, Wagner H, Lohmann-Mattes M-L. Polysaccharides isolated from plant cell cultures of Echinacea purpurea enhance the resistance of immunosuppressed mice against systemic infecions with Candida albicans and Listeria monocytogenes. International Journal of Immunopharmacology. 1993;15(5):605-14.

18. Muller-Jakic B, Breu W, Probstle A, Redl K, Greger H, Bauer R. In vitro inhibition of cyclooxygenase and 5-lipoxygenase by alkamides from Echinacea and Achillea species. Planta Medica. 1994;60:37-40.

19. Bauer R, Khan AI, Wagner H. TLC and HPLC Analysis of Echinacea pallida and E. angustifolia roots. Planta Medica. 1988;54:426-30.

20. Bauer R, et al. Alkamides from the roots of Echinacea angustifolia. Phytochemistry. 1989;28:505-508.

21. Bohlman F, Hoffmann M. Further amides from Echinacea purpurea. Phytochemistry 1983;22:1173-75.

22. Proksch A, Wagner H. Structural analysis of 4-0-methyl-glucuronoarabinoxylan with immuno-stimulating activity from Echinacea purpurea. Phytochemistry. 1987;26(7):1989-93.

23. Wagner H, et al. Immunologically active polysaccharides of Echinacea purpurea cell cultures. Phytochemistry. 1988;27:119-26.

24. Roesler J, Steinmuller C, Kiderlen A, Emmendorffer A, Wagner H, Lohmann-Matthes M-L. Application of purified polysaccharides from cell cultures of the plant Echinacea purpurea to mice mediates protection against systemic infections with Listeria monocytogenes and Candida albicans. International Journal of Immunopharmacology. 1991;13(1):27-37.

25. Roesler J, Emmendorffer A, Steinmuller C, Luettig B, Wagner H, Lohmann-Matthes M-L. Application of purified polysaccharides from cell cultures of the plant Echinacea purpurea to test subjects mediates activation of the phagocyte system. International Journal of Immunopharmacology. 1991;13(7):931-41.

26. Wildfeur A, Mayerhofer D. The effects of plant preparations on cellular functions in body defense [German]. Arzneimittel-Forschung. 1994;44(3):361-66.

27. Vömel T. Der einfluss einen pflanzelische immunostimulans auf die phagozytose von erythozyten durch das retikulohistozytäre system der isoliert perfundierten rattenleber. Arzneimittel-Forschung. 1985;35:1437-39.

28. Bauer R, et al. Immunological in vivo and in vitro examinations of Echinacea extracts. Arzneimittel-Forschung. 1988;38:276-81.

29. Stotzem CD, Hungerland U, Mengs U. Influence of Echinacea purpurea on the phagocytosis of human granulocytes. Medical Science Research. 1992;20:717-20.

30. Bukovsky M, Kostalova D, Magnusova R, Vaverkova S. Testing for immunomodulating effects of ethanol-water extracts of the above-ground parts of the plants Echinaceae (Moench) and Rudbeckia L.J. [Slovak]. Ceskoslovenska Farmacie. 1993;42(5):228-31.

31. Stimpel M, Proksch A, Wagner H, Lohmann-Matthes M-L. Macrophage activation and induction of macrophage cytotoxicity by purified polysaccharide fractions from the plant *Echinacea purpurea*. Infection and Immunity. 1984;46(3):845-49.

32. Mose J. Effect of echinacin on phagocytosis and natural killer cells. Med Welt. 1983;34:1463-67.

33. Bukovsky M, Vaverkova S, Kostalova D. Immunomodulating activity of *Echinacea gloriosa* L., *Echinacea angustifolia* DC. and *Rudbeckia speciosa* Wenderoth ethanol-water extracts. Polish Journal of Pharmacology. 1995;47:175-77.

34. Wagner H, Proksch A. Immunomodulatory drugs of fungi and higher plants. In: Farnsworth N, Hikino H, H. W, ed. Economic and Medicinal Plant Research. Orlando, FL: Academic Press; 1985:113-55.

35. Juricic K, Melchart D, Holzmann M, Martin M, Bauer P, Doenicke A, et al. Zeitschrift fur Phytotherapie. 1989;10:67-70.

36. Fong Y, Moldawer LL, Marano M, Wei H, Tatter SB, Clarick RH, et al. Endotexemia elicits increased circulating B2-IFN/IL-6 in man. Journal of Immunity. 1989;142:2321-40.

37. Berg A, Northoff H, Konig D, Weinstock C, Grathwohl D, Parnham MJ, et al. Influence of Echinacin (EC31) treatment on the exercise-induced immune response in athletes. Journal of Clinical Research. 1998;1:367-80.

38. Melchart D, Linde K, Fischer P, Kaesmayr J. Echinacea for preventing and treating the common cold (Cochrane Review). In The Cochrane Library. 2000; 3rd ed.

39. Braunig B, Dorn M, Limburg E, Knick E. *Echinacea purpurea* radix for stregthening the immune system in flu-like infections [in German]. Zeitschrift fur Phytotherapie. 1992;13:7-13.

40. Braunig B, Knick E. Therapeutische Ergahrungen mit *Echinacea pallida* bei grippalen Infekten. Naturheilpraxis mit Naturmedizin 1993;1:72-75.

41. Reitz HD. Immunmodulatoren mit pflanzlichen Wirkstoffen. 2. Teil: eine wissenschaftliche Studie am Beispiel Esberitox N. Notabene medici. 1990;20:362-66.

42. Vorberg G. Treatment of menopause symptoms. ZFA. 1984;60:626-29.

43. Scaglione F, Lund B. Efficacy in the treatment of the common cold of a preparation containing an Echinacea extract. International Journal of Immunotherapy. 1995;6:163-66.

44. Vorberg G, Schneider B. Pflanzliches Immunstimulans verkurzt grippalen Infekt. Doppelblindstudie belegt die Steigerung der unspezifischen Infektabwehr. Arzneimittal- Forschung. 1989;36:3-8.

45. Dorn M. Milderung grippaler Infekte durch ein pflanzliches Immunstimulans. Natur- und Ganzheitsmedizin. 1989;2:314-19.

46. Barrett B, Vohmann M, Calabrese C. Echinacea for upper respiratory infection [see comments]. Journal of Family Practice. 1999;48(8):628-35.

47. Brinkeborn RM, Shah DV, Degenring FH. Echinaforce and other Echinacea fresh plant preparations in the treatment of the common cold. A randomized, placebo controlled, double-blind clinical trial. Phytomedicine. 1999;6(1):1-6.

48. Henneicke-von Zepelin H, Hentschel C, Schnitker J, Kohnen R, Kohler G, Wustenberg P. Efficacy and safety of a fixed combination phytomedicine in the treatment of the common cold (acute viral respiratory tract infection): results of a randomised, double blind, placebo controlled, multicentre study. Current Medical Research Opinions. 1999;15(3):214-27.

49. Barrett BP, Brown RL, Locken K, Maberry R, Bobula JA, D'Alessio D. Treatment of the common cold with unrefined echinacea. A randomized, double-blind, placebo-controlled trial. Ann Intern Med. 2002;137(12):939-46.

50. Hoheisel O, Sandberg M, Bertram S, M. B, Schafer M. Echinacea treatment shortens the course of the common cold: a double-blind, placebo-controlled clinical trial. Europena Journal of Clinical Research. 1997;9:261-69.

51. Melchart D, Walther E, Linde K, Brandmaier R, Lersch C. Echinacea root extracts for the prevention of upper respiratory tract infections: A double-blind, placebo-controlled randomized trial. Archives of Family Medicine. 1998;7(6):541-45.

52. Schoneberger D. The influence of immune-stimulating effects of pressed juice from *Echinacea purpuraea* on the course and severity of colds. Results of a recent double-blind study [German]. Forum Immunologie. 1992;8:2-12.

53. Schmidt U, Albrecht M, Schenk N. Pflanzliches Immunstimulans senkt Haufigkeit grippaler Infekte. Plazebokontrollierte Doppelblindstudie mit einem kombinierten Echinacea-Praparat mit 646 Studenten der Kolner Universitat. Natur- und Ganzheitsmedizin. 1990;3(9):277-81.

54. Turner RB, Riker DK, Gangemi JD. Ineffectiveness of echinacea for prevention of experimental rhinovirus colds. Antimicrob Agents Chemother. 2000;44(6):1708-09.

55. Grimm W, Muller HH. A randomized controlled trial of the effect of fluid extract of *Echinacea purpurea* on the incidence and severity of colds and respiratory infections. American Journal of Medicine. 1999;106(2):138-43.

56. Busing KH. Inhibition of hyaluronidase by Echinacin [German]. Arzneimittelforsch. 1952;2:467-72.

57. Korting GW, Born W. Beeinflussung des trypanociden salvarson-effekts durch hyaluronidase und einen hyaluronidase- inhibitor (Echinacin). Arzneimittelforsch. 1954;4:424-26.

58. Koch FE, Haase H. Eine modifikation des spreading-testes im tierversuch, gleichzeitig ein beitrag zum wirkungsmechanismus von Echinacin. Arzneimittelforsch. 1953;2:464-67.

59. Koch FE, Uebel H. Experimentelle untersuchungen uber den einfu von *Echinacea purpurea* auf das hypophysen- nebennierenrinden-system. Arzneimittelforsch. 1953;3:133-37.

60. Tunnerhoff FK, Schwabe HK. Studies in human beings and animals on the influence of Echinacea extracts on the formation of connective tissue following the implantation of fibrin (in German). Arzneimittelforsch. 1956;6:330-34.

61. Keller H. German Patent 950 674 (11 October 1956). Chemical Abstracts 1959;53:8550i.

62. Bonadero I, et al. Echinacin B: Active polysaccharide from Echinacea [Italian]. Riv Ita. Essenze Profumi Piante. 1971;53:281-95.

63. Bonadero I, Lavazza M. Echinacina B: suo azione sui fibroblasti (Italian). Rivista Italiana Essenze Profumi. 1972;54:195.

64. Tragni E, et al. Evidence from two classical irritation tests for an anti-inflammatory action of a natural extract, echinacea B. Food and Chem Toxicicology. 1985;23:317-19.

65. Tubaro A, al. e. Anti-inflammatory activity of a polsaccharide fraction of *Echinacea angustifolia*. Journal of Pharmacy and Pharmacology. 1987;39:567-69.

66. Wagner H, Breu W, Willer F, Wierer M, Remiger P, Schwenker G. Planta Medica. 1989;55:566-67.

67. Gaisbauer M, Zimmerman W, Schleich T. Natura. Med. 1986;1:6-10.

68. Coeugniet EG, Elek E. Immunomodulation with *Viscum album* and *Echinacea purpurea* extracts. Onkologie. 1987;10(3 (Supplement)):27-33.

69. Stoll A, Renz J, Brack A. Isolierung und konstitution des echinacosids, eines glykosids aus den wurzeln von *Echinacea angustifolia* D.C. Helvetica Chimica Acta. 1950;33:1877-93.

70. Schulte KE, al. e. Das vorkommen von polyacetylen-verbindungen in *Echinacea purpurea* Mnch. und *Echinacea angustifolia* DC. Arzneimittel-Forschung. 1967;17:825-29.

71. Samochowiec E, Urbanska L, Manka W, Stolarska E. Evaluation of the effect of *Calendula officinalis* and *Echinacea angustifolia* extracts on *Trichemonas vaginalis in vitro* [Polish]. Wiadomosci Parazytologiozne. 1979;25(1):77-81.

72. Orinda D, et.al. Antiviral activity of constituents of the compositae purpurea (in German). Arzneimittelforsch. 1973;23:1119-20.

73. Wacker A, Hilbig W. Virus inhibition by *Echinacea purpurea*. Planta Medica. 1978;33:89-102.

74. May G, Willuhn G. Antiviral effect of aqueous plant extracts in tissue culture [German]. Arzneimittel Forschung. 1978;28(1-4):1-7.

75. Cheminat A, Zawatzky R, Becker H, Brouillard R. Caffeoyl conjugates from *Echinacea* spp: Structures and biological functions. Phytochemistry. 1988;27:2787-94.

76. Lersch C, et.al. Nonspecific immunostimulation with low doses of cyclophosphamide (LDCY), thymostimulin, and *Echinacea purpurea* extracts (echinacin) in patients with far advanced colorectal cancers: preliminary results. Cancer Investig. 1992;10(5):343-48.

77. Voaden DJ, Jacobson M. Tumor inhibitors. 3. Identification and synthesis of an oncolytic hydrocarbon from American coneflower roots. Journal of Medical Chem. 1972;15:619-23.

78. Paranich AV, Pocherniava VF, Dubinskaia GM, Mishchenko VP, Mironova NG, Gugalo P, et al. Effect of supposed radioprotectors on oxidation-reduction of vitamin E in the tissues of irradiated rats [Russian]. Radiatsionnaia Biologiia, Radioecologiia. 1993;33(5):653-57.

79. Melchart D, Clemm C, Weber B, Draczynski T, Worku F, Linde K, et al. Polysaccharides isolated from *Echinacea purpurea* herba cell cultures to counteract undesired effects of chemotherapy—a pilot study. Phytother Res. 2002;16(2):138-42.

80. Facino RM, Carini M, Aldini G, Saibene L, Pietta P, Mauri P. Echinoside and caffeoyl conjugates protect collagen from free-radical-induced degradation: A potential use of Echinacea extracts in the prevention of skin photodamage. Planta Medica. 1995;61:510-14.

81. Vonau B, Chard S, Mandalia S, Wilkinson D, Barton SE. Does the extract of the plant *Echinacea purpurea* influence the clinical course of recurrent genital herpes? International Journal Sexually Transmitted Diseases and AIDS. 2001;12(3):154-58.

82. Beuscher N, Bodinet C, Willigmann I, Satzgitter DE. Immonomudulierende eigenschaften von wurzelextrakten verschiedener Echinacea-arten. Zeitschrift fur Phytotherapie. 1995;16:157-66.

83. Bergner P. Echinacea Species. Medical Herbalism. 1995;7(3):16.

84. Blumenthal M, Brusse WR, Goldberg A, Gruenwald J, Hall T, Riggins CW, et al. The Complete German Commission E Monographs. Austin, TX: American Botanical Council; 1998.

85. Lenk M. Z. Acute toxicity of various polysaccharides from *Echinacea purpurea* in the mouse. Phytotherapie. 1989;10:49-52.

86. Schimmer O, Abel G, Behninger C. Z. Investigations on the geotoxic potency of neural polysaccaride from Echinacea cell cultures in cultured human lymphocytes. Zeitschrift fur Phytotherapie. 1989;10:39-42.

87. Mattocks AR. Chemistry and Toxicology of Pyrrolizidine Alkaloids. London: Academic Press; 1986.

88. Newall C, Anderson L, Philipson J. Herbal Medicines: A Guide for Health Care Professionals. London: The Pharmaceutical Press; 1996.

89. Reynolds JE. Martindale. The Extra Pharmacopoeia. 29th ed. London: The Pharmaceutical Press; 1989.

90. Bergner P. Contraindications for echinacea? Medical Herbalism. 1997;9(1):1,11-14.

91. Tyler VE. Herbs of Choice. The Therapeutic Use of Phytomedicinals. Binghamton, NY: Pharmaceutical Products Press; 1994.

92. Mullins RJ. Echinacea-associated anaphylaxis. Medical Journal of Australia. 1998;168(4):170-71.

93. Mullins RJ, Heddle R. Adverse reactions associated with echinacea: the Australian experience. Annals of Allergy and Asthma Immunology. 2002;88(1):42-51.

94. Soon SL, Crawford RI. Recurrent erythema nodosum associated with Echinacea herbal therapy. J Am Acad Dermatol. 2001;44(2):298-99.

95. von Unruh V. Echinacea angustifolia and Inula helenium in the treatment of tuberculosis. Nat Eclect Med Assoc Quart. 1915;7:63.

96. Heesen W, Schroeder C. Die bedeutung des Echiancin in der tuberculose-therapie. Med Monatssch.r 1960;14:251-56.

97. McLeod D. Case history of chronic lymphatic leukaemia. The Modern Phytotherapist. 1996;2(3):10.

98. Gallo M, Sarkar M, Au W, Pietrzak K, Comas B, Smith M, et al. Pregnancy outcome following gestational exposure to echinacea: A prospective controlled study. Archives of Internal Medicine. 2000;160(20):3141-43.

99. Gilroy CM, Steiner JF, Byers T, Shapiro H, Georgian W. Echinacea and truth in labeling. Arch Intern Med. 2003;163(6):699-704.

100. Bergner P. Echinacea myth: Phagocytosis not diminshed after ten days. Medical Herbalism. 1994;6(1):1.

101. Bone K. Long term use of echinacea. Medical Herbalism. 1995; Spring and Summer(1-2):23.

102. Bradley P. British Herbal Compendium. Bournemouth, UK: The British Herbal Medical Association; 1992.

Elder

1. Stelling K. Sambucus/Elder. Canadian Journal of Herbalism. 1991;12:15-18.

2. Newall C, Anderson L, David Phillipson J. Herbal Medicines: A Guide for Health Care Professionals. London: The Pharmaceutical Press; 1996:296.

3. Hutchens A. Indian Herbology of North America. Boston: Shambhala; 1991:382.

4. Marles RJ, Associate Professor, Department of Botany, Brandon University, Brandon, Manitoba. Review of Medicinal Plant Modules for CCNM; 1997.

5. Leung A, Foster S. Encyclopedia of Common Natural Ingredients in Food, Drugs and Cosmetics. 2nd ed. New York, NY: John Wiley and Sons; 1996:649.

6. Stelling K. Restoring the liver. Canadian Journal of Herbalism. 1991;12:7-10.

7. Chevallier A. The Encyclopedia of Medicinal Plants. London: Reader's Digest; 1996:336.

8. McCutcheon A, Roberts T, Gibbons E, et al. Antiviral screening of British Columbian medicinal plants. Journal of Ethnopharmacology. 1995;49:101-10.

9. Bradley P. British Herbal Compendium. Bournemouth: BHMA; 1992:239.

10. Evans W. Trease and Evans' Pharmacology. 13th ed. London: Bailliere-Tindall; 1989:832.

11. Davidek J. Isolation of chromatographically pure rutin from flowers of elder. Nature. 1961;189:487-88.

12. Willuhn G, Richter W. On the constituents of Sambucus nigra II.The lipophillic components of the flowers. Planta Medica. 1977;31:328-43.

13. Toulemonde B, Richard H. Volatile constituents of dry elder (Sambucus nigra.L) flowers. Journal of Agriculture and Food Chemistry. 1983;31:365-70.

14. Jensen S, Nielsen B. Cyanogenic glucosides in Sambucus nigra L. Acta Chemica Scandinavica. 1973;27:2661-85.

15. Wren R. Potter's New Encyclopedia of Botanical Drugs and Preparations. Saffron Walden: C.W. Daniel Company; 1988:362.

16. Hoffman D. Holistic Herbal. Rockport, MA: Element Books; 1996:256.

17. Mills S. The Essential Book of Herbal Medicine. 2nd ed. London: Penguin; 1991:677.

18. Rebuelta M, et al. Etude de l'effet diuretique de differentes preparations des fleurs du sambucus nigra L. Plantes Medicinales et Phytotherapie. 1983;17:173-81.

19. McCutcheon A, Ellis S, Hancock R, Towers G. Antibiotic screening of medicinal plants of the British Columbian native peoples. Journal of Ethnopharmacology. 1993;37:213-23.

20. McCutcheon A, Ellis S, Hancock R, Towers G. Antifungal screening of medicinal plants of the British Columbian native peoples. Journal of Ethnopharmacology. 1994;44:157-69.

21. Mascolo N, et al. Biological screening of Italian medicinal plants for anti-inflammatory activity. Phytotherapy Research. 1987;1:28-31.

22. Richter A. Changes in the motor activity if smooth muscles of the rat uterus in vitro as the effect of phytohaemag glutins from Sambucus nigra. Folia Biol. 1973;21:33-48.

23. Weiss R. Herbal Medicine. Beaconsfield: Beaconsfield Publishers; 1988:362.

Evening Primrose

1. Wren R. Potter's New Encyclopedia of Botanical Drugs and Preparations. Saffron Walden: C.W. Daniel Company; 1988.

2. Newall CA, Anderson LA, Phillipson JD. Herbal Medicines. A Guide for Health Care Professionals. London: The Pharmaceutical Press; 1996.

3. Leung AY, Foster S. Encyclopedia of Common Natural Ingredients Used in Food, Drugs, and Cosmetics. 2nd ed. Toronto/New York: John Wiley and Sons Inc; 1996.

4. Briggs CJ. Evening primrose. Canadian Pharmaceutical Journal. 1986;119(5):249-54.

5. Hutchens A. Indian Herbology of North America. Boston, MA: Shambhala Press; 1991.

6. MacLennan A, Wilson D, Taylor A. Prevalence and cost of alternative medicine in Australia. Lancet. 1996;347:569-73.

7. Horrobin DF, Manku MS. Clinical biochemistry of essential fatty acids. In: Omega-6 Essential Fatty Acids: Pathophysiology and Roles in Clinical Medicine. New York: Alan R. Liss; 1990:1-54.

8. Horrobin DF. Gammalinolenic acid: an intermediate in essential fatty acid metabolism with potential as an ethical pharmaceutical and as a food. Reviews of Contemporary Pharmacotherapy. 1990;1:1-45.

9. Horrobin D. Loss of delta-6-desaturase activity as a key factor in aging. Medical Hypotheses. 1981;7:1211-20.

10. Jones D, Carter R, Haitas B, Mann J. Low phospholipid arachidonic acid values in diabetic platelets. British Medical Journal. 1983;286:173-75.

11. Tuna N, Frankhausen S, Goetz F. Total serum fatty acids in diabetes: relative and absolute concentrations of individual fatty acids. American Journal of Medical Science. 1968;255:120-30.

12. Brenner R, Peluffo R, Nervi A. Effect of ethanol administration on fatty acid desaturation. Lipids. 1980;15:263-68.

13. Horrobin D. Essential fatty acids, prostaglandins and alcoholism: an overview. Alcoholism, Clinical and Experimental Research. 1987;11:2-9.

14. Behan P, Behan W. Essential fatty acids in the treatment of postviral fatigue syndrome. Pathophysiology and Roles in Clinical Medicine. 1990:275-82.

15. Behan P, Behan W, Horrobin D. Effect of high doses of essential fatty acids on the postviral fatigue syndrome. Acta Neurol Scand. 1990;82(3):209-16.

16. Bettger W, Reeves P, Moscatelli E, O'Dell B. Interaction of zinc and essential fatty acids in the rat. Journal of Nutrition. 1979;109:480-90.

17. Huang Y, Cunnane S, Horrobin D, Davignon J. Most biological effects of zinc deficiency corrected by gamma-linoleic acid but not linoleic acid. Atherosclerosis. 1982;41:193-207.

18. Cunnane S, Manku M, Horrobin D. Accumulation of linoleic and gamma-linolenic acids in tissue lipids of pyridoxine-deficient rats. Journal of Nutrition. 1984;114:1754-61.

19. Leichsenring M, Kochsiek U, Paul K. (n-6)-Fatty acids in plasma lipids of children with atopic bronchial asthma. Pediatr Allergy Immunol. 1995;6(4):209-12.

20. Brown D. Herbal Prescriptions for Better Health. Rocklin, CA: Prima Publishing; 1996.

21. Lovell CR, et al. Treatment of atopic eczema with evening primrose oil. Lancet. 1981(1):278.

22. Wright S, Burton JL. Oral evening primrose seed oil improves atopic eczema. Lancet. 1982(ii):1120-22.

23. Morse PF, Horrobin DF, et al. Meta-analysis of placebo-controlled studies of the efficacy of Epogam in the treatment of atopic eczema. Relationship between plasma essential fatty acid changes and clinical response. British Journal of Dermatology. 1989;121:75-90.

24. Bordoni A, Biagi PL, et al. Evening primrose oil (Efamol) in the treatment of children with atopic eczema. Drugs Exp Clinical Research. 1987;14:291-97.

25. Stewart JCM, et al. Treatment of severe and moderately severe atopic dermatitis with evening primrose oil (Epogam); a multicentre study. Journal of Nutritional Medicine. 1991;2:9-15.

26. Schalin-Karrila M, et al. Evening primrose oil in the treatment of atopic eczema: effect on cliniacal status, plasma phospholipid fatty acids and circulating blood prostaglandins. British Journal of Dermatology. 1987;117:11-19.

27. Anonymous. Oral medication treats symptoms and underlying cause of atopic eczema. Hospital Medicine. 1991;13(4):1-2.

28. Biagi PL, Bordoni A, Hrelia S, Celadon M, Ricci GP, Cannella V, et al. The effect of gamma-linolenic acid on clinical status, red cell fatty acid composition and membrane microviscosity in infants with atopic dermatitis. Drugs under Experimental and Clinical Research. 1994;20(2):77-84.

29. Yoshimoto-Furuie K, Yoshimoto K, Tanaka T, Saima S, Kikuchi Y, Shay J, et al. Effects of oral supplementation with evening primrose oil for six weeks on plasma essential fatty acids and uremic skin symptoms in hemodialysis patients. Nephron. 1999;81(2):151-59.

30. Berth-Jones J, Graham-Brown RA. Placebo-controlled trial of essential fatty acid supplementation in atopic dermatitis [published erratum appears in Lancet, 1993 Aug 28;342(8870):564] [see Comments]. Lancet. 1993;341(8860):1557-60.

31. Bamford JTM, et al. Atopic eczema unresponsive to evening primrose oil (linolenic and gamma-linolenic acids). Journal of the American Academy of Dermatology. 1985;13:959-65.

32. Whitaker DK, Cilliers J, de Beer C. Evening primrose oil (Epogam) in the treatment of chronic hand dermatitis: Disappointing therapeutic results. Dermatology. 1996;193(2):115-20.

33. Hederos CA, Berg A. Epogam evening primrose oil treatment in atopic dermatitis and asthma. Archives of Disease in Children. 1996;75(6):494-97.

34. Berg A. Epogam evening primrose oil treatment in atopic dermatitis and asthma. Archives of Disease in Children. 1996;75(6):494-97.

35. McHenry PM, et al. Management of atopic eczema. British Medical Journal. 1995;310:843-47.

36. Berth-Jones J, Graham-Brown RA. Evening primrose oil. Does not show promise in atopic dermatitis [Letter; Comment]. British Medical Journal. 1994;309(6966):1437.

37. Anon. No therapeutic effect for evening primrose oil in eczema. Pharmaceutical Journal. 1993;250:864.

38. Janosy I, Raguz J, et al. Effects of a cream containing 12.5% evening primrose oil on atopic disposition. H & G Journal. 1995;70:498-502.

39. Oliwiecki S, Armstrong J, Burton JL, Bradfield J. The effect of essential fatty acids on epidermal atrophy due to topical steroids. Clinical and Experimental Dermatology. 1993;18(4):326-28.

40. Oliwiecki S, Burton JL. Evening primrose oil and marine oil in the treatment of psoriasis. Clinical and Experimental Dermatology. 1994;19(2):127-29.

41. Stenius-Aarniala B, Aro A, Hakulinen A, Ahola I, Seppala E, Vapaatalo H. Evening primrose oil and fish oil are ineffective as supplementary treatment of bronchial asthma. Annals of Allergy. 1989;62:534-37.

42. Ebden P, Bevan C, Banks J, Fennerty A, Walters E. A study of evening primrose seed oil in atopic asthma. Prostaglandins Leukot Essent Fatty Acids. 1989;35:69-72.

43. Julu P. Gammalinolenic acid: A novel remedy for diabetic neuropathy in experimental animals. In: Omega 6 Essential Fatty Acids: Pathophysiology and Roles in Clinical Medicine. New York, NY: Alan R Liss Inc; 1990:465-76.

44. Reichert RG. Evening primrose oil and diabetic neuropathy. Quarterly Review of Natural Medicine. 1995(Summer):141-45.

45. Omawari N, Dewhurst M, Vo P, Mahmood S, Stevens E, Tomlinson DR. Deficient nitric oxide responsible for reduced nerve blood flow in diabetic rats: effects of L-NAME, L-arginine, sodium nitroprusside and evening primrose oil. British Journal of Pharmacology. 1996;118(1):186-90.

46. Cameron NE, Cotter MA, Hohman TC. Interactions between essential fatty acid, prostanoid, polyol pathway and nitric oxide mechanisms in the neurovascular deficit of diabetic rats. Diabetologia. 1996;39(2):172-82.

47. Julu PO, Gow JW, Jamal GA. Endogenous cyclo-oxygenase substrates mediate the neuroactivity of evening primrose oil in rats. J Lipid Mediat Cell Signal. 1996;13(2):115-25.

48. Fang C, Jiang Z, Tomlinson DR. Expression of constitutive cyclo-oxygenase (COX-1) in rats with streptozotocin-induced diabetes; effects of treatment with evening primrose oil or an aldose reductase inhibitor on COX-1 mRNA levels. Prostaglandins Leukot Essent Fatty Acids. 1997;56(2):157-63.

49. Julu PO. Latency of neuroactivity and optimum period of treatment with evening primrose oil in diabetic rats. J Lipid Mediat Cell Signal. 1996;13(2):99-113.

50. Cameron NE, Cotter MA. Comparison of the effects of ascorbyl gamma-linolenic acid and gamma-linolenic acid in the correction of neurovascular deficits in diabetic rats. Diabetologia. 1996;39(9):1047-54.

51. Dines CD, Cotter MA, Cameron NE. Nerve function in galactosaemic rats: effects of evening primrose oil and doxazosin. European Journal of Pharmacology. 1995;281(3):303-09.

52. Cameron NE, Cotter MA, Dines KC, Robertson S, Cox D. The effects of evening primrose oil on nerve function and capillarization in streptozotocin-diabetic rats: Modulation by the cyclo-oxygenase inhibitor flurbiprofen. British Journal of Pharmacology. 1993;109(4):972-79.

53. Stevens EJ, Lockett MJ, Carrington AL, Tomlinson DR. Essential fatty acid treatment prevents nerve ischaemia and associated conduction anomalies in rats with experimental diabetes mellitus [see comments]. Diabetologia. 1993;36(5):397-401.

54. Jamal GA, Charmichael H. The effect of gamma-linolenic acid on human diabetic peripheral neuropathy: A double-blind placebo-controlled trial. Diabetic Medicine. 1990;7:319-23.

55. Keen H, Payan J, et al. Treatment of diabetic neuropathy with gamma-linolenic acid. Diabetes Care. 1993;16:8-15.

56. Dines KC, Cotter MA, Cameron NE. Effectiveness of natural oils as sources of gamma-linolenic acid to correct peripheral nerve conduction velocity abnormalities in diabetic rats: modulation by thromboxane A2 inhibition. Prostaglandins Leukot Essent Fatty Acids. 1996;55(3):159-65.

57. Puolakka J, Makarainen L, Viinikka L, Ylikorkala O. Biochemical and clinical effects of treating the premenstrual syndrome with prostaglandin synthesis precursors. Journal of Reproductive Medicine. 1985;30:149-53.

58. Horrobin DF. The role of essential fatty acids and prostaglandins in premenstrual syndrome. Journal of Reproductive Medicine. 1983;28:465-68.

59. Brush MG. Efamol (evening primrose oil) in the treatment of premenstrual syndrome. In: Horrobin DF, ed. Clinical Uses for Essential Fatty Acids. Buffalo, New York, NY: Eden Press; 1982:155.

60. Collins A, Cerin A, et al. Essential fatty acids in the treatment of premenstrual syndrome. Obstetrics and Gynecology. 1993;81:93-98.

61. Steinberg S. The treatment of late luteal phase dysphoric disorder. Life Sciences. 1991;49(11):767-802.

62. Lurie S, Borenstein R. The Premenstrual Syndrome. Obstetrical and Gynecological Survey. 1990;45(4):220-28.

63. Brush MG, Watson SJ, et al. Abnormal essential fatty levels in plasma of women with premenstrual syndrome. American Journal of Obstetrical Gynecology. 1984;150:363-66.

64. Budeiri D, Li Wan Po A, Dornan JC. Is evening primrose oil of value in the treatment of premenstrual syndrome? Control Clin Trials. 1996;17(1):60-68.

65. Pye JK, et.al. Clinical experience of drug treatments for masatalgia. Lancet. 1985(ii):373-77.

66. Mansel R, Pye J, Hughes L. Effects of essential fatty acids on cyclical mastalgia and non-cyclical breast disorders. In: Omega-6 Essential Fatty Acids: Pathophysiology and Roles in Clinical Medicine. New York, NY: Alan R Liss; 1990:557-66.

67. Wetzig NR. Mastalgia: a 3-year Australian study. Australia and New Zealand Journal of Surgery. 1994;64(5):329-31.

68. Gateley CA, Miers M, Mansel R, Hughes L. Drug treatments for mastalgia: 17-year experience in the Cardiff mastalgia clinic. Journal of the Royal Society of Medicine. 1992;85:12-15.

69. Genolet P, Delaloye J, De Grandi P. Diagnosis and treatment of mastodynia (French). Rev Med Suisse Romande. 1995;115(5):385-90.

70. Blommers J, de Lange-De Klerk ES, Kuik DJ, Bezemer PD, Meijer S. Evening primrose oil and fish oil for severe chronic astalgia: A randomized, double-blind, controlled trial. Am J Obstet Gynecol. 2002;187(5):1389-94.

71. Anon. Cyclical breast pain — what works and what doesn't. Drugs and Therapeutics Bulletin. 1992;30(1):1-3.

72. Chenoy R, Hussain S, Tayob Y, O'Brien P, Moss M, Morse P. Effect of oral gamalinolenic acid from evening primrose oil on menopausal flushing. British Medical Journal. 1994;38:501-03.

73. Bassey EJ, Littlewood JJ, Rothwell MC, Pye DW. Lack of effect of supplementation with essential fatty acids on bone mineral density in healthy pre- and postmenopausal women: Two randomized controlled trials of Efacal v. calcium alone. British Journal of Nutrition. 2000;83(6):629-35.

74. Horrobin DF. Nutritional and medical importance of gamma-linolenic acid. Prog Lipid Research. 1992;31:163-94.

75. Joe LA, Hart LL. Evening primrose oil in rheumatoid arthritis. Ann Pharmacother. 1993;27(12):1475-77.

76. Li Wan Po A. Evening primrose oil. Pharmacy Journal. 1991;246:670-76.

77. Belch J, Ansell R, Madhok R, O'Dowd A, Sturrock R. Effects of altering dietary essential fatty acids on requirements for non-steroidal anti-inflammatory drugs in patients with rheumatoid arthritis: a double blind placebo controlled study. Ann Rheum Dis. 1988;47(2):96-104.

78. Hansen T, Lerche A, Kassis V, Lorenzen I, Sondergaard J. Treatment of rheumatoid arthritis with prostaglandin E1 precursors cis-linoleic acid and gamma-linolenic acid. Scandanavian Journal of Rheumatology. 1983;12:85-88.

79. Jantti J, Seppala E, Vapaatalo H, Isomaki H. Evening primrose oil and olive oil in the treatment of rheumatoid arthritis. Clinical Rheumatology. 1989;8:238-44.

80. Veale DJ, Torley HI, Richards IM, O. Dowd A, Fitzsimons C, Belch JJ, et al. A double-blind placebo controlled trial of Efamol Marine on skin and joint symptoms of psoriatic arthritis. British Journal of Rheumatology. 1994;33(10):954-58.

81. Horrobin D. Multiple sclerosis: The rational basis for treatment with colchicine and evening primrose oil. Medical Hypotheses. 1979;5(3):365-78.

82. Mertin H, Meade C. Relevance of fatty acids in Multiple Sclerosis. British Medical Bulletin. 1977;33:67-71.

83. Dworkin R, et al. Linoleic acid and multiple sclerosis: A reanalysis of three double-blind trials. Neurology. 1984;34:1441-45.

84. Barber HJ. Evening primrose oil: A panacea? Pharmacy Journal. 1988;240:723-25.

85. Horrobin D. Essential fatty acid and prostaglandin metabolism in Sjogren's syndrome, systemic sclerosis and rheumatoid arthritis. Scand J Rheumatol Suppl. 1986;61:242-45.

86. Oxholm P, Manthorpe R, Prause J, Horrobin D. Patients with primary Sjogrens syndrome treated for two months with evening primrose oil. Scandanavian Journal of Rheumatology. 1986;15(2):103-08.

87. Theander E, Horrobin DF, Jacobsson LT, Manthorpe R. Gammalinolenic acid treatment of fatigue associated with primary Sjogrens syndrome. Scandanavian Journal of Rheumatology. 2002;31(2):72-79.

88. Werbach M, Murray M. Nutritional Influences on Illness. 2nd ed. Tarzana, CA: Third Line Press; 1993.

89. Mtabaji JP, Manku MS, Horrobin DF. Abnormalities in dihomo-gamma-linolenic acid release in the pathogenesis of hypertension. American Journal of Hypertension. 1993;6(6 Pt 1):458-62.

90. Belch J, Shaw B, O'Dowd A, Saniabadi A, Leiberman P, Sturrock R, et al. Evening primrose oil (Efamol) in the treatment of Raynauld's phenomenon: A double blind study. Thrombosis and Haemostasis. 1985;54(2):490-94.

91. Vaddadi K. The use of gamma-linolenic acid and linoleic acid to differentiate between temporal lobe epilepsy and schizophrenia. Prostaglandins and Medicine. 1981;6:375-79.

92. Vaddadi K, Courtney P, Gilleard C, Manku M, Horrobin D. A double-blind trial of essential fatty acid supplementation in patients with tardive dyskinesia. Psychiatry Research. 1989;27:313-23.

93. Holman C, Bell A. A trial of evening primrose oil in the treatment of chronic schizophrenia. J Orthomolecular Psychiatry. 1983;12:302-04.

94. Stevens L, Zentall S, Abate M, Kuczek A, Burgess J. Omega-3 fatty acids in boys with behaviour, learning and health problems. Physiol Behav. 1996;59(4/5):915-20.

95. Stevens L, Zentall S, Deck J, Abate M, Watkins B, Lipp S, et al. Essential fatty acid metabolism in boys with attention-deficit hyperactivity disorder. American Journal of Clinical Nutrition. 1995;62(4):761-68.

96. Shreeve C. A state of perpetual motion. World Medicine. 1982;5(1):87-93.

97. Manku M, Morse-Fischer N, Horrobin D. Changes in human plasma essential fatty acid levels as a result of administration of linoleic acid and gamma-linolenic acid. European Journal of Clinical Nutrition. 1988;42:55-60.

98. Blackburn M. Use of Efamol (Oil of Evening Primrose) for depression and hyperactivity in children. In: Pathophysiology and Roles in Clinical Medicine. New York, NY: Alan R Liss, Inc; 1990:345-49.

99. Greenfield SM, Green AT, Teare JP, Jenkins AP, Punchard NA, Ainley CC, et al. A randomized controlled study of evening primrose oil and fish oil in ulcerative colitis. Aliment Pharmacol Ther. 1993;7(2):159-66.

100. Chilton SA. Cognitive behaviour therapy for the chronic fatigue syndrome. Evening primrose oil and magnesium have been shown to be effective [Letter; Comment]. British Medical Journal. 1996;312(7038):1098.

101. Lewith G. Chronic fatigue syndrome. Update. 1995(50):765.

102. Warren G, McKendrick M, Peet M. The role of essential fatty acids in chronic fatigue syndrome. A case- controlled study of red-cell membrane essential fatty acids (EFA) and a placebo-controlled treatment study with high dose of EFA. Acta Neurol Scand. 1999;99(2):112-16.

103. Horrobin D. A biochemical basis for alcoholism and alcohol-induced damage including the fetal alcohol syndrome and cirrhosis; Interference with essential fatty acid and prostaglandin metabolism. Med Hypotheses. 1980;6:929-42.

104. Varma P, Persaud T. Protection against ethanol-induced embryonic damage by administering gamma-linolenic acid and linoleic acids. Prostaglandins Leukot Med. 1982;8(6):641-45.

105. Morphake P, Bariety J, Darlametsos I, Tsipas G, Gkikas G, Hornysh A, et al. Alteration of cyclosporine (CsA)-induced nephrotoxicity by gamma linolenic acid (GLA) and eicosapentaenoic acid (EPA) in Wistar rats. Prostaglandins Leukot Essent Fatty Acids. 1994;50(1):29-35.

106. Mills DE, de Antueno R, Scholey J. Interaction of dietary fatty acids and cyclosporine A in the borderline hypertensive rat: tissue fatty acids. Lipids. 1994;29(1):27-32.

107. Burgess NA, Reynolds TM, Williams N, Pathy A, Smith S. Evaluation of four animal models of intrarenal calcium deposition and assessment of the influence of dietary supplementation with essential fatty acids on calcification. Urology Research. 1995;23(4):239-42.

108. Tulloch I, Smellie WS, Buck AC. Evening primrose oil reduces urinary calcium excretion in both normal and hypercalciuric rats. Urol Res. 1994;22(4):227-30.

109. du Toit PJ, van Aswegen CH, Nel JD, Strasheim B, Becker PJ, du Plessis DJ. Pyelonephritis: Renal urokinase activity in rats on essential fatty acid diets. Urology Research. 1994;22(3):127-30.

110. Kenny FS, Pinder SE, Ellis IO, Gee JM, Nicholson RI, Bryce RP, et al. Gamma linolenic acid with tamoxifen as primary therapy in breast cancer. Int J Cancer. 2000;85(5):643-48.

111. Haslett C, Douglas J, Chalmers S, Weighhill A, Munro J. A double-blind evaluation of evening primrose oil as an antiobesity agent. International Journal of Obesity. 1983;7(6):549-53.

112. Garcia C, et al. Gamma linolenic acid causes weight loss and lower blood pressure in overweight patients with family history of obesity. Swedish Journal of Biological Medicine. 1986;4:8-11.

113. Vaddadi K, Horrobin D. Weight loss produced by evening primrose oil administration in normal and schizophrenic individuals. IRCS J Med Sci. 1979;7:52.

114. Kleijnen J. Evening primrose oil [Editorial] [see Comments]. British Medcial Journal. 1994;309(6958):824-25.

115. Everett D, Greenough R, Perry C, McDonald P, Bayliss P. Chronic toxicities studies of Efamol evening primrose oil in rats and dogs. Med. Sci. Res. 1988;16:863-64.

116. Everett D, Perry C, Bayliss P. Carcinogenicity studies of Efamol evening primrose oil in rats and mice. Med. Sci. Res. 1988;16:865-66.

117. Lepik K. Safety of Herbal Medications in Pregnancy. Canadian Pharmaceutical Journal. 1997;130(3):29-33.

118. Cant A, Shay J, Horrobin DF. The effect of maternal supplementation with linolenic and gamma-linolenic acids on the fat composition and content of human milk. Journal of Nutritional Science and Vitaminolology. 1991;37:573-79.

119. Dove D, Johnson P. Oral evening primrose oil: Its effect on length of pregnancy and selected intrapartum outcomes in low-risk nulliparous women. J Nurse Midwifery. 1999;44(3):320-24.

120. Stockley I. Drug Interactions. A Sourcebook of Adverse Interactions, Their Mechanisms, Clinical Importance, and Management. 3rd ed. Cambridge, UK: Blackwell Scientific Press; 1994.

121. Brenner RR. Nutritional and hormonal factors influencing desaturation of essential fatty acids. Progress in Lipid Research. 1982;20:41-48.

122. Lieb J. Linoleic acid in the treatment of lithium toxicty and familial tremor. Prostaglandin and Medicine. 1980;4:275-79.

Feverfew

1. Wren R. Potter's New Encyclopedia of Botanical Drugs and Preparations. Saffron Walden: C.W. Daniel Company; 1988.

2. Hutchens A. Indian Herbology of North America. Boston, MA: Shambhala; 1991.

3. Newall C, Anderson L, David Phillipson J. Herbal Medicines A Guide for Health Care Professionals. London: The Pharmaceutical Press; 1996.

4. Groenewegen W, Knight D, Heptinstall S. Progress in the Medicinal Chemistry of the Herb Feverfew. Progress in Medicinal Chemistry. 1992;29:217-38.

5. Awang D. Herbal Medicine, feverfew. Canadian Pharmaceutical Journal. 1989;122:266-70.

6. Berry M. Feverfew. Pharmaceutical Journal. 1994;253:806-08.

7. Leung A, Foster S. Encylcopedia of Common Natural Ingredients used in Food, Drugs and Cosmetics. 2nd ed. New York, NY: John Wiley and Sons; 1996.

8. Berry M. Feverfew faces the future. Pharmaceutical Journal. 1984;232:611-14.

9. Awang D. Feverfew fever-a headache for the consumer. Herbalgram. 1993;29:34-36,66.

10. Wagner H, Fessler B, Lotter H, et al. New chlorine containing sesquiterpene lactones from Chrysanthemum parthenium. Planta Medica. 1988;54:171-77.

11. Marles RJ, Associate Professor, Department of Botany, Brandon University, Brandon, Manitoba. Review of Medicinal Plant Modules for CCNM; 1997.

12. Collier H, Butt N, McDonald-Gibson W, Saeed S. Extract of feverfew inhibits prostaglandin biosynthesis. Lancet. 1980;ii:922-73.

13. Capasso F. The effect of an aqueous extract of Tanacetum parthenium L. on arachidonic acid metabolism by rat peritoneal leucocytes. J Pharm Pharmacol. 1986;38:71-72.

14. Makheja A, Martyn Bailey J. The active principle in feverfew. Lancet. 1981;11:1054.

15. Makheja A, Bailery J. A platelet phospholipase inhibitor from the medicinal herb feverfew. Prostaglandins, Leukotrienes Med. 1982;8:653-60.

16. Sumner H, Salan U, Knight D, Hoult R. Inhibition of 5-lipoxygenase and cyclooxygenase in leukpcytes by feverfew. Biochemical Pharmacology. 1992;43:2313-20.

17. Groenewegen W, Heptinstall S. A comparison of the effects of an extract of feverfew and parthenolide, a component of feverfew, on human platelt activity in vitro. Journal of Pharmacy and Pharmacology. 1990;42(8):553-57.

18. Pugh W, Sambo K. Prostaglandin synthetase inhibitors in feverfew. Journal of Pharmacy and Pharmacology. 1988;40:743-45.

19. Heptinstall S, White A, Williamson L, Mitchell J. Extracts of feverfew inhibit granule secretion in blood platelets and polymorphnuclear leukocytes. Lancet. 1985;i:1071-74.

20. Loesche W, Mazurov A, Voyno-Yasenetskaya A, Groenewegen W, Heptinstall S, Repin V. Feverfew — an antithrombotic drug. Folia Haematol. 1988;115(1-2):181-84.

21. Groenewegen W, Knight D, Heptinstall S. Compounds extracted from feverfew that have anti-secretory activity contain an alpha-methylene butyrolactone unit. Journal of Pharmacy and Pharmacology. 1986;38(9):709-12.

22. Losche W, Mitchel E, Heptinstall S, Krause S, Groenewegen W, Pescarmona G, et al. Inhibition of the behaviour of human polynuclear leukocytes by an extract of Chrysanthemum parthenium. Planta Medica. 1988;54:381-84.

23. Heptinstall S, Groenewegen W, Spangenberg P, Loesche W. Extracts of feverfew may inhibit platelet behaviour via neutralization of sulphydryl groups. Journal of Pharmacy and Pharmacology. 1987;39:459-65.

24. Voyno-Yasenetskaya T, Loesche W, hepistall S, Repin V, Till U. Effects of an extract of feverfew on endothelial cell integrity and on cAMP in rabbit perfused aorta. Journal of Pharmacy and Pharmacology. 1988;40(7):501-02.

25. Hayes N, Foreman J. The activity of compounds extracted from feverfew on histamine release from rat mast cells. Journal of Pharmacy and Pharmacology. 1987;39:466-70.

26. O'Neill LA, Barrett ML, Lewis GP. Extracts of feverfew inhibit mitogen induced human peripheral blood mononuclear cell proliferation and cytokine mediated responses: a cytotoxic effect. British Journal of Clinical Pharmacology. 1987;23(1):81-83.

27. Brown D. Herbal Prescriptions for Better Health. Rocklin, CA: Prima Publishing; 1995.

28. Diamond S. Herbal therapy for migraine. An unconventional approach. Postgraduate Medicine. 1987;July:197-98.

29. Johnson E. Patients who chew chrysanthemum leaves. MIMS Magazine. 1983;May 15:32-35.

30. Johnson ES, Kadam NP, Hylands DM, Hylands PJ. Efficacy of feverfew as prophylactic treatment of migraine. British Medical Journal. 1985;291:569-73.

31. Waller P, Ramsay L. Efficacy of feverfew as prophylactic treatment of migraine. British Medical Journal. 1985;291:1128.

32. Murphy JJ, Hepinstall S, Mitchell JRA. Randomized double-blind placebo-controlled trial of feverfew in migraine prevention. Lancet. 1988;ii:189-92.

33. De Weerdt CJ, Bootsma HPR, Hendriks H. Herbal medicines in migraine prevention. Randomised double-blind placebo-controlled crossover trial of a feverfew preparation. Phytomedicine. 1996;3(3):225-30.

34. Brown D. Feverfew-Disappointing Results in Migraine Study. Quarterly Review of Natural Medicine. 1997;4(2):89-90.

35. Pfaffenrath V, Diener HC, Fischer M, Friede M, Henneicke-von Zepelin HH. The efficacy and safety of *Tanacetum parthenium* (feverfew) in migraine prophylaxis—a double-blind, multicentre, randomized placebo-controlled dose-response study. Cephalalgia. 2002;22(7):523-32.

36. Vogler BK, Pittler MH, Ernst E. Feverfew as a preventive treatment for migraine: A systematic review. Cephalalgia. 1998;18(10):704-08.

37. Pittler MH, Vogler BK, Ernst E. Feverfew for preventing migraine. Cochrane Database Syst Rev. 2000;3.

38. Pattrick M, Hepinstall S, Doherty M. Feverfew in rheumatoid arthritis:A double blind, placebo controlled study. Annals of Rheumatic Disease. 1989;48:547-49.

39. Kalodera Z, Pepeljnjak S, Petrak T. The antimicrobial activity of *Tanacetum parthenium* extract. Pharmazie. 1996;51(12):995-96.

40. Blakeman J, Atkinson P. Antimicrobial properties and possible role in host pathogen interactions of parthenolide, a sesquiterpene lactone isolated from glands of *Chrysanthemum parthenium*. Physiol Plant Pathol. 1979;15:183-92.

41. Tyler V. Herbs of Choice. The Therapeutic Use of Phytomedicinals. Binghampton, NY: Pharmaceutical Products Press; 1994.

42. Paulsen E, Christensen L, Andersen K. Do monoterpenes released from feverfew plants cause airborne Compositae dermatitis? Contact Dermatitis. 2002;47:14-18.

43. Schmidt R, Kingston T. Chrysanthemum dermatitis in South Wales; diagnosis by patch testing with feverfew (*Tanacetum parthenium*) extract. Contact Dermatitis. 1985;13:120-27.

44. Rodriguez E, Epstein W, Mitchell J. The role of sesquiterpene lactones in contact hypersensitivity to some North and South American species of Feverfew (Parthenium-compositae). Contact Dermatitis. 1977;3:155-62.

45. Mensing H, Kimming W, Hausen B. Airborne contact dermatitis. Der Hautarzt. 1985;36(7):398-402.

46. Hausen B. Occupational contact allergy to feverfew *Tanacetum pathenium*. Dermatosen in Beruf and Umwelt. 1981;29(1):18-21.

47. Hausen B, Osmundsen P. Contact allergy to parthenolide in *Tanacetum parthenium* schulz-Bip (feverfew, Asteraceae) and cross-reactions to related sesquiterpene lactone containing compositae species. Acta Dermato-Venereologica. 1983;63(4):308-14.

48. Anderson D, Jenkinson P, Dewdney R, Blowers S, Johnson E, Kadam N. Investigation of possible genotoxic effects of feverfew in migraine patients. Human Toxicology. 1987;6:533-54.

49. Lepik K. Safety of Herbal Medications in Pregnancy. Canadian Pharmaceutical Journal. 1997;130(3):29-33.

50. Farnsworth N, Bingel A, Cordell G, Crane F, Fong H. Potential value of plants as sources of new antifertility agents I. Journal of Pharmaceutical Sciences. 1975;64(4):535-98.

51. Heptinstall S, Awang DVC, Dawson BA, et al. Parthenolide content and bioactivity of feverfew (*Tanacetum parthenium*). Estimation of commercial and authenticated feverfew products. Journal of Pharmaceutical Pharmacology. 1992;44:391-95.

52. Awang D, Dawson B, Kindack D. Parthenolide content of Feverfew (*Tanacetum parthenium*) assessed by HPLC and H-NMR spectroscopy. Journal of Natural Products. 1991;Nov-Dec 54(6):1516-21.

53. Groenewegen W, Hepinstall S. Amounts of feverfew in commercial preparations of the herb. Lancet. 1986;ii:44-45.

54. Smith R, Burford M. Supercritical fluid extraction and gas chromatographic determination of the sesquiterpene lactone parthenolide in the medicinal herb feverfew (Tanacetum parthenium). Journal of Chromatogy. 1992;627:255-61.

55. Marles R, Heptinstall J, Kaminski J, Arnason J, T., Pazos-Sanou L, Fischer N, et al. A bioassay for inhibition of serotonin release from bovine platelets. Journal of Natural Products. 1992;55(8):1044-56.

56. Bradley P. British Herbal Compendium. Bournemouth, UK: The British Herbal Medical Association; 1992.

Garlic

1. Augusti KT. Therapeutic values of onion (Allium cepa L.) and garlic (*Allium sativum* L.) [Review]. Indian Journal of Experimental Biology. 1996;34(7):634-40.

2. Foster S. Garlic, *Allium sativum*. Austin, TX: The American Botanical Council; 1991: Botanical Series No. 311.

3. Agarwal KC. Therapeutic actions of garlic constituents. [Review]. Medicinal Research Reviews. 1996;16(1):111-24.

4. Fenwick GR, Hanley AB. The Genus Alllium Part 1. CRC Critical Review in Food Science and Nutrition. 1985;22:199.

5. Fenwick GR, Hanley AB. The Genus Alllium Part 2. CRC Critical Review in Food Science and Nutrition. 1985;22:273.

6. Fenwick GR, Hanley AB. The Genus Alllium Part 3. CRC Critical Review in Food Science and Nutrition. 1985;23:1.

7. Lawson LD, Wood SG, Hughes BG. Planta Medica. 1991;57:263q.

8. Tyler VE. Herbs of Choice. The Therapeutic Use of Phytomedicinals. Binghamton, NY: Pharmaceutical Products Press; 1994.

9. Block E. The chemistry of garlic and onions. Scientific American. 1985;252(3):94-99.

10. Nagae S, Ushijima M, Hatono S, Imai J, Kasuga S, Matsuura H, et al. Pharmacokinetics of the garlic compound S-allylcysteine. Planta Medica. 1994;60(3):214-17.

11. Larner AJ. How does garlic exert its hypocholesterolaemic action? The tellurium hypothesis. Medical Hypotheses. 1995;44(4):295-97.

12. Ackermann RT, Mulrow CD, Ramirez G, Gardner CD, Morbidoni L, Lawrence VA. Garlic shows promise for improving some cardiovascular risk factors. Archives of Internal Medicine. 2001;161(6):813-24.

13. Bordia A, Bansal HC. Essential oil of garlic in the prevention of atherosclerosis. Lancet. 1973;II:1491-92.

14. Jain RC. Effect of garlic on serum lipids, coagulability, and fibrinolytic activity of blood. American Journal of Clinical Nutrition. 1977;30:1380-81.

15. Bordia A. Effect of garlic on blood lipids in patients with coronary heart disease. American Journal of Clinical Nutrition. 1981;34:2100-03.

16. Lau B, Adetumbia MA, Sanchez A. *Allium sativum* (Garlic) and athersclerosis: A review. Nutrition Research. 1983;3:119-28.

17. Harenberg J, Giese C, Zimmermann R. Effect of dried garlic on blood coagulation, fibrinolysis, platelet aggregation and serum cholesterol levesl in patients with hyperlipoproteinemia. Athersclerosis. 1988;74:247-49.

18. Mader FH. Treatment of hyperlipidaemia with garlic powder tablets. Evidence from the German Association of General Practitioner's multicentric placebo-controlled double-blind study[German]. Arzneimittelforschung. 1990;40:1111-16.

19. Auer W, Eiber A, Hertkorn E, Hoehfeld E, Koehrie U, Lorenz A, et al. Hypertension and hyperlipidemia: Garlic helps in mild cases. British Journal of Clinical Practice. 1990;44(8) (Supplement 69):3-6.

20. Vorberg G, Schneider B. Therapy with garlic: Results of a placebo-controlled, double-blind study. British Journal of Clinical Practice. 1990;44(8 (Supplement 69)):7-11.

21. Brosche T, Platt D, Dorner H. The effect of a garlic preparation on the composition of plasma lipoproteins and erythrocyte membranes in geriatric subjects. British Journal of Clinical Practice. 1990;44(supplement 69):12-19.

22. Zimmermann W, Zimmerman B. Reduction in elevated blood lipids in hospitalized patients by a standardized garlic preparation. British Journal of Clinical Practice. 1990;44(supplement 69):20-23.

23. Mansell P, Reckless JPD. Garlic: Effects on serum lipids, blood pressure, coagulation, platelet aggregation, and vasodilation. British Medical Journal. 1991;303:379-80.

24. Barrie SA, Wright JV, Pizzarno JE. Effects of garlic oil on platelet aggregation, serum lipids, and blood pressure in humans. Journal of Orthomolecular Medicine. 1987;2:15-21.

25. Mathew BC, Daniel RS, Augusti KT. Hypolipidemic effect of garlic protein substituted for casein in diet of rats compared to those of garlic oil. Indian Journal of Experimental Biology. 1996;34(4):337-40.

26. Mathew BC, Augusti KT. Biochemical effects of garlic protein diet and garlic oil on glycosaminoglycan in cholesterol fed rats. Indian Journal of Experimental Biology. 1996;34(4):346-50.

27. Steiner M, Khan AH, Holbert D, Lin RI. A double-blind crossover study in moderately hypercholesterolemic men that compared the effects of aged garlic extract and placebo administration on blood lipids. American Journal of Clinical Nutrition. 1996;64(6):866-70.

28. Adler AJ, Holub BJ. Effect of garlic and fish-oil supplementation on serum lipid and lipoprotein concentrations in hypercholesterolemic men [see Comments]. American Journal of Clinical Nutrition. 1997;65(2):445-50.

29. Gupta NK. Modification of radiation induced changes in murine hepatic lipid profiles by garlic (*Allium sativum* Linn.) unsaturated oils. Indian Journal of Experimental Biology. 1996;34(9):851-53.

30. Ali M, Thomson M. Consumption of a garlic clove a day could be beneficial in preventing thrombosis. Prostaglandins Leukotrienes & Essential Fatty Acids.1995;53(3):211-12.

31. Sainani GS, Desai DB, Gorhe NH, Nath SM, Pise DV, Sainani PG. Indian Journal of Medical Research. 1979;69:776.

32. Kannar D, Wattanapenpaiboon N, Savige GS, Wahlqvist ML. Hypocholesterolemic effect of an enteric-coated garlic supplement. J Am Coll Nutr. 2001;20(3):225-31.

33. Luley C, Lehmann-Leo W, Moller B, Martin I, Schwartzkopff W. Lack of efficacy of dried garlic in patients with hyperlipoproteinemia. Arzneim Forsch./Drug Research. 1986;36:766-68.

34. Arora RC, Arora S, Gupta RK. The long-term use of garlic in ischemic heart disease. Athersclerosis. 1981;40:175-79.

35. Berthold HK, Sudhop T, von Bergmann K. Effect of a garlic oil preparation on serum lipoproteins and cholesterol metabolism: a randomized controlled trial. Journal of the American Medical Association. 1998;279(23):1900-02.

36. McCrindle BW, Helden E, Conner WT. Garlic extract therapy in children with hypercholesterolemia. Archives of Pediatric and Adolescent Medicine. 1998;152(11):1089-94.

37. Isaacsohn JL, Moser M, Stein EA, Dudley K, Davey JA, Liskov E, et al. Garlic powder and

plasma lipids and lipoproteins: a multicenter, randomized, placebo-controlled trial. Archives of Internal Medicine. 1998;158(11):1189-94.

38. Gardner CD, Chatterjee LM, Carlson JJ. The effect of a garlic preparation on plasma lipid levels in moderately hypercholesterolemic adults. Atherosclerosis. 2001;154(1):213-20.

39. Superko HR, Krauss RM. Garlic powder, effect on plasma lipids, postprandial lipemia, low-density lipoprotein particle size, high-density lipoprotein subclass distribution and lipoprotein(a). J Am Coll Cardiol. 2000;35(2):321-26.

40. Zhang XH, Lowe D, Giles P, Fell S, Board AR, Baughan JA, et al. A randomized trial of the effects of garlic oil upon coronary heart disease risk factors in trained male runners. Blood Coagul Fibrinolysis. 2001;12(1):67-74.

41. Ernst E. Cardiovascular effects of garlic (*Allium sativum*): A review. Pharmatherapeutica. 1987;5(2):83-89.

42. Kendler BS. Garlic (*Allium sativum*) and onion (*Allium cepa*): A review of their relationship to cardiovascular disease. Preventative Medicine. 1987;16:670-85.

43. Kleijnen J, Knipschild P, ter Riet G. Garlic, onions and cardiovascular risk factors. A review of the evidence from human experiments with emphasis on commercially available preparations. British Journal of Clinical Pharmacology. 1989;28:535-44.

44. Bordai A, Bansal HC, Arora SK, Singh SV. Effect of the essential oils of garlic and onion on alimentary hyperlipemia. Atherosclerosis. 1975;21:15-19.

45. Bordia A, Joshi HK, Sanadhya YK, Bhu N. Effect of essential oil of garlic on serum fibrinolytic activity in patients with coronary artery disease. Atherosclerosis. 1977;28:155-59.

46. Bordia A, Sharma KD, Parmar YK, Verma SK. Protective effect of garlic oil on the changes produced by 3 weeks of fatty diet on serum cholesterol, serum triglycerides, fibrinolytic activity and platelet adhesiveness in man. Indian Heart J. 1982;34:86-8.

47. Bhushan S, Sharma SP, Singh SP, Agrawal S, Indrayan A, Seth P. Effect of garlic on normal blood cholesterol level. Indian Journal of Physiol. Pharmac. 1979;23:211-14.

48. Sucur M. Effect of garlic on serum lipids and lipoproteins in patients suffering from hyperlipoproteinemia. Diabetologia Croatica. 1980;9:323-28.

49. Chutani SK, Bordia A. The effect of fried versus raw garlic on fibinolytic activity in man. Athersclerosis. 1981;38:417-21.

50. Arora RC, Arora S. Comparative effect of clofibrate, garlic and onion on alimentary hyperlipemia. Athersclerosis. 1981;39:447-52.

51. Lutomski J. Klinische untersuchungen zur therapeutischen wirksamkeit von ilja rogoff knoblauchpillen mit rutin. Zeitschrift fur Phytotherapie. 1984;5:938-42.

52. Ernst E, Weihmayr T, Matrai A. Garlic and blood lipids. British Medical Journal. 1985;291:139.

53. Sitprija S, Plengvidhya C, Kangkaya V, Bhuvapanich S, Tunkayoon M. Garlic and diabetes mellitus phase II clinical trial. Journal of the Medical Association of Thailand. 1987;70 (Supplement #2):223-27.

54. Turner M. Garlic and circulatory disorders. Journal of the Royal Society of Health. 1990;110:90-93.

55. Warshafsky S, Kamer RS, Sivak SL. Effect of garlic on total serum cholesterol. A meta-analysis [see Comments]. Annals of Internal Medicine. 1993;119(7 Pt 1):599-605.

56. Plengvidhya C, Sitprija S, Chinayon S, Pasatrat S, Tankeyoon M. Effects of spray dried garlic preparation on primary hyperlipoproteinemia. Journal of the Medical Assoc Thailand. 1988;71:248-52.

57. Lau BH, Lam F, Wang-Cheng R. Effect of an odor modified garlic preparation on blood lipids. Nutrition Research. 1987;7:139-49.

58. Silagy C, Neil A. Garlic as a lipid lowering agent—a meta-analysis. Journal of the Royal College of Physicians of London. 1994;28(1):2-8.

59. Stevinson C. Garlic for treating hypercholesterolemia: A meta-analysis of randomized clinical trials. Annals of Internal Medicine. 2000;133(6):420-29.

60. Simons LA, Balasubramaniam S, von Konigsmark M, Parfitt A, Simons J, Peters W. On the effect of garlic on plasma lipids and lipoproteins in mild hypercholesterolaemia. Atherosclerosis. 1995;113(2):219-25.

61. Jain AK, Vargas R, Gotzkowsky S, McMahon FG. Can garlic reduce levels of serum lipids? A controlled clinical study. American Journal of Medicine. 1993;94(6):632-35.

62. Holzgartner H, Schmidt U, Kuhn U. Comparison of the efficacy and tolerance of a garlic preparation vs. bezafibrate. Arzneimittelforschung / Drug Research. 1992;42:1473-77.

63. Koscielny J, Klussendorf D, Latza R, Schmitt R, Radtke H, Siegel G, et al. The antiatherosclerotic effect of *Allium sativum*. Atherosclerosis. 1999;144(1):237-49.

64. Chi MS, Koh ET, Steward TJ. Effects if garlic on lipid metabolism in rats fed cholesterol or lard. Journal of Nutrition. 1982;112:241-48.

65. Qureshi AA, Din ZZ, Abuirmeileh N, Burger WC, Ahmad Y, Elson CE. Suppression of avian hepatic lipid metabolism by solvent extracts of garlic: Impact on serum lipids. Journal of Nutritin. 1983;113:1746-55.

66. Qureshi AA, Crenshaw TD, Abuirmeileh N, Peterson N, Elson CE. Influence of minor plant constituents on porcine hepatic lipid metabolism. Impact on serum lipids. Atherosclerosis. 1987;64:109-15.

67. Qureshi AA, Abuirmeileh N, Din ZZ, Elson CE, Burger WC. Inhibition of cholesterol and fatty acid biosynthesis in liver enzymes and chicken hepatocytes by polar fractions of garlic. Lipids. 1983;18:343-48.

68. Gebhardt R, Beck H. Differential inhibitory effects of garlic-derived organosulfur compounds on cholesterol biosynthesis in primary rat hepatocyte cultures. Lipids. 1996;31(12):1269-76.

69. Byrne DJ, Neil HA, Vallance DT, Winder AF. A pilot study of garlic consumption shows no significant effect on markers of oxidation or sub-fraction composition of low-density lipoprotein including lipoprotein(a) after allowance for non-compliance and the placebo effect. Clin Chim Acta. 1999;285(1-2):21-33.

70. Bordia A. Effect of garllic on human platelet aggregation *in vitro*. Athersclerosis. 1978;30:355.

71. Vanderhoek JY, Makheja AN, Bailey JM. Inhibition of fatty acid oxegenases by onion and garlic oils. Biochemical Pharmacology. 1980;29:3169.

72. Samson RR. Effects of dietary garlic and temporal drift on platelet aggregation. Athersclerosis. 1982;44:199.

73. Mohammad SM, Woodward SC. Characterization of a potent inhibitor of platelet aggregation and release reaction isolated ffrom *Allium sativum* (garlic).Thrombosis Research. 1986;44:793.

74. Lawson LD, Ransom DK, Hughes BG. Inhibition of whole blood platelet aggregation by compounds in garlic clove extracts and commercial garlic products. Thrombosis Research. 1992;65:141.

75. Das I, Khan NS, Sooranna SR. Potent activation of nitric oxide synthase by garlic: a basis for its therapeutic applications. Current Medical Research & Opinion. 1995;13(5):257-63.

76. Makeja AN, Bailey JM. Antiplatelet constituents of garlic and onions. Agents Actions. 1990;29:360-63.

77. Kiesewetter H, Jung F, Mrowietz C, Wenzel E. Hemorrheological and circulatory effects of Gincosan. International Journal of Clinical Pharmacology, Therapy, & Toxicology. 1992.

78. Kiesewetter H, Jung F, Jung EM, Mroweitz C, Koscielny J, Wenzel E. Effect of garlic on platelet aggregation in patients with increased risk of juvenile ischaemic attack. European Journal of Clinical Pharmacology. 1993;45(4):333-36.

79. Bordia A, Verma SK, Srivastava KC. Effect of garlic on platelet aggregation in humans: A study in healthy subjects and patients with coronary artery disease. Prostaglandins Leukotrienes & Essential Fatty Acids. 1996;55(3):201-05.

80. Steiner M, Lin RS. Changes in platelet function and susceptibility of lipoproteins to oxidation associated with administration of aged garlic extract. J Cardiovasc Pharmacol. 1998;31(6):904-08.

81. Steiner M, Li W. Aged garlic extract, a modulator of cardiovascular risk factors: a dose- finding study on the effects of AGE on platelet functions. Journal of Nutrition. 2001;131(3s):980S-4S.

82. Legnani C, Frascaro M, Guazzaloca G, Ludovici S, Cesarano G, Coccheri S. Effects of a dried garlic preparation on fibrinolysis and platelet aggregation in healthy subjects. Arzneimittel Forschung Drug Research. 1993;43(2):119-22.

83. Ali M. Mechanism by which garlic (*Allium sativum*) inhibits cyclooxygenase activity. Effect of raw versus boiled garlic extract on the synthesis of prostanoids. Prostaglandins Leukotrienes & Essential Fatty Acids. 1995;53(6):397-400.

84. Bordia T, Mohammed N, Thomson M, Ali M. An evaluation of garlic and onion as antithrombotic agents. Prostaglandins Leukotrienes & Essential Fatty Acids. 1996;54(3):183-86.

85. Block E, Ahmad S, Jain MK, Crecely RW, Apitz-Castro R, Ross MR. American Journal of Clinical Nutrition. 1984;34:2100-03.

86. Villar R, Alvarino MT, Flores R. Inhibition by ajoene of protein tyrosine phosphatase activity in human platelets. Biochimica et Biophysica Acta. 1997;1337(2):233-40.

87. Apitz-Castro R, Escalante J, Vargas R, Jain MK. Ajeone, the antiplatelet principle of garlic, synergistically potentiates the antiaggregatory action of prostacyclin, forskolin, indomethacin and dypiridamole on human platelets. Thrombosis Research. 1986;42:303-11.

88. Apitz-Castro R, Badimon JJ, Badimon L. A garlic derivative, ajoene, inhibits platelet deposition on severely damaged vessel wall in an in vivo porcine experimental model. Thrombosis Research. 1994;75(3):243-49.

89. Jain MK, Apitz-Castro R. Trends Biol Sci. 1987;12:252.

90. Block E. Antithrombotic agent of garlic: A lesson from 5,000 years of folk medicine. In: Steiner RP, ed. Folk Medicine: The Art and the Science. Washington, D.C.: American Chemical Society; 1986:125-38.

91. Jain M, KaA-C, R. Garlic — a product of spilled ambrosia. Current Science. 1993;65:148.

92. Jamaluddin MP, Krishnan LK, Thomas A. Biochem Biophy Res Commun. 1988;153:479.

93. Boullin DJ. Garlic as a platelet inhibitor. Lancet. 1981;I:776.

94. Das I, Hirani J, Sooranna S. Arginine is not responsible for the activation of nitric oxide synthase by garlic. Journal of Ethnopharmacology. 1996;53(1):5-9.

95. Pantoja CV, Norris BC, Contreras CM. Diuretic and natriuretic effects of chromatographically purified fraction of garlic (*Allium sativum*). Journal of Ethnopharmacology. 1996;52(2):101-05.

96. Kandziora J. Antihypertensive effectiveness and tolerance of a garlic medication [German]. Arzliche Forschung. 1988;1:1-8.

97. Kandziora J. The blood pressure lowering and lipid lowering effect of a garlic preparation in combination with a diuretic. Arzliche Forschung. 1988;3:1-8.

98. Kiesewetter H, Jung F, Pinder G, Jung EM, Mrowietz C, Wenzel E. Effect of garlic on thrombocyte aggregation, microcirculation, and other risk factors. International Journal of Clinical Pharmacol Ther Toxicol. 1991;29:151-55.

99. Santos OS, Grunwald J. Effect of garlic powder tablets on blood lipids and blood pressure. A six month placebo-controlled double-blind study. British Journal of Clinical Research. 1993;4:37-44.

100. Silagy CA, Neil HA. A meta-analysis of the effect of garlic on blood pressure. Journal of Hypertension. 1994;12(4):46368.

101. Melzig MF, Krause E, Franke S. Inhibition of adenosine deaminase activity of aortic endothelial cells by extracts of garlic (*Allium sativum* L.). Pharmazie. 1995;50(5):359-61.

102. Koch HP, Jager W, Hysek J, Korpert B. Phytotherapy Research. 1992;6:50.

103. Adetumbi MA, Lau BH. *Allium sativum* (garlic) — a natural antibiotic. Medical Hypothesis. 1983;12:227-37.

104. Fulder S. Scorn not Garlicke. Pharmacy Update. 1988;October:327-29.

105. Sharma VD, Sethi MS, Kumar PS, Rarotra JR. Antibacterial property of *Allium sativum* Linn.:

In vivo and *in vitro* studies. Indian Journal of Experimental Biology. 1977;15:466-68.

106. Elnima EI, Ahmed SA, Mekkawi A, Mossa JS. The antimicrobial activity of garlic and onion extracts. Pharmazie. 1983;38:747-48.

107. Sivam GP, Lampe JW, Ulness B, Swanzy SR, Potter JD. Helicobacter pylori — *in vitro* susceptibility to garlic (*Allium sativum*) extract. Nutrition & Cancer. 1997;27(2):118-21.

108. Amer M, Taha M, Tosson Z. The effect of aqueous garlic extract on the growth of dermatophytes. International Journal of Dermatology. 1980;19:285-87.

109. Davis LE, Shen J, Royer RE. *In vitro* synergism of concentrated *Allium sativum* extract and amphotericin B against Cryptococcus neoformans. Planta Medica. 1994;60(6):546-49.

110. You WC, Blot WJ, Chang YS, Ershow ZAG, Yang QT, An B, et al. Cancer Research. 1988;48:3518.

111. Dausch JG, Nixon DW. Garlic: A review of its relationship to malignant disease. Preventive Medicine. 1990;19:346-61.

112. Buiatti E, Palli D, Decarli A, Amadori D, Avellini C, Bianchi S, et al. International Journal of Cancer. 1989;44:611.

113. Haenszel W, Kurihara M, Segi M. Stomach cancer among Japanese in Hawaii. Journal of the National Cancer Institute.1972;49:969.

114. Sumiyoshi H, Wargovich MJ. Garlic (*Allium sativum*): A review of its relationship to cancer. Asia Pacific Journal of Pharmacology. 1989;4:133.

115. Lau BHS, Tadi PP, Tosk JM. *Allium sativum* (garlic) and cancer prevention. Nutrition Research. 1990;10:937-44.

116. Dorant E, van den Brandt PA, Goldbohm RA, Hermus RJ, Sturmans F. Garlic and its significance for the prevention of cancer in humans: A critical review. [Review]. British Journal of Cancer. 1993;67(3):424-29.

117. Ernst E. Can Allium vegatables prevent cancer? Phytomedicine 1997;4(1):79-83.

118. Wang Z, Boice JD, Wei L, Beebe GW, Zha Y, Kaplan MM, et al. Thyroid nodularity and chromosone aberrations among women in areas of high background radiation in China. Journal of the National Cancer Institute. 1990;82:478-85.

119. You W, Blot WJ, Chang Y, Ershow AG, Yang Z, An Q, et al. Allium vegetables and reduced risk of stomach cancer. Journal of the National Cancer Institute. 1989;81:162-64.

120. Palli D, Bianchi S, Decarli A, Cipriani F, Avellini C, Cocco P, et al. A case-control study of cancer of the gastric cardia in Italy. British Journal of Cancer. 1992;65:263-66.

121. Tuyns AJ, Kaaks R, Haelterman M, Riboli E. Diet and gastric cancer. A case control study in Belgium. International Journal of Cancer. 1992;51:1-6.

122. Zheng W, Blot WJ, Shu X-O, Diamond EL, Gao Y-T, Ji B-T, et al. A population-based case-control study of cancers of the nasal cavity and paranasal sinuses in Shanghai. International Journal of Cancer. 1992;52:557-61.

123. Zheng W, Blot WJ, Shu X-O, Gao Y-T, Ji B-T, Zieler RG, et al. Diet and other risk factors for laryngeal cancer in Shanghai. American Journal of Epidemiology 1992;136:178-91.

124. Hasson LE. Diet and risk of cancer. A population-based case-control study in Sweden. International Journal of Cancer. 1993;55:181-89.

125. Steinmetz KA, Kushi LH, Bostick RM, Folsom AR, Potter JD. Vegetables, fruit, and colon cancer in the Iowa Women's Health Study [see Comments]. American Journal of Epidemiology. 1994;139(1):1-15.

126. Dorant E, van den Brandt PA, Goldbohm RA. A prospective cohort study on the relationship between onion and leek consumption, garlic supplement use and the risk of colorectal carcinoma in The Netherlands. Carcinogenesis. 1996;17(3):477-84.

127. Dorant E, van den Brandt PA, Goldbohm RA. Allium vegetable consumption, garlic supplement intake, and female breast carcinoma incidence. Breast Cancer Research & Treatment. 1995;33(2):163-70.

128. You WC, Chang YS, Heinrich J, Ma JL, Liu WD, Zhang L, et al. An intervention trial to inhibit the progression of precancerous gastric lesions: compliance, serum micronutrients and S-allyl cysteine levels, and toxicity. Eur J Cancer Prev. 2001;10(3):257-63.

129. Belman S. Onion and garlic oils inhibit tumour progression. Carcinogenesis. 1983;4:1063-65.

130. Schaffer EM, Liu JZ, Green J, Dangler CA, Milner JA. Garlic and associated allyl sulfur components inhibit N-methyl-N- nitrosourea induced rat mammary carcinogenesis. Cancer Letters. 1996;102(1-2):199-204.

131. Cheng JY, Meng CL, Tzeng CC, Lin JC. Optimal dose of garlic to inhibit dimethylhydrazine-induced colon cancer. World Journal of Surgery. 1995;19(4):621-25.

132. Sundaram SG, Milner JA. Diallyl disulfide suppresses the growth of human colon tumor cell xenografts in athymic nude mice. Journal of Nutrition. 1996;126(5):1355-61.

133. Das T, Choudhury AR, Sharma A, Talukder G. Effects of crude garlic extract on mouse chromosomes *in vivo*. Food & Chemical Toxicology. 1996;34(1):43-47.

134. RoyChoudhury A, Das T, Sharma A, Talukder G. Dietary garlic extract in modifying clastogenic effects of inorganic arsenic in mice: two-generation studies. Mutation Research. 1996;359(3):165-70.

135. Ip C, Lisk DJ, Thompson HJ. Selenium-enriched garlic inhibits the early stage but not the late stage of mammary carcinogenesis. Carcinogenesis. 1996;17(9):1979-82.

136. Schaffer EM, Liu JZ, Milner JA. Garlic powder and allyl sulfur compounds enhance the ability of dietary selenite to inhibit 7,12-dimethylbenz [a]anthracene-induced mammary DNA adducts. Nutrition & Cancer. 1997;27(2):162-68.

137. Amagase H, Schaffer EM, Milner JA. Dietary components modify the ability of garlic to suppress 7,12-dimethylbenz(a) anthracene-induced mammary DNA adducts. Journal of Nutrition. 1996;126(4):817-24.

138. Singh SP, Abraham SK, Kesavan PC. *In vivo* radioprotection with garlic extract. Mutation Research. 1995;345(3-4):147-53.

139. Sundaram SG, Milner JA. Diallyl disulfide inhibits the proliferation of human tumor cells in culture. Biochimica et Biophysica Acta. 1996;1315(1):15-20.

140. Maurya AK, Singh SV. Differential induction of glutathione transferase isoenzymes of mice stomach by diallyl sulfide, a naturally occuring anticarcinogen. Cancer Letters. 1991;57:1212-9.

141. Hatono S, Jimenez A, Wargovich MJ. Chemopreventive effect of S-allylcysteine and its relationship to the detoxification enzyme glutathione S-transferase. Carcinogenesis. 1996;17(5):1041-44.

142. Hu X, Benson PJ, Srivastava SK, Mack LM, Xia H, Gupta V, et al. Glutathione S-transferases of female A/J mouse liver and forestomach and their differential induction by anti-carcinogenic organosulfides from garlic. Archives of Biochemistry & Biophysics. 1996;336(2):199-214.

143. Shenoy NR, Choughuley ASU. Inhibitory effect of diet related sulphydryl compounds on the formation of carcinogenic nitrosamines. Cancer Letters. 1992;65:227-32.

144. Cellini L, Di Campli E, Masulli M, Di Bartolomeo S, Allocati N. Inhibition of Helicobacter pylori by garlic extract (*Allium sativum*). FEMS Immunology & Medical Microbiology. 1996;13(4):273-77.

145. Ishikawa K, Naganawa R, Yoshida H, Iwata N, Fukuda H, Fujino T, et al. Antimutagenic effects of ajoene, an organosulfur compound derived from garlic. Bioscience, Biotechnology & Biochemistry. 1996;60(12):2086-88.

146. Sheela CG, Kumud K, Augusti KT. Anti-diabetic effects of onion and garlic sulfoxide amino acids in rats [Letter]. Planta Medica 1995;61(4):356-57.

147. Bever BO, Zahnd GR. Plants with oral hypoglycaemic action. Quarterly Journal of Crude Drug Research. 1979;17:139-96.

148. Abdullah TH, Kirkpatrick DV, Carter J. Enhancement of natural killer cell activity in AIDS with garlic [German]. Deutsche Zeitschrift Onkologie (German Journal of Oncology). 1989;21:52-53.

149. Moriguchi T, Saito H, Nishiyama N. Aged garlic extract prolongs longevity and improves spatial memory deficit in senescence-accelerated mouse. Biological & Pharmaceutical Bulletin. 1996;19(2):305-07.

150. Moriguchi T, Takashina K, Chu PJ, Saito H, Nishiyama N. Prolongation of life span and improved learning in the senescence accelerated mouse produced by aged garlic extract. Biological & Pharmaceutical Bulletin. 1994;17(12):1589-94.

151. Wei-cheng H. Garlic slice in repairing eardrum perforation. Chinese Medical Journal. 1977;3:204-05.

152. Numagami Y, Sato S, Ohnishi ST. Attenuation of rat ischemic brain damage by aged garlic extracts: A possible protecting mechanism as antioxidants. Neurochemistry International. 1996;29(2):135-43.

153. Batirel HF, Aktan S, Aykut C, Yegen BC, Coskun T. The effect of aqueous garlic extract on the levels of arachidonic acid metabolites (leukotriene C4 and prostaglandin E2) in rat forebrain after ischemia-reperfusion injury. Prostaglandins Leukotrienes & Essential Fatty Acids. 1996;54(4):289-92.

154. Prasad K, Laxdal VA, Yu M, Raney BL. Evaluation of hydroxyl radical-scavenging property of garlic. Molecular & Cellular Biochemistry. 1996;154(1):55-63.

155. Prasad K, Laxdal VA, Yu M, Raney BL. Antioxidant activity of allicin, an active principle in garlic. Molecular & Cellular Biochemistry. 1995;148(2):183-89.

156. Rekka EA, Kourounakis PN. Investigation of the molecular mechanism of the antioxidant activity of some *Allium sativum* ingredients. Pharmazie. 1994;49(7):539-40.

157. Wang EJ, Li Y, Lin M, Chen L, Stein AP, Reuhl KR, et al. Protective effects of garlic and related organosulfur compounds on acetaminophen-induced hepatotoxicity in mice. Toxicology & Applied Pharmacology. 1996;136(1):146-54.

158. Hu JJ, Yoo JS, Lin M, Wang EJ, Yang CS. Protective effects of diallyl sulfide on acetaminophen-induced toxicities. Food & Chemical Toxicology. 1996;34(10):963-69.

159. Stjernberg L, Berglund J. Garlic as an insect repellent. Journal of the American Medical Association. 2000;284(7):831.

160. McHugh C. Garlic as a tick repellent. Journal of the American Medical Association. 2001;285(1):41.

161. Burden AD, Wilkinson SM, Beck MH, Chalmers RJ. Garlic-induced systemic contact dermatitis. Contact Dermatitis. 1994;30(5):299-300.

162. Garty BZ. Garlic burns. Pediatrics. 1993;91(3):658-59.

163. Lembo G, Balato N, Patruno C, Auricchio L, Ayala F. Allergic contact dermatitis due to garlic (*Allium sativum*). Contact Dermatitis. 1991;25(5):330-31.

164. McFadden JP, White IR, Rycroft RJ. Allergic contact dermatitis from garlic. Contact Dermatitis. 1992;27(5):333-34.

165. Farrell AM, Staughton RC. Garlic burns mimicking herpes zoster [Letter]. Lancet. 1996;347(9009):1195.

166. Parish RA, McIntire S, Heimbach DM. Garlic burns: A naturopathic remedy gone awry. Pediatric Emergency Care. 1987;3:258-60.

167. Kaplan B, Schewach-Miller M, Yorav S. Factitial dermatitis induced by application of garlic. International Journal of Dermatology. 1990;29:75-76.

168. Canduela V, Mongil I, Carrascosa M, Docio S, Cagigas P. Garlic: always good for the health? [Letter]. British Journal of Dermatology. 1995;132(1):161-62.

169. Jappe U, Bonnekoh B, Hausen BM, Gollnick H. Garlic-related dermatoses: Case report and review of the literature. Am J Contact Dermat. 1999;10(1):37-39.

170. Asero R, Mistrello G, Roncarolo D, Antoniotti PL, Falagiani P. A case of garlic allergy. J Allergy Clin Immunol. 1998;101(3):427-28.

171. Perez-Pimiento AJ, Moneo I, Santaolalla M, de Paz S, Fernandez-Parra B, Dominguez-Lazaro AR. Anaphylactic reaction to young garlic. Allergy. 1999;54(6):626-29.

172. German K, Kumar U, Blackford HN. Garlic and the risk of TURP bleeding. British Journal of Urology. 1995;76(4):518.

173. Burnham BE. Garlic as a possible risk for postoperative bleeding [Letter] [see Comments]. Plastic & Reconstructive Surgery. 1995;95(1):213.

174. Petry JJ. Garlic and postoperative bleeding [Letter; Comment]. Plastic & Reconstructive Surgery.1995;96(2):483-84.

175. Falleroni A. Occupational asthma secondary to inhalation of garlic dust. Journal of Allergy and Clinical Immunology. 1981;68:159-60.

176. Seuri M, Taivanen A, Ruoppi P, Tukiaimen H. Three cses of occupational asthma and rhinitis caused by garlic. Clin Exp Allergy. 1993;23:1011-14.

177. Lybarger J, Gallagher J, Pulver A, Litwin A, Books S, Bernstein L. Occupational ashtma induced by inhalation and ingestion of garlic. Journal of Allergy and Clinical Immunology. 1982;69:448-54.

178. Brewster JL, Rabinowitch, eds. Onions and Allied Crops. Boca Raton, FL: CRC Press, Inc.; 1990.

179. Alnaqeeb MA, Thomson M, Bordia T, Ali M. Histopathological effects of garlic on liver and lung of rats. Toxicology Letters. 1996;85(3):157-64.

180. Newall C, Anderson L, Phillipson J. Herbal Medicines. A Guide for Health Care Professionals. London: The Pharmaceutical Press; 1996.

181. Brenner S, Wolf R. Possible nutritional factors in induced pemphigus. [Review]. Dermatology. 1994;189(4):337-39.

182. Sunter W. Warfarin and garlic. The Pharmaceutical Journal. 1991;246:72.

183. Fulder S. Garlic and the prevention of cardiovascular disease. Cardiology in Practice. 1989;March:30,34-35.

184. Laroche M, Choudhri S, Gallicano K, Foster B. Severe gastrointestinal toxicity with concomittant ingestion of ritonavir and garlic. Canadian Journal of Infectious Diseases. 1998;9(Supplement A):417P.

185. Gallicano K, Foster B, Choudhri S. Effect of short-term administration of garlic supplements on single-dose ritonavir pharmacokinetics in healthy volunteers. British Journal of Clinical Pharmacoly. 2003;55:199-202.

186. Blumenthal M. Therapeutic Monographs on Medicinal Plants for Human Use of Special Expert Committee, Federal Health Agency, Germany. Austin, TX: American Botanical Council; 1998.

187. Murray MT. The Healing Power of Herbs. Rocklin, CA: Prima Publishing; 1992.

188. Bradley P. British Herbal Compendium. Bournemouth, UK: The British Herbal Medical Association; 1992.

189. Marles RJ, Associate Professor, Department of Botany, Brandon University, Brandon, Manitoba. Review of Medicinal Plant Modules for CCNM; 1997.

Ginger

1. Newall C, Anderson L, Phillipson J. Herbal Medicines. A Guide for Health Care Professionals. London: The Pharmaceutical Press; 1996.

2. Foster S, Chongxi Y. Herbal Emissaries. Bringing Chinese Herbs to the West. Rochester, VT: Healing Arts Press; 1992.

3. Mascolo N, Jain R, Jain SC, Capasso F. Ethnopharmacologic investigation of ginger (*Zingiber officinalis*). Journal of Ethnopharmacology. 1989;27:129-40.

4. Awang DVC. Ginger. Canadian Pharmaceutical Journal. 1992;125:309-11.

5. Leung AY, Foster S. Encyclopedia of Common Natural Ingredients Used in Food, Drugs and Cosmetics. 2nd ed. New York: John Wiley and Sons; 1996.

6. Bradley P. British Herbal Compendium. Bournemouth, UK: The British Herbal Medical Association; 1992.

7. Fulder S, Tenne M. Ginger as anti-nausea remedy in pregnancy. The issue of safety. Herbalgram. 1996;38:47-50.

8. Platel K, Srinivasan K. Influence of dietary spices or their active principles on digestive enzymes of small intestinal mucosa in rats. International Journal of Food Sciences & Nutrition. 1996;47(1):55-59.

9. Pengelly A. Ginger extracts prevent ulcers. Australian Jouranl of Medical Herbalism. 1993;59(2):73.

10. Yamahara J, Mochizuki M, Rong HQ, Matsuda H, Fujimura H. The anti-ulcer effect in rats of ginger constituents. Journal of Ethnopharmacology. 1988;23:299-304.

11. Al-Yahya MA, Rafatullah S, Mossa JS, Ageel AM, Parmar NS, Tariq M. Gastroprotective activity of ginger *Zingiber officinale* Rosc., in albino rats. American Journal of Chinese Medicine. 1989;17(1-2):51-56.

12. Sertie J, Basile A, Oshiro T, Mazella A. Preventative anti-ulcer activity of the rhizome extract of *Zingiber officinale*. Fitoterapia. 1992;63:55-59.

13. Sakai K, Miyazaki Y, Yamane T, Saitoh Y, Ikawa C, Nishihata T. Effect of extracts of Zingiberaceae herbs on gastric secretion in rabbits. Chemical and Pharmaceutical Bulletin. 1989;37(1):215-17.

14. Yamahara J, Miki K, Chisaka T, Sawada T, Fujimura H, Tomimatsu T, et al. Cholagogic effect of ginger and its active constituents. Journal of Ethnopharmacology. 1985;13:217-25.

15. Verma S, Singh J, Khamesra R, Bordia A. Effect of ginger on platelet aggregation in man. Indian Journal of Medical Research. 1993;98:240-42.

16. Srivastava KC. Effects of aqueous extracts of onion, garlic and ginger on the platelet aggregation and metabolism of arachidonic acid in the blood vascular system: *In vitro* study. Prostaglandins, Leukotrienes and Medicine. 1984;13:277-35.

17. Lumb AB. Effect of dried ginger on human platelet function. Thrombosis & Haemostasis. 1994;71(1):110-11.

18. Gujral S, Bhumra H, Swaroop M. Effect of ginger (*Zingibar officinale* roscoe) oleoresin on serum and hepatic cholesterol levels in cholesterol fed rats. Nutr Rep Intl. 1978;17:183-89.

19. Giri J, Devi STK, Meerarani S. Effect of ginger on serum cholesterol levels. The Indian Journal of Dietetics. 1984;21:433-36.

20. Tanabe M, Chen Y-D, Saito K-i, Kano Y. Cholesterol biosynthesis inhibitory component from *Zingiber officinale* Roscoe. Chemical & Pharmaceutical Bulletin. 1993;41(4):710-13.

21. Brown D. Anti-Inflammatory potential of ginger. Quarterly Review of Natural Medicine. 1993;Spring:17.

22. Srivastava KC, Mustafa T. Ginger (*Zingiber officinale*) and rheumatic disorders. Medical Hypotheses. 1989;29:25-28.

23. Srivastava KC, Mustafa T. Ginger (*Zingiber officinale*) in rheumatism and musculoskeletal disorders. Medical Hypotheses. 1992;39:342-48.

24. Sharma JN, Srivastava KC, Gan EK. Suppressive effects of eugenol and ginger oil on arthritic rats. Pharmacology. 1994;49(5):314-18.

25. Altman RD, Marcussen KC. Effects of a ginger extract on knee pain in patients with osteoarthritis. Arthritis Rheum. 2001;44(11):2531-38.

26. Bliddal H, Rosetzsky A, Schlichting P, Weidner MS, Andersen LA, Ibfelt HH, et al. A randomized, placebo-controlled, cross-over study of ginger extracts and ibuprofen in osteoarthritis. Osteoarthritis Cartilage. 2000;8(1):9-12.

27. Kiuchi F, Shibuyu M, Sankawa U. Inhibitors of prostaglandin biosynthesis from ginger. Chemical and Pharmaceutical Bulletin. 1982;30:754-57.

28. McCaleb R. Ginger and atractylodes as an anti-inflammatory. Herbalgram. 1993;29:19.

29. Mowrey DB, Clayson DE. Motion sickness, ginger, and psychophysics. Lancet. 1982;I:655-57.

30. Stewart JJ, Wood MJ, D. WC, Mims ME. Effects of ginger on motion sickness susceptibility and gastric function. Pharmacology. 1991;42:111-20.

31. Grøntved A, Brask T, Kambskard J, Hentzer E. Ginger root against seasickness. A controlled trial on the open sea. Acta Otolaryngol (Stockholm). 1988;105(1-2):45-49.

32. Wood CD, Manno JE, Wood MJ, Manno BR, Mims ME. Comparison of efficacy of ginger with various antimotion sickness drugs. Clinical Research Practices and Drug Regulatory Affairs. 1988;6(2):129-36.

33. Lien HC, Sun WM, Chen YH, Kim H, Hasler W, Owyang C. Effects of ginger on motion sickness and gastric slow-wave dysrhythmias induced by circular vection. Am J Physiol Gastrointest Liver Physiol. 2003;284(3):G481-89.

34. Tyler VE. Herbs of Choice. The Therapeutic Use of Phytomedicinals. Binghamton, NY: Pharmaceutical Products Press; 1994.

35. Brown D. Antimotion sickness action of ginger questioned. Quarterly Review of Natural Medicine. 1993;Spring:15-16.

36. Bone ME, Wilkinson DJ, Young JR, McNeil J, Charlton S. Ginger Root — a new antiemetic. The effect of ginger root on postoperative nausea and vomiting after major gynaecological surgery. Anaesthesia. 1990;45(8):669-71.

37. Phillips S, Ruggier R, Hutchinson S. *Zingiber officinale* (ginger) — an antiemetic for day case surgery. Anaesthesia. 1993;48(8):715-17.

38. Arfeen Z, Owen H, Plummer J, Ilsley A, Sorby-Adams R, Doecke C. A double-blind randomized controlled trial of ginger for the prevention of postoperative nausea and vomiting. Anaesthesia & Intensive Care. 1995;23(4):449-52.

39. Eberhart LH, Mayer R, Betz O, Tsolakidis S, Hilpert W, Morin AM, et al. Ginger does not prevent postoperative nausea and vomiting after laparoscopic surgery.

Anesth Analg. 2003;96(4):995-98, table of contents.

40. Visalyaputra S, Petchpaisit N, Somcharoen K, Choavaratana R. The efficacy of ginger root in the prevention of postoperative nausea and vomiting after outpatient gynaecological laparoscopy. Anaesthesia. 1998;53(5):506-10.

41. Fischer-Rasmussen W, Kjær SK, Dahl C, Asping U. Ginger treatment of hyperemesis gravidarum. European Journal of Obstetrics and Gynecology and Reprodroductive Biology. 1990;38:19-24.

42. Vutyavanich T, Kraisarin T, Ruangsri R. Ginger for nausea and vomiting in pregnancy: Randomized, double-masked, placebo-controlled trial. Obstet Gynecol. 2001;97(4):577-82.

43. Keating A, Chez RA. Ginger syrup as an antiemetic in early pregnancy. Altern Ther Health Med. 2002;8(5):89-91.

44. Yamahara J, Rong HQ, Naitoh Y, Kitani T, Fujimura H. Inhibition of cytotoxic drug-induced vomitting in suncus by a ginger constituent. Journal of Ethnopharmacology. 1989;27:353-55.

45. Holtmann S, Clarke AH, Scherer H, Hohn M. The anti-motion sickness mechanism of ginger. A comparative study with placebo and Dimenhydrinate. Acta Oto-Laryngologica (Stockholm). 1989;198(3-4):168-74.

46. Kawai T, Kinosita K. Antiemetic principle of *Magnolia obovata* and *Zingiber officinale* rhizome. Planta Medica. 1994;60:17-20.

47. Lumb A. Mechanism of antiemetic effect of ginger [Letter; Comment]. Anaesthesia. 1993;48(12):1118.

48. Yamahara J, Rong H, Iwamoto M, Kobayashi G, Matsuda H, Fujimura H. Active components of ginger exhibiting antiserotonergic action. Phytotherapy Research. 1989;3(2):70-71.

49. Mills S. Essential Book of Herbal Medicine. London: Penguin Books Limited; 1991.

50. Shoji N, Iwasa A, Takemoto T, Ishida Y, Ohizumi Y. Cardiotonic principles of ginger (*Zingiber officiniale* Roscoe). Journal of Pharmaceutical Sciences. 1982;71(10):1174-75.

51. Mustafa T, Srivastava KC. Ginger (*Zingiber officinale*) in migraine headaches. Journal of Ethnopharmacology. 1990;29(3):267-73.

52. Chang HM, But PPH. Pharmacology and Application of Chinese Materia Medica. Hong Kong: World Scientific Publishing; 1987.

53. Nagabhushan M, Amonkar AJ, Bhide SV. Mutagenicity of gingerol and shogaol and antimutagenicity of zingerone in salmonella/microsome assay. Cancer Letters. 1987;36:221-33.

54. Nakamura H, Yamamoto T. Mutagen and anti-mutagen in ginger, *Zingiber officinale*. Mutation Research. 1982;103:119-26.

55. Qureshi S, Shah AH, Tariq M, Ageel AM. Studies on herbal aphrodisiacs used in Arab system of medicine. American Journal of Chinese Medicine. 1989;17(1-2):57-63.

56. Backon J. Ginger as an antiemetic: Possible side effects due to its thromboxane synthetase activity (letter/comment). Anaesthesia. 1991;46(8):669-71.

57. Brown D. Herbal Prescriptions for Better Health. Rocklin, CA: Prima Publishing; 1996.

Ginkgo

1. Tyler VE. Herbs of Choice. The Therapeutic Use of Phytomedicinals. Binghamton, NY: Pharmaceutical Products Press; 1994.

2. Wren RC. Potter's New Encyclopaedia of Botanical Drugs and Preparations. Saffron Waldon, UK: C.W. Daniel Company; 1988.

3. Kleijnen J, Knipschild P. *Ginkgo biloba*. Lancet. 1992;340:1136-39.

4. Murray MT. The Healing Power of Herbs. Rocklin, CA: Prima Publishing; 1992.

5. Michel PF. The doyen of trees: The *Ginkgo biloba*. [French]. Presse Medicale 1986;15(31):1450-4.

6. Major RT. The ginkgo, the most ancient living tree. Science. 1967;157:1270-3.

7. Foster S. Ginkgo, *Ginkgo biloba*. Austin, TX: American Botanical Council; 1990: Botanical Series No. 304.

8. Gaby AR. *Ginkgo biloba* extract: A review. Alternative Medicine Review. 1996;1(4):236-42.

9. Houghton PJ. Ginkgo. Pharmacy Journal. 1994;253:122-23.

10. Braquet P. The ginkgolides: Potent platelet-activating afactor antagonists isolated from *Ginkgo biloba* L.: Chemistry, pharmacology and clinical applications. Drugs of the Future. 1987;12:643-99.

11. van Beek TA, Rantio HA, Melger WC, Lelyveld GP. Determination of ginkolides and bilobalide in *Ginkgo biloba* leaves and phytopharmaceuticals. Journal of Chromotography. 1991;543:375-87.

12. Sticher O. Quality of Ginkgo preparations. [Review]. Planta Medica. 1993;59(1):2-11.

13. Newall CA, Anderson LA, Phillipson JD. Herbal Medicines. A Guide for Health Care Professionals. London: The Pharmaceutical Press; 1996.

14. Briancon-Scheid F, et al. HPLC separation and quantitative determination of biflavones in leaves from *Ginkgo biloba*. Planta Medica. 1983;49:204-20.

15. Jung F, Mrowietz C, Kiesewetter H, Wenzel E. Effect of *Ginkgo biloba* on fluidity of blood and peripheral microcirculation in volunteers. Arzneimittel Forschung. 1990;40(5):589-93.

16. Liberti. Ginkgo. The Lawrence Review of Natural Products. 1988;February.

17. Le Poncin Lafitte M, Rapin J, Rapin JR. Effects of *Ginkgo biloba* on changes induced by quantitative cerebral microembolization in rats. Archives Internationales de Pharmacodynamie et de Therapie. 1980.

18. Chatterjee SS, et al. Studies on the mechanism of action of an extract of *Ginkgo biloba*, a drug used for treatment of ischemic vascular disease. Arch Pharmacol. 1988;320:R52.

19. Krieglstein J, Beck T, Seibert A. Influence of an extract of *Ginkgo biloba* on cerebral blood flow and metabolism. Life Sciences. 1986;39(24):2327-34.

20. Tighilet B, Lacour M. Pharmacological activity of the *Ginkgo biloba* extract (EGb 761) on equilibrium function recovery in the unilateral vestibular neurectomized cat. Journal of Vestibular Research. 1995;5(3):187-200.

21. Smith PF, Maclennan K, Darlington CL. The neuroprotective properties of the *Ginkgo biloba* leaf: a review of the possible relationship to platelet-activating factor (PAF). [Review]. Journal of Ethnopharmacology. 1996;50(3):131-9.

22. Stucker O, Pons C, Duverger JP, Drieu K. Effects of *Ginkgo biloba* extract (EGb 761) on arteriolar spasm in a rat cremaster muscle preparation. International Journal of Microcirculation: Clinical & Experimental. 1996.

23. DeFeudis FV. *Ginkgo biloba* Extract (EGb 761): Pharamacological Activities and Clinical Applications. Paris: Elsevier; 1991.

24. Vilain B, DeFeudis FV, Clostre F. Effect of an extract of *Ginkgo biloba* on the isolated ileum of the guinea pig. General Pharmacology. 1982;13(5):401-05.

25. Puglisi L, Salvadori S, Gabrielli G, Pasargiklian R. Pharmacology of natural compounds. I. Smooth muscle relaxant activity induced by a *Ginkgo biloba* L. extract on guinea-pig trachea. Pharmacological Research Communications. 1988;20(7):573-89.

26. Delaflotte S, Auguet M, DeFeudis FV, Baranes J, Clostre F, Drieu K, et al. Endothelium-dependent relaxations of rabbit isolated aorta produced by carbachol and by *Ginkgo biloba* extract. Biomedica Biochimica Acta. 1984;43(8-9):S212-16.

27. Auguet M, DeFeudis FV, Clostre F. Effects of *Ginkgo biloba* on arterial smooth muscle responses to vasoactive stimuli. General Pharmacology. 1982;13(2):169-71.

28. Auguet M, DeFeudis FV, Clostre F, Deghenghi R. Effects of an extract of *Ginkgo biloba* on rabbit isolated aorta. General Pharmacology. 1982;13(3):225-30.

29. Hellegouarch A, Baranes J, Clostre F, Drieu K, Braquet P, DeFeudis FV. Comparison of the contractile effects of an extract of *Ginkgo biloba* and some neurotransmitters on rabbit isolated vena cava. General Pharmacology. 1985;16(2):129-32.

30. Pincemail J, Dupuis M, Nasr C, Hans P, Haag-Berrurier M, Anton R, et al. Superoxide anion scavenging effect and superoxide dismutase activity of *Ginkgo biloba* extract. Experientia. 1989;45(8):708-12.

31. Robak J, Gryglewski RJ. Flavonoids are scavengers of superoxide anions. Biochemical Pharmacology. 1988;37:837-41.

32. Chung KF, G. D, Mccusker M, P. G, et.al. Effect of a gingkolide mixture (BN 52063) in antagonising skin and platelet responses to platelet activating factor in man. Lancet. 1987;1:248-51.

33. Braquet P. Proofs of involvement of PAF-acether in various immune disorders using BN 52021 (ginkgolide B): a powerful PAF-acether antagonist isolated from *Ginkgo biloba* L. Advances in Prostaglandin, Thromboxane, and Leukotriene Research. 1986;16.

34. Braquet P, Hosford D. Ethnopharmacology and the development of natural PAF antagonists as therapeutic agents. Journal of Ethnopharmacology. 1991;32:135-39.

35. Markey AC, et al. Platelet activating factor-induced clinical and histopathologic responses in atopic skin and their modification by the platelet activating factor antagonist BN52063. Journal of the American Academy of Dermatology. 1990;23(2):263-68.

36. Wilkens JH, et al. Effects of a PAF-antagonist (BN 52063) on bronchoconstriction and platelet activation during excercise induced asthma. British Journal of Clinical Pharmacology. 1990;29(1):85-91.

37. Guinot P, et al. Inhibition of PAF-acether induced wheal and flare reaction in man bt a specific PAF antagonist. Prostaglandins. 1986;32(1):160-63.

38. Guinot P, et al. Effect of BN 52063, a specific PAF-acether antagonist, on bronchial provocation test to allergens in asthmatic patients. A preliminary study. Prostaglandins. 1987;34(5):723-31.

39. Guinot P, et al. Tanakan inhibits platelet-activating-factor-induced platelet aggregation in healthy male volunteers. Haemostasis. 1989;19(4):219-23.

40. Bourgain RH, Andries R, Braquet P. Effect of ginkgolide PAF-acether antagonists on arterial thrombosis. Advances in Prostaglandin, Thromboxane, & Leukotriene Research. 1987.

41. Koltai M, et al. Effect of BN 52021, a specific PAF-acether antagonist, on cardiac anaphylaxis in langendorff hearts isolated from passively sensitized guinea pigs. European Journal of Pharmacology. 1986;130:133-36.

42. Kurihara K, Wardlaw AJ, Moqbel R, Kay AB. Inhibition of platelet-activating factor (PAF)-induced chemotaxis and PAF binding to human eosinophils and neutrophils by the specific ginkgolide-derived PAF antagonist, BN 52021. Journal of Allergy & Clinical Immunology. 1989;83(1):83-90.

43. Lamant V, Mauco G, Braquet P, et al. Inhibition of the metabolism of platelet activating factor (PAF-acether) by three specific antagonists from *Ginkgo biloba*. Biochemical Pharmacology. 1987;36:2749-52.

44. Harczy M, Maclouf J, Pradelles P, Braquet P, Borgeat P, Sirois P. Inhibitory effects of a novel platelet activating factor (PAF) antagonist (BN 52021) on antigen-induced prostaglandin and thromboxane formation by the guinea pig lung. Pharmacological Research Communications 1986;18:111-17.

45. Dhainaut J-FA, Tenaillon A, Le Tulzo Y, Schlemmer B, Solet J-P, et al. Platelet activating factor receptor antagonist BN 52021 in treatment of severe sepsis: A randomized, double-blind, placebo-controlled, multicentre clinical trial. Critical Care Medicine. 1994;22(11):1720-28.

46. Bourgain RH, Maes L, Andries R, Braquet P. Thrombus induction by endogenic paf-acether and its inhibition by *Ginkgo biloba* extracts in the guinea pig. Prostaglandins. 1986;32(1):142-44.

47. Belougne E, Aguejouf O, Imbault P, Azougagh Oualane F, Doutremepuich F, Droy-Lefaix MT, et al. Experimental thrombosis model induced by laser beam. Application of aspirin and an extract of *Ginkgo biloba*: EGb 761. Thrombosis Research. 1996;82(5):453-58.

48. Clostre F. From the body to the cell membrane: The different levels of pharmacological action of *Ginkgo biloba* extract. [Review] [French]. Presse Medicale. 1986;15(31):1529-38.

49. Rapin JR, Le Poncin Lafitte M. Cerebral glucose consumption. The effect of *Ginkgo biloba* extract. [French]. Presse Medicale. 1986;15(31):1494-97.

50. Spinnewyn B, Blavet N, Clostre F. Effects of *Ginkgo biloba* extract on a cerebral ischemia model in gerbils. [French]. Presse Medicale. 1986;15(31):1511-15.

51. Spinnewyn B, Blavet N, Clostre F, Bazan N, Braquet P. Involvement of platelet-activating factor (PAF) in cerebral post-ischemic phase in Mongolian gerbils. Prostaglandins. 1987;34(3):337-49.

52. Koc RK, Akdemir H, Kurtsoy A, Pasaoglu H, Kavuncu I, Pasaoglu A, et al. Lipid peroxidation in experimental spinal cord injury. Comparison of treatment with *Ginkgo biloba*, TRH and methylprednisolone. Research in Experimental Medicine. 1995;195(2):117-23.

53. Otamiri T, Tagesson C. *Ginkgo biloba* extract prevents mucosal damage associated with small-intestinal ischaemia. Scandinavian Journal of Gastroenterology. 1989;24(6):666-70.

54. Seif-El-Nasr M, El-Fattah AA. Lipid peroxide, phospholipids, glutathione levels and superoxide dismutase activity in the rat brain after ischemia: effect of *Ginkgo biloba* extract. Pharmacological Research. 1995;32(5):273-78.

55. Birkle DL, Kurian P, Braquet P, Bazan NG. Platelet-activating factor antagonist BN52021 decreases accumulation of free polyunsaturated fatty acid in mouse brain during ischemia and electroconvulsive shock. Journal of Neurochemistry. 1988;51:1900-05.

56. Panetta T, Marcheselli VL, Braquet P, Spinnewyn B, Bazan NG. Effects of a platelet activating factor antagonist (BN 52021) on free fatty acids, dicylglycerols, polyphosphoinositides and blood flow in the gerbil brain: Inhibition of ischemia-reperfusion induced cerebral injury. Biochemical and Biophysical Research Communications. 1987;149:580-87.

57. Kose K, Dogan P. Lipoperoxidation induced by hydrogen peroxide in human erythrocyte membranes. 2. Comparison of the antioxidant effect of *Ginkgo biloba* extract (EGb 761) with those of water-soluble and lipid-soluble antioxidants. Journal of International Medical Research. 1995;23(1):9-18.

58. Kose K, Dogan P. Lipoperoxidation induced by hydrogen peroxide in human erythrocyte membranes. 1. Protective effect of *Ginkgo biloba* extract (EGb 761). Journal of International Medical Research. 1995;23(1):1-8.

59. Maitra I, Marcocci L, Droy-Lefaix MT, Packer L. Peroxyl radical scavenging activity of *Ginkgo biloba* extract EGb 761. Biochemical Pharmacology. 1995;49(11):1649-55.

60. Ni Y, Zhao B, Hou J, Xin W. Preventive effect of *Ginkgo biloba* extract on apoptosis in rat cerebellar neuronal cells induced by hydroxyl radicals. Neuroscience Letters. 1996;214(2-3):115-18.

61. Oyama Y, Fuchs PA, Katayama N, Noda K. Myricetin and quercetin, the flavonoid constituents of *Ginkgo biloba* extract, greatly reduce oxidative metabolism in both resting and Ca(2+) - loaded brain neurons. Brain Research. 1994;635(1-2):125-29.

62. Oyama Y, Chikahisa L, Ueha T, Kanemaru K, Noda K. *Ginkgo biloba* extract protects brain neurons against oxidative stress induces by hydroden peroxide. Brain Research. 1996;712(2):349-52.

63. Rong Y, Geng Z, Lau BH. *Ginkgo biloba* attenuates oxidative stress in macrophages and endothelial cells. Free Radical Biology & Medicine. 1996;20(1):121-27.

64. Haramaki N, Aggarwal S, Kawabata T, Droy-Lefaix MT, Packer L. Effects of natural antioxidant *Ginkgo biloba* extract (EGB 761) on myocardial ischemia-reperfusion injury. Free Radical Biology & Medicine. 1994;16(6):789-94.

65. Shen JG, Zhou DY. Efficiency of *Ginkgo biloba* extract (EGb 761) in antioxidant protection against myocardial ischemia and reperfusion injury. Biochemistry & Molecular Biology International.l 1995;35(1):125-34.

66. Szabo ME, Droy-Lefaix MT, Doly M, Braquet P. Free radical-mediated effects in reperfusion injury: A histologic study with superoxide dismutase and EGb 761 in rat retina. Ophthalmic Research. 1991;23(4):225-34.

67. Pincemail J, Deby C. Antiradical properties of *Ginkgo biloba* extract. [French]. Presse Medicale. 1986;15(31):1475-79.

68. Schaffler K, Reeh PW. Double blind study of the hypoxia protective effect of a standardized *Ginkgo biloba* preparation after repeated administration in healthy subjects [German]. Arzneimittel Forschung. 1985;35(8):1283-86.

69. Oberpichler H, Beck T, Abdel-Rahman MM, Bielenberg GW, Krieglstein J. Effects of *Ginkgo biloba* constituents related to protection against brain damage caused by hypoxia. Pharmacological Research Communications. 1988;20(5):349-68.

70. Karcher L, Zagermann P, Krieglstein J. Effect of an extract of *Ginkgo biloba* on rat brain energy metabolism in hypoxia. Naunyn Schmiedebergs Archives of Pharmacology. 1984;327(1):31-35.

71. Punkt K, Welt K, Schaffranietz L. Changes of enzyme activities in the rat myocardium caused by experimental hypoxia with and without *Ginkgo biloba* extract EGb 761 pretreatment. A cytophotometrical study. Acta Histochemica. 1995;97(1):67-79.

72. Janssens D, Michiels C, Delaive E, Eliaers F, Drieu K, Remacle J. Protection of hypoxia-induced ATP decrease in endothelial cells by *Ginkgo biloba* extract and bilobalide. Biochemical Pharmacology. 1995;50(7):991-99.

73. Arrigo A, Cattaneo S. Clinical and psychometric evaluation of *Ginkgo biloba* extract in chronic cerebro-vascular diseases. In: Agnoli A, et.al., eds. Effects of *Ginkgo biloba* Extracts on Organic Cerebral Impairment. John Libbey Eurotext Ltd.; 1985:71-76.

74. Augustin P. *Ginkgo biloba* extract in geriatrics. Clinical and psychometric study of 189 patients [French]. Psychologie Mediacale. 1976;8:123-30.

75. Eckmann VF, Schlag H. Knotrollierte doppelblind-studie zum wirksamkeitsnachweis von Tebonin forte bei patienten mit zerebrovakularer insuffizienz. Fortschrift der Medizin. 1982;31:1474-78.

76. Gessner B, Voelp A, Klasser M. Study of the long-term action of a *Ginkgo biloba* extract on vigilance and mental performance as determined by means of quantitative pharmaco-EEG and psychometric measurements. Arzneimittel Forschung. 1985;35(9):1459-65.

77. Hofferberth B. The effect of *Ginkgo biloba* extract on neurophysiological and psychometric measurement results in patients with psychotic organic brain syndrome. A double-blind study against placebo [German]. Arzneimittel Forschung. 1989;39(8):918-22.

78. Vorberg G. *Ginkgo biloba* extract (GBE): A long term study of cerebral insufficiency in geriatric patients. Clinical Trials Journal. 1985;22:149-57.

79. Schmidt U, Rabinovici K, Lande S. EifluB eines Ginkgo-biloba-spezialextraktes auf die befindlichkeit bei zerebraler insufizienz. Munch Med Wochenschr. 1991;133(Supplement 1):S15-8.

80. Bruchert E, Heinrich SE, Ruf-Kohler P. Wirksamkeit von LI 1370 bei alteren patienten mit hirnleistungsschwache. Multizentrische doppelblindstudie des fachverbandes deutscher allgemeinarzte. Munch Med Wochenschr. 1991;133(Supplement 1):S9-14.

81. Meyer B. Multicenter randomized double-blind drug vs. placebo study of the treatment of tinnitus with *Ginkgo biloba* extract [French]. Presse Medicale. 1986;15(31):1562-64.

82. Taillander J, et.al. *Ginkgo biloba* extract in the treatment of cerebral disorders due to aging. A longitudinal multicenter double-blind drug vs. placebo study [French]. Presse Medicale. 1986;15(31):1583-87.

83. Haguenauer JP, Cantenot F, Koskas H, Pierart H. Treatment of equilibrium disorders with *Ginkgo biloba* extract. A multicenter double-blind drug vs. placebo study [French]. Presse Medicale. 1986;15(31):1569-72.

84. Eckmann F. Cerebral insufficiency—treatment with Ginkgo-biloba extract. Time of onset of effect in a double-blind study with 60 inpatients [German]. Fortschritte der Medizin. 1990;108(29):557-60.

85. Wesnes K, et al. A double-blind placebo-controlled trial of Gingko Biloba extract in the treatment of idiopathic cognitive impairment in the elderly. Human Psychopharmacology. 1987;2:159-69.

86. Hartmann A, Frick M. Wirkung eines Ginkgo-spezialextraktes auf psychometrische parameter bei patienten mit caskular bedingter demenz. Munch Med Wochenschr. 1991;133(Supplement 1):S23-5.

87. Vesper J, Hansgen KD. Efficacy of *Ginkgo biloba* in 90 outpatients with cerebral insufficiency caused by old age. Results of a placebo-controlled double-blind trial. Phytomedicine. 1994;1:9-16.

88. Pittler MH, Ernst E. *Ginkgo biloba* extract for the treatment of intermittent claudication: a meta-analysis of randomized trials. American Journal of Medicine. 2000;108(4):276-81.

89. Blume J, Kieser M, Holscher U. Placebo-controlled double-blind study of the effectiveness of *Ginkgo biloba* special extract EGb 761 in trained patients with intermittent claudication [German]. Vasa. 1996;25(3):265-74.

90. Natali J, Boissier P. Internal Report: Schwabe; 1985.

91. Bauer U. 6-Month double-blind randomised clinical trial of *Ginkgo biloba* extract versus placebo in two parallel groups in patients suffering from peripheral arterial insufficiency. Arzneimittel Forschung. 1984;34(6):716-20.

92. Thomson GJa. A clinical trial of *Ginkgo biloba* extract in patients with intermittent claudication. Int Angio.l 1990;9(2):75-78.

93. Salz H. Zur wirksamkeit eines Ginkgo-biloba-Praparats bei arteriellen durchblutungstorungen der unteren extremitaten. Therapie Gegenwart. 1980;119:1345-56.

94. Drabaek H, Petersen JR, Winberg N, Hansen KF, Mehlsen J. The effect of *Ginkgo biloba* extract in patients with intermittent claudication [Danish]. Ugeskrift for Laeger. 1996;158(27):3928-31.

95. Peters H, Kieser M, Holscher U. Demonstration of the efficacy of *Ginkgo biloba* special extract EGb 761 on intermittent claudication—a placebo-controlled, double-blind multicenter trial. Vasa. 1998;27(2):106-10.

96. Blume J, Kieser M, Holscher U. Ginkgo-spezialextrakt EGb 761 bei periherer arterieller verschluBkrankheit. Fortschrift der Medizin. 1998;116:137-43.

97. Saudreau F, Serise JM, Pillet J, Maiza D, Mercier V, Kretz JG, et al. Efficacy of an extract of *Ginkgo biloba* in the treatment of chronic obliterating arteriopahies of the lower limbs in stage III of Fontaine's classification [French]. Journal des Maladies Vasculaires. 1989;14(3):177-82.

98. Schweizer J, Hautmann C. Comparison of two dosages of *Ginkgo biloba* extract EGb 761 in patients with peripheral arterial occlusive disease Fontaine's stage IIb. A randomised, double-blind, multicentric clinical trial. Arzneimittelforschung. 1999;49(11):900-04.

99. Mouren X, Calliard PH, Schwarz F. Study of the anti-ischemic action of EGb 761 in the treatment of peripheral arterial occlusive disease by TcPO2 determination. Angiology. 1994;45:413-17.

100. Bauer U. *Ginkgo biloba* extract in the treatment of arteriopathy of the lower extremities. A 65-week trial [French]. Presse Medicale. 1986;15(31):1546-49.

101. Tosaki A, Engelman DT, Pali T, Engelman RM, Droy-Lefaix MT. *Ginkgo biloba* extract (EGb 761) improves postischemic function in isolated preconditioned working rat hearts. Coronary Artery Disease. 1994;5(5):443-50.

102. Koltai M, et.al. Ginkgolide B protects isolated hearts agaist arrhythmias induced by ischaemia but not reperfusion. European Journal of Pharmacology. 1989;164:293-302.

103. Huguet F, Drieu K, Piriou A. Decreased cerebral 5-HT1A receptors during aging: Reversal by *Ginkgo biloba* extract (EGb761). Journal of Pharmaceutical Pharmacology. 1994;46:316-18.

104. Racagni G, Brunello N, Paoletti R. Neuromediator changes during cerebral aging. The effect of *Ginkgo biloba* extract [Review] [French]. Presse Medicale. 1986;15(31):1488-90.

105. Huguet F, Tarrade T. Alpha 2-adrenoceptor changes during cerebral ageing. The effect of *Ginkgo biloba* extract. Journal of Pharmacy & Pharmacology. 1992;44(1):24-27.

106. Ramassamy C, Naudin B, Christen Y, Clostre F, Costentin J. Prevention by *Ginkgo biloba* extract (EGb 761) and trolox C of the decrease in synaptosomal dopamine or serotonin uptake following incubation. Biochemical Pharmacology. 1992;44(12):2395-401.

107. Brunello N, Racagni G, Clostre F, Drieu K, Braquet P. Effects of an extract of *Ginkgo biloba* on noradrenergic systems of rat cerebral cortex. Pharmacological Research Communications. 1985;17(11):1063-72.

108. Taylor JE. Neuromediator binding to receptors in the rat brain. The effect of chronic administration of *Ginkgo biloba* extract [French]. Presse Medicale. 1986;15(31):1491-93.

109. Ramassamy C, Christen Y, Clostre F, Costentin J. The *Ginkgo biloba* extract, EGb761, increases synaptosomal uptake of 5-hydroxytryptamine: *In-vitro* and *ex-vivo* studies. Journal of Pharmacy & Pharmacology. 1992;44(11):943-45.

110. Bruno C, Cuppini R, Sartini S, Cecchini T, Ambrogini P, Bombardelli E. Regeneration of motor nerves in bilobalide-treated rats. Planta Medica. 1993;59(4):302-07.

111. Ramassamy C, Clostre F, Christen Y, Costentin J. Prevention by a *Ginkgo biloba* extract (GBE 761) of the dopaminergic neurotoxicity of MPTP. Journal of Pharmacy & Pharmacology. 1990;42(11):785-89.

112. Amri H, Ogwuegbu SO, Boujrad N, Drieu K, Papadopoulos V. *In vivo* regulation of peripheral-type benzodiazepine receptor and glucocorticoid synthesis by *Ginkgo biloba* extract EGb 761 and isolated ginkgolides. Endocrinology. 1996;137(12):5707-18.

113. Braquet P, Bourgain RH. Anti-anaphylactic properties of BN52021: A potent platelet activating factor antagonist. Advances in Experimental Medicine and Biology. 1987;215:215-33.

114. Brailowsky S, Montiel T, Medina-Ceja L. Acceleration of functional recovery from motor cortex ablation by two *Ginkgo biloba* extracts in rats. Restorative Neurology and Neuroscience. 1995;8:163-67.

115. Sancesario G, Kreutzberg GW. Stimulation of astrocytes affects cytotoxic brain edema. Acta Neuropathologica. 1986;72(1):3-14.

116. Auguet M, Delaflotte S, Hellegouarch A, Clostre F. Pharmacological bases of the vascular impact of *Ginkgo biloba* extract [Review] [French]. Presse Medicale. 1986;15(31):1524-28.

117. Drieu K. Preparation and definition of *Ginkgo biloba* extract [French]. Presse Medicale. 1986;15(31):1455-57.

118. Bruel A, Gardette J, Berrou E, Droy-Lefaix MT, Picard J. Effects of *Ginkgo biloba* extract on glucose transport and glycogen synthesis of cultured smooth muscle cells from pig aorta. Pharmacological Research. 1989;21(4):421-29.

119. Duverger D, DeFeudis FV, Drieu K. Effects of repeated treatments with an extract of *Ginkgo biloba* (EGb 761) on cerebral glucose utilization in the rat: an autoradiographic study. General Pharmacology. 1995;26(6):1375-83.

120. Weitbrecht WU, Jansen W. Primary degenerative dementia: Therapy with *Ginkgo biloba* extract. Placebo-controlled double-blind and comparative study [German]. Fortschritte der Medizin. 1986;104(9):199-202.

121. Halama P, et al. Disturbances in cerebral performance of vascular origin. Randomized, double blind study on the efficacy of *Ginkgo biloba* extract [German]. Fortschritte der Medizin. 1988;106:408-12.

122. Kanowski S, Herrman WM, Stephan K, et.al. Proof of efficacy of the *Ginkgo biloba* special

extract EGb 761 in outpatients suffering from mild to moderate primary degenerative dementia of the Alzheimer type or multi-infarct dementia. Pharmacopsychiatry. 1996;29:47-56.

123. Warburton DM. Clinical psychopharmacology of *Ginkgo biloba* extract [Review] [French]. Presse Medicale. 1986;15(31):1595-604.

124. Hofferberth B. The efficacy of EGb 761 in patients with senile dementia of the Alzheimer type - a double-blind, placebo-controlled study on different levels of investigation. Human Psychopharmacolog.y 1994;9:215-22.

125. Funfgeld EW. A natural and broad spectrum nootropic substance for treatment of SDAT — the *Ginkgo biloba* extract. Progress in Clinical & Biological Research. 1989;317:1247-60.

126. Le Bars PL, Katz MM, Berman N, Turan M, Freedman AM, Schatzberg AF. A placebo-controlled, double-blind, randomized trail of an extract of *Ginkgo biloba* for dementia. Journal of the American Medical Association. 1997;278:1327-32.

127. Le Bars PL, Kieser M, Itil KZ. A 26-week analysis of a double-blind, placebo-controlled trial of the *Ginkgo biloba* extract EGb 761 in dementia. Dement Geriatr Cogn Disord. 2000;11(4):230-37.

128. Wettstein A. Cholinesterase inhibitors and Gingko extracts—are they comparable in the treatment of dementia? Comparison of published placebo-controlled efficacy studies of at least six months' duration. Phytomedicine. 2000;6(6):393-401.

129. Rai GS, Shovlin C, Wesnes KA. A double-blind, placebo controlled study of *Ginkgo biloba* extract ('tanakan') in elderly outpatients with mild to moderate memory impairment. Current Medical Research & Opinion. 1991;12(6):350-55.

130. Allain H, Raoul P, Lieury A, LeCoz F, Gandon JM, d'Arbigny P. Effect of two doses of *Ginkgo biloba* extract (EGb 761) on the dual-coding test in elderly subjects. Clinical Therapeutics. 1993;15(3):549-58.

131. Subhan Z, Hindmarch I. The psychopharmacological effects of *Ginkgo biloba* extract in normal healthy volunteers. International Journal of Clinical Pharmacology Research 1984;4(2):89-93.

132. Hindmarch I. Activity of *Ginkgo biloba* extract on short-term memory [French]. Presse Medicale. 1986;15(31):1592-94.

133. Petkov VD, Kehayov R, Belcheva S, Konstantinova E, Petkov V, Getova D, et al. Memory effects of standardized extracts of *Panax ginseng* (G115), *Ginkgo biloba* (GK 501) and their combination Gincosan (PHL-00701). Planta Medica. 1993;59(2):106-14.

134. Semlitsch HV, Anderer P, Saletu B, Binder GA, Decker KA. Cognitive psychophysiology in nootropic drug research: Effects of *Ginkgo biloba* on event-related potentials (P300) in age-associated memory impaiment. Pharmacopsychiatry. 1995;28(4):134-42.

135. Stoll S, Scheuer K, Pohl O, Muller WE. *Ginkgo biloba* extract (EGb 761) independently improves changes in passive avoidance learning and brain membrane fluidity in the aging mouse. Pharmacopsychiatry. 1996;29(4):144-49.

136. Winter E. Effects of an extract of *Ginkgo biloba* on learning and memory in mice. Pharmacology, Biochemistry & Behavior. 1991;38(1):109-14.

137. Rigney U, Kimber S, Hindmarch I. The effects of acute doses of standardized *Ginkgo biloba* extract on memory and psychomotor performance in volunteers. Phytotherapy Research. 1999;13(5):408-15.

138. Kennedy DO, Scholey AB, Wesnes KA. The dose-dependent cognitive effects of acute administration of *Ginkgo biloba* to healthy young volunteers. Psychopharmacology (Berl). 2000;151(4):416-23.

139. Mix JA, Crews WD, Jr. An examination of the efficacy of *Ginkgo biloba* extract EGb761 on the neuropsychologic functioning of cognitively intact older adults. Journal of Alternative and Complementary Medicine. 2000;6(3):219-29.

140. Mix JA, Crews WD, Jr. A double-blind, placebo-controlled, randomized trial of *Ginkgo biloba* extract EGb 761 in a sample of cognitively intact older adults: neuropsychological findings. Hum Psychopharmacol. 2002;17(6):267-77.

141. Kennedy DO, Scholey AB, Wesnes KA. Modulation of cognition and mood following administration of single doses of *Ginkgo biloba*, ginseng, and a ginkgo/ginseng combination to healthy young adults. Physiol Behav. 2002;75(5):739-51.

142. Porsolt RD, Martin P, Lenegre A, Fromage S, Drieu K. Effects of an extract of *Ginkgo biloba* (EGB 761) on "learned helplessness" and other models of stress in rodents. Pharmacology, Biochemistry & Behavior. 1990;36(4):963-71.

143. Solomon PR, Adams F, Silver A, Zimmer J, DeVeaux R. Ginkgo for memory enhancement: a randomized controlled trial. Journal of the American Medical Association. 2002;288(7):835-40.

144. Wesnes KA, Ward T, McGinty A, Petrini O. The memory enhancing effects of a *Ginkgo biloba/Panax ginseng* combination in healthy middle-aged volunteers. Psychopharmacology (Berl). 2000;152(4):353-61.

145. Scholey AB, Kennedy DO. Acute, dose-dependent cognitive effects of *Ginkgo biloba, Panax ginseng* and their combination in healthy young volunteers: differential interactions with cognitive demand. Hum Psychopharmaco.l 2002;17(1):35-44.

146. Schubert H, Halama P. Depressive episode primarily unresponsive to therapy in elderly patients: Efficacy of *Ginkgo biloba* extract (EGb 761) in combination with antidepressants. Geriatric Forschung. 1993;3:45-53.

147. Lingjaerde O, Foreland AR, Magnusson A. Can winter depression be prevented by *Ginkgo biloba* extract? A placebo- controlled trial. Acta Psychiatr Scand. 1999;100(1):62-66.

148. Rodriguez de Turco EB, Droy-Lefaix MT, Bazan NG. EGb 761 inhibits stress-induced polydipsia in rats. Physiology & Behavior. 1993;53(5):1001-02.

149. White HL, Scates PW, Cooper BR. Extracts of *Ginkgo biloba* leaves inhibit monoamine oxidase. Life Sciences. 1996;58(16):1315-21.

150. Burschka MA, Hassan HA, Reineke T, van Bebber L, Caird DM, Mosges R. Effect of treatment with *Ginkgo biloba* extract EGb 761 (oral) on unilateral idiopathic sudden hearing

loss in a prospective randomized double-blind study of 106 outpatients. Eur Arch Otorhinolaryngol. 2001;258(5):213-19.

151. Reisser CH, Weidauer H. *Ginkgo biloba* extract EGb 761 or pentoxifylline for the treatment of sudden deafness: A randomized, reference-controlled, double-blind study. Acta Otolaryngol. 2001;121(5):579-84.

152. Attella MJ, Hoffman SW, Stasio MJ, Stein DG. *Ginkgo biloba* extract facilitates recovery from penetrating brain injury in adult male rats. Experimental Neurology. 1989;105(1):62-71.

153. Rodriguez de Turco EB, Droy-Lefaix MT, Bazan NG. Decreased electroconvulsive shock-induced diacylglycerols and free fatty acid accumulation in the rat brain by *Ginkgo biloba* extract (EGb 761): selective effect in hippocampus as compared with cerebral cortex. Journal of Neurochemistry. 1993;61(4):1438-44.

154. Zhang XY, Zhou DF, Su JM, Zhang PY. The effect of extract of *Ginkgo biloba* added to haloperidol on superoxide dismutase in inpatients with chronic schizophrenia. J Clin Psychopharmacol. 2001;21(1):85-88.

155. Doly M, Braquet P, Droy MT, Bonhomme B, Vennat JC. Effects of oxygenated free radicals on the electrophysiological activity of the isolated retina of the rat [French]. Journal Francais d Ophtalmologie. 1985;8(3):273-77.

156. Droy-Lefaix MT, Bonhomme B, Doly M. Protective effect of *Ginkgo biloba* extract (EGB 761) on free radical-induced changes in the electroretinogram of isolated rat retina. Drugs Under Experimental & Clinical Research. 1991;17(12):571-74.

157. Apaydin C, Oguz Y, Agar A, Yargicoglu P, Demir N, Aksu G. Visual evoked potentials and optic nerve histopathology in normal and diabetic rats and effect of *Ginkgo biloba* extract. Acta Ophthalmologica. 1993;71(5):623-28.

158. Pritz-Hohmeier S, Chao TI, Krenzlin J, Reichenbach A. Effect of in vivo application of the *Ginkgo biloba* extract EGb 761(Rokan) on the susceptibility of mammalian retinal cells to proteolytic enzymes. Ophthalmic Research. 1994;26(2):80-86.

159. Lebuisson DA, Leroy L, Rigal G. Treatment of senile macular degeneration with *Ginkgo biloba* extract. A preliminary double-blind drug vs. placebo study [French]. Presse Medicale. 1986;15(31):1556-58.

160. Chung HS, Harris A, Kristinsson JK, Ciulla TA, Kagemann C, Ritch R. *Ginkgo biloba* extract increases ocular blood flow velocity. J Ocul Pharmacol Ther. 1999;15(3):233-40.

161. Quaranta L, Bettelli S, Uva M, Semeraro F, Turano R, Gandolfo E. Effect of *Ginkgo biloba* extract on preexisting visual field damage in normal tension glaucoma. Ophthalmology. 2003;110:359-64.

162. Dubreuil C. Therapeutic trial in acute cochlear deafness. A comparative study of *Ginkgo biloba* extract and nicergoline [French]. Presse Medicale. 1986;15(31):1559-61.

163. Meyer B. A multicenter study of tinnitus. Epidemiology and therapy [French]. Annales d Oto Laryngologie et de Chirurgie Cervico Faciale. 1986:Cervico-Faciale.

164. Holgers KM, Axelsson A, Pringle I. Gingko biloba extract for the treatment of tinnitus. Audiology. 1994;33:85-92.

165. Juretzck W. Zusmmenfass und der ergebnisse einer plazebokontrollierten doppelblindstudie zur therapie des tinnitus mit dem ginkgo-extrakt Egb 761: Schwabe Arzneimittel Internal Report 21.7; 1998.

166. Morgenstern C, Biermann E. Ginkgo-spezialextrakt Egb 761 in der behandlung des tinnitus aurium. Fortschr Med. 1997;115:7-11.

167. Ernst E, Stevinson C. *Ginkgo biloba* for tinnitus: a review. Clin Otolaryngol. 1999;24(3):164-67.

168. Drew S, Davies E. Effectiveness of *Ginkgo biloba* in treating tinnitus: Double blind, placebo controlled trial. British Medical Journal. 2001;322(7278):73.

169. Morgenstern C, Biermann E. The efficacy of Ginkgo special extract EGb 761 in patients with tinnitus. Int J Clin Pharmacol Ther. 2002;40(5):188-97.

170. Coles R. Trial of an extract of *Ginkgo biloba* (EGB) for tinnitus and hearing loss [Letter]. Clinical Otolaryngology. 1988;13(6):501-02.

171. Lacour M, Ez-Zaher L, Raymond J. Plasticity mechanisms in vestibular compensation in the cat are improved by an extract of *Ginkgo biloba* (EGb 761). Pharmacology, Biochemistry & Behavior. 1991;40(2):367-79.

172. Yabe T, Chat M, Malherbe E, Vidal PP. Effects of *Ginkgo biloba* extract (EGb 761) on the guinea pig vestibular system. Pharmacology, Biochemistry & Behavior 1992;42(4):595-604.

173. Sikora R, Sohn M, et al. *Ginkgo biloba* extract in the therapy of erectile dysfunction. Journal of Urolog.y 1989;141:Abstract 73.

174. Kang BJ, Lee SJ, Kim MD, Cho MJ. A placebo-controlled, double-blind trial of *Ginkgo biloba* for antidepressant-induced sexual dysfunction. Hum Psychopharmacol. 2002;17(6):279-84.

175. Paick JS, Lee JH. An experimental study of the effect of *Ginkgo biloba* extract on the human and rabbit corpus cavernosus tissue. Journal of Urology. 1996;156(5):1876-80.

176. Emerit I, Oganesian N, Sarkisian T, Arutyunyan R, Pogosian A, Asrian K, et al. Clastogenic factors in the plasma of Chernobyl accident recovery workers: Anticlastogenic effect of *Ginkgo biloba* extract. Radiation Research. 1995;144(2):198-205.

177. Emerit I, Arutyunyan R, Oganesian N, Levy A, Cernjavsky L, Sarkisian T, et al. Radiation-induced clastogenic factors: Anticlastogenic effect of *Ginkgo biloba* extract. Free Radical Biology & Medicine. 1995;18(6):985-91.

178. Dumont E, Petit E, Tarrade T, Nouvelot A. UV-C irradiation-induced peroxidative degradation of microsomal fatty acids: Protection by an extract of Ginko biloba (EGb 761). Free Radical Biology & Medicine. 1992;13(3):197-203.

179. Barth SA, Inselmann G, Engemann R, Heidemann HT. Influences of *Ginkgo biloba* on cyclosporin A induced lipid peroxidation in human liver microsomes in comparison to vitamin E, gluthathione and N-acetylcysteine. Biochemical Pharmacology. 1991;41(10):1521-26.

180. Itokawa H, Totsuka N, Nakahara K, Takeya K, Lepoittevin JP, Asakawa Y. Antitumor principles from *Ginkgo biloba* L. Chemical & Pharmaceutical Bulletin. 1987;35(7):3016-20.

181. Lagrue G, Behar A, Kazandjian M, Rahbar K. Idiopathic cyclic edema. The role of capillary hyperpermeability and its correction by *Ginkgo biloba* extract [French]. Presse Medicale. 1986;15(31):1550-53.

182. Tamborini A, Taurelle R. Value of standardized *Ginkgo biloba* extract (EGb 761) in the management of congestive symptoms of premenstrual syndrome [French]. Revue Francaise de Gynecologie et d Obstetrique. 1993.

183. Hauns B, Haring B, Kohler S, Mross K, Robben-Bathe P, Unger C. Phase II study with 5-fluorouracil and *Ginkgo biloba* extract (GBE 761 ONC) in patients with pancreatic cancer. Arzneimittelforschung. 1999;49(12):1030-34.

184. Lepoittevin JP, Benezra C, Asakawa Y. Allergic contact dermatitis to *Ginkgo biloba* L.: Relationship with urushiol. Archives of Dermatological Research. 1989;281(4):227-30.

185. Mitchell JC, Maibach HI, Guin J. Leaves of *Ginkgo biloba* not allergenic for Toxicodendron-sensitive subjects. Contact Dermatitis. 1981;7(1):47-48.

186. Davydov L, Stirling AL. Stevens-Johnson Syndrome with *Ginkgo biloba*. Journal of Herbal Pharmacotherapy. 2001;1(3):65-69.

187. Rowin J, Lewis SL. Spontaneous bilateral subdural hematomas associated with chronic *Ginkgo biloba* ingestion. Neurology. 1996;46(6):1775-76.

188. Vale S. Subarachnoid haemorrhage associated with *Ginkgo biloba*. Lancet. 1998;352(9121):36.

189. Skogh M. Extracts of *Ginkgo biloba* and bleeding or haemorrhage. Lancet. 1998;352(9134):1145-46.

190. Matthews MK, Jr. Association of *Ginkgo biloba* with intracerebral hemorrhage. Neurology. 1998;50(6):1933-34.

191. Rosenblatt M, Mindel J. Spontaneous hyphema associated with ingestion of *Ginkgo biloba* extract [Letter]. New England Journal of Medicine. 1997;336(15):1108.

192. Wojcicki J, Gawronska-Szklarz B, Bieganowski W, Patalan M, Smulski HK, Samochowiec L, et al. Comparative pharmacokinetics and bioavailability of flavonoid glycosides of *Ginkgo biloba* after a single oral administration of three formulations to healthy volunteers. Materia Medica Polona. 1995;27(4):141-46.

Ginseng (Asian and American/Canadian)

1. Wren R. Potter's New Encyclopedia of Botanical Drugs and Preparations. Saffron Walden: C.W. Daniel Company; 1988.

2. Bradley P. British Herbal Compendium. Bournemouth, UK: The British Herbal Medical Association; 1992.

3. Mills S. Essential Book of Herbal Medicine. London: Penguin Books Limited; 1991.

4. Foster S. American Ginseng: *Panax quinquefolium.*. Austin, TX: American Botanical Association; 1991: Botanical Series No. 308.

5. Foster S. Asian Ginseng: *Panax ginseng*. Austin, TX: American Botanical Council; 1991 1991: Botanical Series No. 303.

6. Shibata S, Tanaka O, Shoji J, Saito H. Chemistry and Pharmacology of Panax. Economic and Medicinal Plant Research. 1985;1:217-84.

7. Leung AY, Foster S. Encyclopedia of Common Natural Ingredients Used in Food, Drugs, and Cosmetics. 2nd ed. Toronto, ON/New York, NY: John Wiley and Sons Inc; 1996.

8. Bahrke MS, Morgan WP. Evaluation of the ergogenic properties of ginseng. Sports Medicine. 1994;18(4):229-48.

9. Baek NI, Kim DS, Lee YH, Park JD, Lee CB, Kim SI. Ginsenoside Rh4, a genuine dammarane glycoside from Korean red ginseng. Planta Medica. 1996;62(1):86-7.

10. Baranov AI. Medicinal uses of ginseng and related plants in the Soviet Union: Recent trends in Soviet literature. Journal of Ethnopharmacology. 1982;6(3):339-53.

11. Murray MT. The Healing Power of Herbs. Rocklin, CA: Prima Publishing; 1992.

12. Tyler VE. Herbs of Choice. The Therapeutic Use of Phytomedicinals. Binghamton, NY: Pharmaceutical Products Press; 1994.

13. Lewis WH. Chapter 15. In: Etkin NL, ed. Plants in Indigenous Medicine and Diet: Biobehavioral Approaches. Bedford Hills, NY: Regrave Publishing; 1986:290-305.

14. Vogler BK, Pittler MH, Ernst E. The efficacy of ginseng. A systematic review of randomised clinical trials. European Journal of Clinical Pharmacology. 1999;55(8):567-75.

15. Chang H-M, But PP-H. Pharmacology and Applications of Chinese Materia Medica. Singapore: World Scientific Press; 1986.

16. Teegarden R. Chinese Tonic Herbs. New York, NY: Japan Publishing Inc; 1985.

17. Bensky D, Gamble A. Chinese Herbal Materia Medica. Seattle, WA: Eastland Press; 1986.

18. Kumar R, Grover SK, Divekar HM, Gupta AK, Shyam R, Srivastava KK. Enhanced thermogenesis in rats by *Panax ginseng*, multivitamins and minerals. Int J Biometeorol. 1996;39(4):187-91.

19. Caso Marasco A, Vargas Ruiz R, Salas Villagomez A, Begona Infante C. Double-blind study of a multivitamin complex supplemented with ginseng extract. Drugs under Experimental and Clinical Research. 1996;22(6):323-29.

20. Avakia EV, Evonuk E. Effects of *Panax ginseng* extract on tissue glycogen and adrenal cholesterol depeletion during prolonged exercise. Planta Medica. 1979;36:43-48.

21. Fulder SJ. Ginseng and the hypothalamic-pituitary control of stress. American Journal of Chinese Medicine. 1981;9:112-18.

22. Wagner H, Norr H, Winterhoff H. Plant adaptogens. Phytomedicine 1994;1:63-76.

23. Hiai S, Yokoyama H, Oura H. Features of ginseng saponin-induced corticosterone secretion. Endocrinol Japan. 1979;26:737-40.

24. Hiai S, Yokoyama H, Oura H, Kawashima Y. Evaluation of corticosterone secretion-inducing effects of ginsenosides and their prosapogenins and sapogenins. Chem Pharm Bull. 1983;31:168-74.

25. Gaffney BT, Hugel HM, Rich PA. The effects of *Eleutherococcus senticosus* and *Panax ginseng* on steroidal hormone indices of stress and lymphocyte subset numbers in endurance athletes. Life Sciences. 2001;70(4):431-42.

26. Popov IM, Goldwag WJ. A review of the properties and clinical effects of ginseng. American Journal of Chinese Medicine. 1973;1(2):263-70.

27. Brekhman II, Dardymov IV. Pharmacological investigation of glycosides from Ginseng and Eleutherococcus. Lloydia. 1969;32(1):46-51.

28. Filaretov AA, Bogdanova TS, Podvigina TT, et al. Role of pituitary-adrenocortical system in body adaptation abilities. Exper Clin Endocrinol. 1988;92:129-36.

29. Martinez B, Staba EJ. The physiological effects of Aralia, Panax and Eleutherococcus on exercised rats. Japan Journal of Pharmacology. 1984;35(2):79-85.

30. Lewis WH, Zenger VE, Lynch RG. No adaptogen response of mice to ginseng and Eleutherococcus infusions. Journal of Ethnopharmacology. 1983;8(2):209-14.

31. Hallstrom C, Fulder S, Carruthers M. Effect of ginseng on the performance of nurses on night duty. Comparat Med East West. 1982;6(4):277-82.

32. Knapik JJ, Wright JE, Welch MJ, et al. The influence of *Panax ginseng* on indices of substrate utilization during repeated exhaustive exercise in man [Abstract]. Federation Proceedings. 1983;42:336.

33. Pieralisi G, Ripari P, Vecchiet L. Effects of a standardized ginseng extract combined with dimethylaminoethanol bitartrate, vitamins, minerals and trace elements on physical performance during exercise. Clin Ther. 1991;13(3):373-82.

34. Van Schepdael P. Les effects dy ginseng G115 sur la capacite physique de sportifs d'endurance. Acta Therapeutica. 1993;19:337-47.

35. Allen JD, McLung J, Nelson AG, Welsch M. Ginseng supplementation does not enhance healthy young adults' peak aerobic exercise performance. Journal of the American College of Nutrition. 1998;17(5):462-66.

36. Ziemba AW, Chmura J, Kaciuba-Uscilko H, Nazar K, Wisnik P, Gawronski W. Ginseng treatment improves psychomotor performance at rest and during graded exercise in young athletes. Int J Sport Nutr. 1999;9(4):371-77.

37. Brekman II, Dardymov IV. New substances of plant origin which increase nonspecific resistance. Ann Rev Pharmacol. 1969;9:419-30.

38. Avakian EV, Sugimoto RB, Taguchi S, et al. Effect of *Panax ginseng* extract on energy metabolism during exercise in rats. Planta Medica. 1984;50:151-4.

39. Brown D. Herbal Prescriptions for Better Health. Rocklin, CA: Prima Publishing; 1996.

40. D'Angelo L, Grimwaldi R, Caravaggi M, et al. A double-blind, placebo-controlled clinical study on the effect of a standardized ginseng extract on psychomotor performance in healthy volunteers. Journal of Ethnopharmacology. 1986;16:15-22.

41. Petkov W. The mechanism of action of *P. ginseng*. Arzeniumittel Forschung. 1961;11:288-95.

42. Samira MMH, Attia MA, Allam M, Elwan O. Effect of standardized ginseng extract G115 on the metabolism and electrical activity of the rabbit's brain. Journal of International Medical Research. 1985;13:342-48.

43. Petkov VD, Kehayov R, Belcheva S, Konstantinova E, Petkov V, Getova D, et al. Memory effects of standardized extracts of *Panax ginseng* (G115), *Ginkgo biloba* (GK 501) and their combination Gincosan (PHL-00701). Planta Medica. 1993;59(2):106-14.

44. Xiao PG, Xing ST, Wang LW. Immunological aspects of Chinese medicinal plants as antiageing drugs [Review]. Journal of Ethnopharmacology. 1993;38(2-3):167-75.

45. Jeong TC, Kim HJ, Park JI, Ha CS, Park JD, Kim SI, et al. Protective effects of red ginseng saponins against carbon tetrachloride-induced hepatotoxicity in Sprague Dawley rats. Planta Medica. 1997;63(2):136-40.

46. Park HJ, Park KM, Rhee MH, Song YB, Choi KJ, Lee JH, et al. Effect of ginsenoside Rb1 on rat liver phosphoproteins induced by carbon tetrachloride. Biological and Pharmaceutical Bulletin. 1996;19(6):834-48.

47. Kim MY, Lee KY, Lee SK. Inductive effect of ginsenoside-Rg1 on tyrosine aminotransferase gene expression in rat primary hepatocyte cultures. Biochem Mol Biol Int. 1994;34(4):845-51.

48. Lin JH, et al. Effects of ginseng on the blood chemistry profile od dexamethasone treated male rats. American Journal of Chinese Medicine. 1995;13:167-172.

49. Oura H, et al. Effect of *Radix ginseng* on serum protein synthesis. Chemical and Pharmaceutical Bulletin. 1972;20:980-86.

50. Oura H, et al. Effect of ginseng on endoplastic reticulum and ribosome. Planta Medica. 1975;28:76-88.

51. Hikino H, Kiso Y, Sanada S, Shoji J. Antihepatotoxic actions of ginsenosides from *Panax ginseng* roots. Planta Medica. 1985;52:62-64.

52. Oh JS, et al. The effect of ginseng on experimental hypertension. Korean Journal of Pharmacology. 1968;4:27-31.

53. Siegel RK. Ginseng and high blood pressure [Letter]. Journal of the American Medical Association. 1980;243:32.

54. Wood WB, Roh BL, White RP. Cardiovascular actions of *Panax ginseng* in dogs. Japanese Journal of Pharmacology. 1964;14:284-94.

55. Lee DC, Lee MO, Kim CY, et al. Effect of ether, ethanol and aqueous extracts of ginseng on cardiovascular functions in dogs. Can J Comparat Med. 1981;45:182-87.

56. Baldwin CA, Anderson LA, Phillipson JD. What pharmacists should know about ginseng. The Pharmaceutical Journal. 1986;November 8:583-86.

57. Han KH, Choe SC, Kim HS, Sohn DW, Nam KY, Oh BH, et al. Effect of red ginseng on blood pressure in patients with essential hypertension and white coat hypertension. American Journal of Chinese Medicine. 1998;26(2):199-209.

58. Caron MF, Hotsko AL, Robertson S, Mandybur L, Kluger J, White CM. Electrocardiographic and hemodynamic effects of *Panax ginseng*. Annals of Pharmacotherapy. 2002;36(5):758-63.

59. Sung J, Han KH, Zo JH, Park HJ, Kim CH, Oh BH. Effects of red ginseng upon vascular endothelial function in patients with essential hypertension. American Journal of Chinese Medicine. 2000;28(2):205-16.

60. Kimura Y, Okuda H, Arichi S. Effects of various ginseng saponins on 5-hydroxytryptamine release and aggregation in human platelets. J Pharm Pharmacol. 1988;40:838-43.

61. Matsuda H, Namba K, Fukuda S, et al. Pharmacological study on *Panax ginseng* C.A.

Meyer. III. Effects of red ginseng on experimental disseminated intrvascular coagulation. (2) Effects of ginsenosides on blood coagulation and fibrinolytic systems. Chem Pharm Bull. 1986;34(3):1153-57.

62. Matsuda H, Namba K, Fukuda S, et al. Pharmacological study on *Panax ginseng* C.A. Meyer. IV. Effects of red ginseng on experimental disseminated intravascular coagulation. (3) Effect of ginsenoside-R_0 on the blood coagulative and fibrinolytic systme. Chemical and Pharmaceutical Bulletin. 1986;34(5):2100-04.

63. Kuo SC, Tenagg CM, Lee JC, Ko FN, Chen SC, Wu TS. Antiplatelet components of *Panax ginseng*. Planta Medica. 1990;56:164-67.

64. Park HJ, Lee JH, Song YB, Park KH. Effects of dietary supplementation of lipophilic fraction from *Panax ginseng* on cGMP and cAMP in rat platelets and on blood coagulation. Biological and Pharmaceutical Bulletin. 1996;19(11):1434-39.

65. Park HJ, Rhee MH, Park KM, Nam KY, Park KH. Effect of non-saponin fraction from *Panax ginseng* on cGMP and thromboxane A2 in human platelet aggregation. Journal of Ethnopharmacology. 1995;49(3):157-62.

66. Toh HT. Improved isolated heart contractility and mitochondrial oxidation after chronic treatment with *Panax ginseng* in rats. American Journal of Chinese Medicine. 1994;22(3-4):275-84.

67. Yamamoto M, et al. Serum HDL-cholesterol-increasing and fatty liver-improving action of *Panax ginseng* in High cholesterol diet-fed rats with clinical effect on hyperlipidemia in man. American Journal of Chinese Medicine. 1983;11:96-101.

68. Chen X. Cardiovascular protection by ginsenosides and their nitric oxide releasing action [Review]. Clinical and Experimental Pharmacology and Physiology. 1996;23(8):728-32.

69. Choi SR, Saji H, Iida Y, Magata Y, Yokoyama A. Ginseng pretreatment protects against transient global cerebral isdhemia in the rat: Measurement of local cerebral glucose utilization by [14C] deoxyglucose autoradiography. Biological and Pharmaceutical Bulletin. 1996;19(4):644-66.

70. Wen TC, Yoshimura H, Matsuda S, Lim JH, Sakanaka M. Ginseng root prevents learning disability and neuronal loss in gerbils with 5-minute forebrain ischemia. Acta Neuropathol. 1996;91(1):15-22.

71. Scaglione F, Cattaneo G, Alessandria M, Cogo R. Efficacy and safety of the standardised Ginseng extract G115 for potentiating vaccination against the in [corrected] [published erratum appears in Drugs Exp Clin Res 1996;22(6):338]. Drugs under Experimental and Clinical Research. 1996;22(2):65-72.

72. See DM, Broumand N, Sahl L, Tilles JG. *In vitro* effects of echinacea and ginseng on natural killer and antibody-dependent cell cytotoxicity in healthy subjects and chronic fatigue syndrome or acqired immunodeficiency syndrome patients. Immunopharmacology 1997;35(3):229-35.

73. Jin R, Wan LL, Mitsuishi T, Sato S, Akuzawa Y, Kodama K, et al. Effect of shi-ka-ron and Chinese herbs on cytokine production of macrophage in immunocompromised mice.

American Journal of Chinese Medicine. 1994;22(3-4):255-66.

74. Akagawa G, Abe S, Tansho S, Uchida K, Yamaguchi H. Protection of C3H/HE J mice from development of *Candida albicans* infection by oral administration of Juzen-taiho-to and its component, *Ginseng radix*: Possible roles of macrophages in the host defense mechanisms. Immunopharmacol Immunotoxicol. 1996;18(1):73-89.

75. Lee YS, Chung IS, Lee IR, Kim KH, Hong WS, Yun YS. Activation of multiple effector pathways of immune system by the antineoplastic immunostimulator acidic polysaccharide ginsan isolatedfron *Panax ginseng*. Anticancer Research. 1997;17(1A):323-31.

76. Liu J, Wang S, Liu H, Yang L, Nan G. Stimulatory effect of saponin from *Panax ginseng* on immune function of lymphocytes in the elderly. Mech Ageing Dev. 1995;83(1):43-53.

77. Tomoda M, Hirabayashi K, Shimizu N, Gonda R, Ohara N, Takada K. Characterization of two novel polysaccharides having immunological activities from the root of *Panax ginseng*. Biological and Pharmaceutical Bulletin.l 1993;16(11):1087-90.

78. Tomoda M, Takeda K, Shimizu N, Gonda R, Ohara N, Takada K, et al. Characterization of two acidic polysaccharides having immunological activities from the root of *Panax ginseng*. Biological and Pharmaceutical Bulletin. 1993;16(1):22-25.

79. Gupta S, et al. Panax: A new mitogen and interferon producer. Clinical Research 1980;28:504A.

80. Jie YH, Cammisuli S, Baggiolini M. Immunomodulatory effects of *Panax ginseng* C.A. Meyer in the mouse. Agents and Actions. 1984;15:386-91.

81. Singh VK, et al. Immunomodulatory activity of *Panax ginseng* extract. Planta Medica. 1984;51:462-65.

82. Yun TK, Yun YS, Han IW. Anti-carcinogenic effect of long-term oral administration of newborn mice exposed to various chemical carcinogens. Cancer Detection and Prevention. 1983;6:515-25.

83. Yeung HW, et al. Immunopharmacology of Chinese medicine. I. Ginseng-induced immunosuppression in virus infected mice. American Journal of Chinese Medicine. 1982;10:44-54.

84. Kang SY, Lee KY, Lee SK. Ginsenoside-Rg1 regulates the induction of tyrosine aminotransferase gene transcription in rat hepatocyte cultures. Biochem Biophys Res Commun. 1994;205(3):1696-701.

85. Yoshimura H, Watanabe K, Ogawa N. Psychotropic effects of ginseng saponins on agonistic behaviour between resident and intruder mice. European Journal of Pharmacology. 1988;146:291-97.

86. Yoshimura H, Watanabe K, Ogawa N. Acute and chronic effects of ginseng saponins on maternal aggression in mice. European Journal of Pharmacology. 1988;150:319-24.

87. Bhattacharya SK, Mitra SK. Anxiolytic activity of *Panax ginseng* roots: An experimental study. Journal of Ethnopharmacology. 1991;34:87-92.

88. Nguyen TT, Matsumoto K, Yamasaki K, Nguyen MD, Nguyen TN, Watanabe H. Effects of majonoside-R2 on pentobarbital sleep and gastric lesion in psychologically stressed mice. Pharmacol Biochem Behav. 1996;53(4):957-63.

89. Mitra SK, Chakraborti A, Bhattacharya SK. Neuropharmacological studies on *Panax ginseng*. Indian J Exp Biol. 1996;34(1):41-47.

90. Kim H-S, Oh K, Park WK, Yamano S, Toki S. Effects of *Panax ginseng* on the development of morphine tolerance and dependence. Korean Journal of Ginseng Science. 1987;11:182-90.

91. Kim H-S, Jang CG, Lee MK. Antinarcotic effects of the standardized ginseng extract G115 on morphine. Planta Medica 1990;56:158-63.

92. Kim HS, Kang JG, Seong YH, Nam KY, Oh KW. Blockade by ginseng total saponin of the development of cocaine induced reverse tolerance and dopamine receptor supersensitivity in mice. Pharmacol Biochem Behav. 1995;50(1):23-27.

93. Tokuyama S, Takahashi M, Kaneto H. The effect of ginseng extract on locomotor sensitization and conditioned place preference induced by methamphetamine and cocaine in mice. Pharmacol Biochem Behav. 1996;54(4):671-76.

94. Kim HS, Kang JG, Rheu HM, Cho DH, Oh KW. Blockade by ginseng total saponin of the development of methamphetamine reverse tolerance and dopamine receptor supersensitivity in mice. Planta Medica. 1995;61(1):22-25.

95. Nishiyama N, Cho SI, Kitagawa I, Saito H. Malonylginsenoside Rb1 potentiates nerve growth factor (NGF)-induced neurite outgrowth of cultured chick embryonic dorsal root ganglia. Biological and Pharmaceutical Bulletin. 1994;17(4):509-13.

96. Okamura N, Kobayashi K, Akaike A, Yagi A. Protective effect of ginseng saponins against impaired brain growth in neonatal rats exposed to ethanol. Biological and Pharmaceutical Bulletin. 1994;17(2):270-74.

97. Abe K, Cho SI, Kitagaw I, Nishiyama N, Saito H. Differential effects of ginsenoside Rb1 and malonylginsenoside Rb1 on long-term potentiation in the dentate gyrus of rats. Brain Res. 1994;649(1-2):7-11.

98. Vuksan V, Sievenpiper J, Wong J, Xu Z, et al. American ginseng qu(*Panax inquefolius* L.) attenuates postprandial glycemia in a time-dependent but not dose-dependent manner in healthy indviduals. The American Journal of Clinical Nutrition. 2001;73(4):753-58.

99. Vuksan V, Stavro M, Sievenpiper JL, Beljan-Zdravkovic U, Leiter L, Josse R, et al. Similar postprandial glycemic reductions with escalation of dose and administration time of American ginseng in type 2 diabetes. Diabetes Care. 2000;23(9):1221-26.

100. Vuksan V, Sievenpiper JL, Koo VY, Francis T, Beljan-Zdravkovic U, Xu Z, et al. American ginseng (*Panax quinquefolius* L) reduces postprandial glycemia in nondiabetic subjects and subjects with type 2 diabetes mellitus. Arch Intern Med. 2000;160(7):1009-13.

101. Vuksan V, Sievenpiper JL, Xu Z, Wong E, Jenkins Al, Beljan-Zdravkovic U, et al. Konjac-Mannan and American ginseng: Emerging alternative therapies for ype 2 diabetes mellitus. Journal of the American College of Nutrition. 2001;20(5):370S-380S.

102. Sievenpiper JL, Arnason JT, Leiter L, Vuksan V. Variable effects of American ginseng: A batch of American ginseng (*Panax quinquefolius* L.) with a depressed ginsenoside profile does not affect postprandial glycemia. European Journal of Clinical Nutrition. 2003;57:243-48.

103. Ng TB, Yeung HW. Hypoglycemic constituents of *Panax ginseng*. Gen Pharmacol. 1985;6:549-52.

104. Konno C, et al. Isolation and hypoglycemic activity of panaxans A,B,C,D, and E, glycans of *Panax ginseng* roots. Planta Medica. 1984;51:4343-6.

105. Waki I, et al. Effects of a hypoglycemic component of ginseng radix on insulin biosynthesis in normal and diabetic animals. J Pharm Dyn. 1982;5:547-44.

106. Oshima Y, Sato K, Hikino H. Isolation and hypoglycemic activity of quinquefolans A, B, C, glycans of *Panax quinquefolium* roots. Journal of Natural Products. 1987;50(2):188-90.

107. Kim C, et al. Influence of ginseng on mating behaviour of male rats. American Journal of Chinese Medicine. 1976;4(2):163-68.

108. Salvati G, Genovesi G, Marcellini L, Paolini P, De Nuccio I, Pepe M, et al. Effects of *Panax ginseng* C.A. Meyer saponins on male fertility. Panminerva Med. 1996;38(4):249-54.

109. Chen X, Lee TJ. Ginsenosides-induced nitric oxide-mediated relaxation of the rabbit corpus cavernosum. British Journal of Pharmacology. 1995;115(1):15-18.

110. Punnonen R, Lukola A. Oestrogen-like effects of ginseng. British Medical Journal. 1980;281:1110.

111. Palmer BV, Montgomery ACV, Monteiro JC. Ginseng and mastalgia [Letter]. British Medical Journal. 1978;1:1284.

112. Koriech OM. Ginseng and mastaglia. British Medical Journal. 1978;1:1556.

113. Ben-Hur E, Fulder S. Effect of *P. ginseng* saponins and *Eletherococcus senticosus* on survival of cultured mammalian cells after ionizing radiation. American Journal of Chinese Medicine. 1981;9:48-56.

114. Yun TK, Shoi SY. A Case controlled study of ginseng intake in cancer. International Journal of Epidemiology. 1990;19(4):871-76.

115. Sato K, Mochizuki M, Saiki I, Yoo YC, Samukawa K, Azuma I. Inhibition of tumor angiogenesis and metastasis by a saponin of *Panax ginseng*, ginsenoside-Rb2. Biological and Pharmaceutical Bulletin. 1994;17(5):635-39.

116. Mochizuki M, Yoo YC, Matsuzawa K, Sato K, Saiki I, Tono-oka S, et al. Inhibitory effect of tumor metastasis in mice by saponins, ginsenoside-Rb2, 20(R)- and 20(S)-ginsenoside-Rg3, of red ginseng. Biological and Pharmaceutical Bulletin. 1995;18(9):1197-202.

117. Tode T, Kikuchi Y, Kita T, Hirata J, Imaizumi E, Nagata I. Inhibitory effects by oral administration of ginsenoside Rh2 on the growth of human ovarian cancer cells in nude mice. J Cancer Res Clin Oncol. 1993;120(1-2):24-26.

118. Lee YN, Lee HY, Chung HY, Kim SI, Lee SK, Park BC, et al. *In vitro* induction of differentiation by ginsenoides in F9 teratocarcinoma cells. Eur J Cancer. 1996;8:1420-28.

119. Yun TK. Experimental and epidemiological evidence of the cancer-preventive effects of *Panax ginseng* C.A. Meyer [Review]. Nutr Rev. 1996;54(11 Pt 2):S71-81.

120. Wiklund IK, Mattsson LA, Lindgren R, Limoni C. Effects of a standardized ginseng extract on quality of life and physiological parameters in symptomatic postmenopausal women: A double- blind, placebo-controlled trial. Swedish Alternative Medicine Group. Int J Clin Pharmacol Res. 1999;19(3):89-99.

121. Cardinal BJ, Engels HJ. Ginseng does not enhance psychological well-being in healthy, young adults: Results of a double-blind, placebo-controlled, randomized clinical trial. J Am Diet Assoc. 2001;101(6):655-60.

122. Ellis JM, Reddy P. Effects of *Panax ginseng* on quality of life. Annals of Pharmacotherapy. 2002;36(3):375-79.

123. Foster S, Chongxi Y. Herbal Emissaries. Bringing Chinese Herbs to the West. Rochester, VT: Healing Arts Press; 1992.

124. Dega H, Laporte JL, Frances C, Herson S, Chosidow O. Ginseng as a cause for Stevens-Johnson syndrome? [Letter] [see Comments]. Lancet. 1996;347(9011):1344.

125. Gonzalez-Seijo JC, Ramos YM, Lastra I. Manic episode and ginseng: report of a possible case [Letter]. Journal of Clinical Psychopharmacology. 1995;15(6):447-48.

126. Ryu SJ, Chien YY. Ginseng-associated cerebral arteritis. Neurology. 1995;45(4):829-30.

127. Faleni R, Soldati F. Ginseng as cause of Stevens-Johnson syndrome? [Letter; Comment]. Lancet. 1996;348(9022):267.

128. Sonnenborn U, Hansel R, De Smit. Adverse Effects of Herbal Drugs. Berlin: Springer; 1992.

129. Siegel RK. Ginseng Abuse Syndrome. Journal of the American Medical Association. 1979;241:1644-45.

130. Stockley I. Drug Interactions. A Sourcebook of Adverse Interactions, Their Mechanisms, Clinical Importance, and Management. 3rd ed. Cambridge, UK: Blackwell Scientific Press; 1994.

131. Shader RI, Greenblat DJ. Phenelzine and the dream machine-ramblings and reflections. J Clin Psychopharmacol. 1985;5(2):65.

132. Shader RI, Greenblatt DJ. Bees, ginseng and MAOIs revisited. J Clin Psychopharmacology. 1988;8(4):235.

133. Jones B, Runikis A. Interaction of Ginseng with Phenelzine. Journal of Clinical Psychopharmacology. 1987;7(3):201-02.

134. Liberti LE, der Marderosian A. Evaluation of commercial ginseng products. Journal of Pharmaceutical Sciences. 1978;67:1487-89.

135. Cui JF, Garle M, Bjorkhem I, Eneroth P. Determination of aglycones of ginsenosides in ginseng preparations sold in Sweden and in urine samples from Swedish athletes consuming ginseng. Scand J Clin Lab Invest. 1996;56(2):151-60.

136. Cui J, Garle M, Eneroth P, I B. What do commercial ginseng preparations contain? Lancet. 1994;344:134.

137. Walker AF. What is in ginseng? [Letter; Comment]. Lancet. 1994;344(8922):619.

138. Watt J, Bottomley MB, Read MTF. Olympic athletics medical experience, Seoul — personal views. British Journal of Sports Medicine. 1989;23(2):76-79.

Ginseng (Siberian)

1. Foster S. Siberian Ginseng: *Eleuthercoccus senticosus*. Austin, TX: American Botanical Council; 1991:7

2. Farnsworth NR, Kinghorn AD, Soejarto D, Waller DP. Siberian ginseng (*Eleutherococcus senticosus*): Current tatus as an adaptogen. In: Wagner H, Hikino H, Farnsworth NR, eds. Economic and Medicinal Plant Research. Orlando, Florida: Academic Press; 1985:155-215.

3. Halstead BW, Hood LL. *Eleutherococcus senticosus* Siberian Ginseng: An Introduction to the Concept of Adaptogenic Medicine. Long Beach, CA: Oriental Healing Arts Institute; 1984:240

4. Leung A, Foster S. Encyclopedia of Common Natural Ingredients Used in Food, Drugs and Cosmetics. 2nd ed. New York, NY: John Wiley and Sons; 1996:649.

5. Tyler VE. Herbs of Choice. The Therapeutic Use of Phytomedicinals. Binghamton, NY: Pharmaceutical Products Press; 1994:209.

6. Brown D. Herbal Prescriptions for Better Health. Rocklin, CA: Prima Publishing; 1996:349.

7. Baldwin CA, Anderson LA, Phillipson JD. What pharmacists should know about ginseng. The Pharmaceutical Journal. 1986;November 8:583-86.

8. Newall CA, Anderson LA, Phillipson JD. Herbal Medicines: A Guide for Health Care Professionals. London: The Pharmaceutical Press; 1996:296.

9. Shibata S, Tanaka O, Shoji J, Saito H. Chemistry and Pharmacology of Panax. Economic and Medicinal Plant Research. 1985;1:217-84.

10. Bahrke MS, Morgan WP. Evaluation of the ergogenic properties of ginseng. Sports Medicine. 1994;18(4):229-48.

11. Fulder S. The drug that builds Russians. New Science. 1980;21:576-79.

12. Brekhman II, Kirillov OI. Effect of eleutherococcus on alarm-phase of stress. Life Sciences. 1969;8(3):113-21.

13. Lewis WH, Zenger VE, Lynch RG. No adaptogen response of mice to ginseng and Eleutherococcus infusions. Journal of Ethnopharmacology. 1983;8(2):209-14.

14. Martinez B, Staba EJ. The physiological effects of Aralia, Panax and Eleutherococcus on excised rats. Japanese Journal of Pharmacology. 1984;35(2):79-85.

15. Asano K, Takahashi T, Miyashita M, et al. Effect of *Eleutherococcus senticosus* extract on human physical working capacity. Planta Medica. 1986;3:175-77.

16. Dowling EA, Redondo DR, Branch JD, et al. Effect of *Eleutherococcus senticosus* on submaximal and maximal exercise performance. Medicine and Sciences in Sports and Exercise. 1996;28(4):482-89.

17. Bohn B, Nebe CT, Birr C. Flow-cytometric studies with *Eleutherococcus senticosus* extract as an immunomodulatory agent. Arzneimittelforschung. 1987;37(10):1193-96.

18. Hikino H, Takahashi M, Otake K, Konno C. Isolation and hypoglycemic activity of eleutherans A, B, C, D, E, F, and G: Gycans of Eleutherococcus senticosus roots. Journal of Natural Products. 1986;49(2):293-97.

19. Medon PJ, Thompson EB, Farnsworth NR. Hypoglycemic effect and toxicity of *Eleutherococcus senticosus* following acute and chronic administration in mice. Chung Kuo Yao Li Hsueh Pao. 1981;2(4):281-85.

20. Yun-Choi HS, Kim J, Lee J. Potential inhibitors of platelet aggregation from plant sources III. Journal of Natural Products. 1987;50:1059-64.

21. Hacker B, Medon PJ. Cytotoxic effects of *Eleutherococcus senticosus* aqueous extracts in combination with N6-(delta 2-isopentenyl)-adenosine and 1-beta-D-arabinofuranosylcytosine against L1210 leukemia cells. Journal of Pharmaceutical Sciences. 1984;73(2):270-72.

22. Ben-Hur E, Fulder S. Effect of P. ginseng saponins and *Eletherococcus senticosus* on survival of cultured mammalian cells after ionizing radiation. American Journal of Chinese Medicine. 1981;9:48-56.

23. Barnanov AI. Medicinal uses of ginseng and related plants in the Soviet Union: Recent trends in the Soviet literature. Journal of Ethnopharmacology. 1982;6:339-53.

24. Koren G, Randor S, Martin S, Danneman D. Maternal ginseng use associated with neonatal androgenization. Journal of the American Medical Association. 1990;264(22):2866.

25. Awang DVC. Maternal use of ginseng and neonatal androgenization [Comment]. Journal of the American Medical Association. 1991;265:1839.

26. Waller DP, Martin AM, Farnsworth NR, Awang DVC. Lack of androgenicity of Siberian ginseng [Letter]. Journal of the American Medical Association. 1992;267(17):2329.

27. Bradley P. British Herbal Compendium. Bournemouth, UK: The British Herbal Medical Association; 1992:239.

28. Medon PJ, Ferguson PW, Watson CF. Effects of *Eleutherococcus senticosus* extracts on hexobarbital metabolism *in vivo* and *in vitro*. Journal of Ethnopharmacology. 1984;10(2):235-41.

29. McRae S. Elevated serum digoxin levels in a patient taking digoxin and Siberian ginseng [see Comments]. Canadian Medical Association Journal. 1996;155(3):293-95.

30. Awang DV. Siberian ginseng toxicity may be case of mistaken identity [Comment]. Canadian Medical Association Journal. 1996;155(9):1237.

Goldenseal

1. Marie Snow J. *Hydrastis canadensis*. The Protocol Journal of Botanical Medicine. 1997;2(2):25-28.

2. Hutchens A. Indian Herbology of North America. Boston, MA: Shambhala Press; 1991:382.

3. Bradley P. British Herbal Compendium. Bournemouth, UK: BHMA; 1992:239.

4. Leung A, Foster S. Encylcopedia of Common Natural Ingredients Used in Food, Drugs and Cosmetics. 2nd ed. New York, NY: John Wiley and Sons; 1996:649.

5. Murray M, J P. *Hydrastis canadensis, Berberis vulgaris, Berberis aquifolium*, and other Berberine-containing Plants. In: Murray M, Pizzorno J, eds. The Textbook of Natural Medicine. Seattle, WA: Bastyr University; 1992.

6. Newall C, Anderson L, Philipson JD. Herbal Medicines: A Guide for Health Care Professionals. London: The Pharmaceutical Press; 1996:296.

7. Gleye J, et al. La canadaline: Nouvel alcaloide d'Hydrastic canadensis. Phytochemistry. 1974;13:675-76.

8. El-Masry S, et al. Colorimetric and spectrophotometric determination of Hydrastsis alkaloids in pharmaceutical preparations. Journal of Pharmaceutical Sciences. 1980;69:597-98.

9. Genest K, Hughes DW. Natural products in Canadian pharmaceuticals iv. *Hydrastis canadensis*. Canadian Journal of Pharmaceutical Science. 1969;4:41-45.

10. Wisniewski W, Furmanczyk Z, Zapasnik M. Determination of hydrastine, hydrastinine and berberine in the liquid extract of hydrastis. Acta Poloniae Pharmaceutica. 1970;27(5):487-91.

11. Mills S. The Essential Book of Herbal Medicine. 2nd ed. London: Penguin; 1991:677.

12. Hoffmann D. Holistic Herbal. Rockport, CA: Element Books; 1996:256.

13. Chevallier A. The Encyclopedia of Medicinal Plants. London: Reader's Digest; 1996:336.

14. Bove M. An Encylopedia of Natural Healing For Children and Infants. New Canaan, CT: Keats; 1996:303.

15. Bergner P. Goldenseal and the common cold: The antibiotic myth. Medical Herbalism. 1996-97;8(4):1-10.

16. Tyler V. The Honest Herbal. 3rd ed. Binghamton, NY: Pharmaceutical Products Press; 1993:375.

17. Nebelkopf E. Herbal therapy in the treatment of drug abuse. International Journal of the Addictions. 1987;22(8):695-717.

18. Crombie J, Nugent T, Tobin T. Inability of goldenseal to interfere with the detection of morphine in urine. Equine Veterinary Science. 1982;Jan/Feb:16-21.

19. Foster S. Goldenseal masking of drug tests. Herbalgram. 1989;21:7.

20. Amin A, Subbaiah T, Abbasi K. Berberine sulphate: Antimicrobial activity, bioassay, and mode of action. Canadian Journal of Microbiology. 1969;15(9):1067-76.

21. Kaneda Y, Torii M, Tanaka T, Aikawa M, et al. *In vitro* effects of berberine sulphate on the growth of *Entamoeba histolytica, Giardia lamblia* and *Trichomonas vaginalis*. Annals of Tropical Medicine and Parasitology. 1991;85:417-25.

22. Mahajan V, Sharma A, Rattan A. Antimycotic activity of berberine sulphate: An alkaloid from an Indian medicinal herb. Sabouraudia. 1982;20:79-81.

23. Subbaiah T, Amin A. Effect of berberine sulphate on Entamoeba histolytica. Nature. 1967;215(100):527-8.

24. Sabir M, Mahajan V, Mohapatra L, Bhide N. Experimental study of the antitrachoma action of berberine. Indian Journal of Medical Research. 1976;64(8):1160-67.

25. Sun D, Courtney H, Beachey E. Berberine sulfate blocks adherence of *Streptococcus pyogenes* to epithelial cells, fibronectin, and hexadecane. Antimicrobial Agents and Chemotherapy. 1988;32(9):1370-74.

26. Rabbani GH, Butler T, Knight J, et al. Randomised controlled trial of berberine sulphate therapy for diarrhoea due to enterotoxigenic *Escherichia coli* and *Vibrio cholerae*. Journal of Infectious Diseases. 1987;155:979-84.

27. Khin-Maung U, Myo-Kin, Nyunt-Nyaunt-Wai, Aye-Kyaw, Tin-U. Clinical trial of berberine in acute watery diarrhoea. British Medical Journal. 1985;291:1601-05.

28. Gupte S. Use of berberine in the treatment of giardiasis. American Journal of Diseases of Children. 1975;129:866.

29. Nishino H, Kitagawa K, Fujiki H, Iwashima A. Berberine sulphate inhibits tumour-promoting activity of telecidin in two stage carcinogenesis on mouse skin. Oncology. 1986;43:131-34.

30. Zhang R, Dougherty D, Rosenblum M. Laboratory studies of berberine used alone and in combination with 1,3-Bis (2-chloroethyl-1-nitrosurea) to treat malignant brain tumours. Chinese Medicine Journal. 1990;103(8):658-65.

31. Swanston-Flatt S, Day C, Bailey C, Flatt P. Evaluation of traditional plant treatments for diabetes: Studies in streptozotocin diabetic mice. Acta Diabetologica Latina. 1989;26(1):51-55.

32. Brinker F. Toxicology of Botanical Medicine. 2nd ed. Portland, OR: National College of Naturopathic Medicine; 1983:141.

33. Murray M. The Healing Power of Herbs. Rocklin, CA: Prima Publishing; 1992:410.

34. De Smet P.A.G.M, Keller K, Hansel R, Chandler R. Adverse Effects of Herbal Drugs. Berlin: Springer-Verlag; 1997:250.

35. Farnsworth N, Bingel A, Cordell G, et al. Potential Value of Plants as Sources of New Antifertility Agents I. Journal of Pharmaceutical Sciences. 1975;64(4):535-98.

36. Murray M, Werbach M. Botanical Influences on Illness. Tarzana, CA: Third Line Press; 1994:344.

Hawthorn

1. Chandler F, ed. Herbs: Everyday Reference for Health Professionals. 1st ed. Ottawa: Canadian Pharmacists' Association; 2000.

2. Barnes J, Anderson L, David Phillipson J. Herbal Medicines. 2nd ed. London: The Pharmaceutical Press; 2002.

3. Pharmacopeia AH. Hawthorn Berry. Santa Cruz, CA: American Herbal Pharmacopeia; 1999:19.

4. Djumilija L. Crataegus oxycantha. Australian Journal of Medical Herbalism. 1994;6(2):37-42.

5. Mills S, Bone K. Practice and Practice of Modern Phytotherapy. London: Churchill Livingstone; 2000.

6. Pharmacopeia AH. Hawthorn Leaf and Flower. Santa Cruz, CA: American Herbal Pharmacopeia; 1999:19.

7. Stelling K. Crataegus — Hawthorn. Canadian Journal of Herbalism 1993;xiv(iii):11-17.

8. Rigelsky J, Sweet B. Hawthorn: Pharmacology and therapeutic uses. American Journal of Health-Systems Pharmacy. 2002;59(5):417-22.

9. Holubarsch C, Colucci W, Meinertz T, Gaus W, Tendera M. Survival and prognosis: Investigation of crataegus extract WS 1442 in congestive heart failure. European Journal of Heart Failure. 2000;2(4):431-37.

10. Naturalstandard. Hawthorn: Naturalstandard; 2002.

11. Morelli V, Zoorob R. Alternative Therapies: Part II. Congestive Heart Failure and Hypercholesteremia. American Family Physician. 2000;62(6):1325-26.

12. Zapatero J. Selections from current literature: effects of hawthorn on the cardiovascular system. Family Practice. 1999;16:534-38.

13. Fong H, Bauman J. Hawthorn. Journal of Cardiovascular Nursing 2002;16(4):1-8.

14. Weihmayr T, Ernst E. Die therapeutische wirksamkeit von Crataegus. Forschr Med. 1996;114:27-29.

15. Pittler M, Schmidt K, Ernst E. Hawthorn extract for treating chronic heart failure: meta-analysis of randomised trials. American journal of Medicine. 2003;114(8):665-74.

16. Chang Q, Zuo Z, Harrison F, Chow M. Hawthorn. Journal of Clinical Pharmacology. 2002;42(6):605-12.

17. Zhang Z, Ho W, Huang Y, James A, Lam L, Chen Z. Hawthorn fruit is hypolipidemic in rabbits fed a high cholesterol diet. Journal of Nutrition. 2002;132(1):5-10.

18. Walker A, Marakis G, Morris A, Robinson P. Promising hypotensive effect of hawthorn extract: A randomized double-blind pilot study of mild, essential hypertension. Phytotherapy Research. 2002;16(1):48-54.

19. Ammon H, Handel M. Crataegus, toxicology and pharmacology. Part I: Toxicity. Planta Medica. 1981;43:105-20.

20. Ammon H, Handel M. Crataegus, toxicology and pharmacology. Part II: Pharmacodynamics. Planta Medica. 1981;43:209-39.

21. Ammon H, Handel M. Crataegus, toxicology and pharmacology. Part III: Pharmacodynamics and Pharmacokinetics. Planta Medica. 1981;43:313-22.

22. Bradley P, ed. British Herbal Compendium. Bournemouth: British Herbal Medical Association; 1992.

23. Ernst E, ed. The Desktop Guide to Complementary and Alternative Medicine. London: Mosby; 2001:444.

Hops

1. Bradley P. British Herbal Compendium. Bournemouth, UK: BHMA; 1992:239.

2. Leung A, Foster S. Encylcopedia of Common Natural Ingredients Used in Food, Drugs and Cosmetics. 2nd ed. New York, NY: John Wiley and Sons; 1996:649.

3. Newall C, Anderson L, Philipson JD. Herbal Medicines: A Guide for Health Care Professionals. London: The Pharmaceutical Press; 1996:296.

4. Weiss R. Herbal Medicine. 6th ed. Gothenburg, Sweden: AB Arcanum; 1988:362.

5. Mills S. The Essential Book of Herbal Medicine. 2nd ed. London: Penguin; 1991:677.

6. Wren R. Potter's New Encyclopaedia of Botanical Drugs and Preparations. Saffron Walden: C.W Daniel Company; 1988:362.

7. Hansel R, et al. The sedative-hypnotic principle of hops. 3. Communication: Contents of 2-methyl-3-butene-2-ol in hops and hop preparations. Planta Medica. 1982;45:224-28.

8. Fenselau C, Talalay P. Is oestrogenic activity present in hops? Food Cosmetics and Toxicology. 1973;11:597-603.

9. Tyler V. Herbs of Choice.The Therapeutic Use of Phytomedicinals. Binghampton, NY: Pharmaceutical Products Press; 1994:208.

10. Wohlfart R, Wurm R, Hansel R, Schmidt H.Nachweis sedativ-hypnotischer wirkstofe im hopfen, 5. mitt. Der abbau der bitterssauren zum 2-methyl-3-buten-2-ol, einem hopfeninhaltsstoff mit sedative-hypnotischer wirkung. Archiv der Pharmazie. 1983;316(2):132-37.

11. Hoffmann D. Holistic Herbal. Rockport, CA: Element Books; 1996:256.

12. Chevallier A. The Encyclopedia of Medicinal Plants. London: Reader's Digest; 1996:336.

13. Bove M. An Encyclopedia of Natural Healing for Children and Infants. New Canaan, CT: Keats; 1996:303.

14. Langezaal CR, Chandra A, Scheffer JJ. Antimicrobial screening of essential oils and extracts of some *Humulus lupulus* L. cultivars. Pharmaceutisch Weekblad. 1992;14(6):353-56.

15. Schmalreck AF, Teuber M. Structural features determining the antibiotic potencies of natural and synthetic hop bitter resins, their precursors and derivatives. Canadian Journal of Microbiology. 1975;21:205-12.

16. Mizobuchi S, Sato Y. Antifungal activities of hop bitter resins and related compounds. Agric Biol Chem. 1985;49:399-405.

17. Hansel R, Wohlfart R. Narcotic action of 2-methyl-3-butene-2-ol contained in the exhalation of hops. Zeitschrift fur Naturforschung. 1980;35(11-12):1096-97.

18. Wohlfart R, Hansel R, Schmidt H. The sedative-hypnotoc principle of hops. 4. Communication: Pharmacology of 2-methyl-3-buten-2-ol. Planta Medica. 1983;48:120-23.

19. Muller-Limmroth W, Ehrenstein W. Experimental studies of the effects of Seda-Kneipp on the sleep of sleep disturbed subjects; implications for the treatment of different sleep disturbances. Medizinische Klinik. 1977;72(25):1119-25.

20. Gerhard U, Linnenbrink N, Georghaidou C, Hobi V. Vigilance-decreasing effects of 2 plant-derived sedatives. Schweizerische Rundschau fur Medizin Praxis. 1996;85(15):473-81.

21. Houghton P. Valerian. Pharmaceutical Journal. 1994;253:95-96.

22. Hobbs C. Valerian. Herbalgram. 1989;21:19-34.

23. Mannering GJ, Shoeman JA, Deloria LB. Identification of the antibiotic hops component, colupulone, as an inducer of hepatic cytochrome P-4503A in the mouse. Drug Metabolism and Disposition. 1992;20(2):142-47.

24. Mannering GJ, Shoeman JA, Shoeman DW. Effects of colupulone, a component of hops and brewer's yeast, and chromium on glucose tolerance and hepatic cytochrome P450 in ondiabetic and spontaneously diabetic mice.

Biochemical and Biophysical Research Communications. 1994;200(3):1455-62.

25. Mannering GJ, Shoeman JA. Murine cytochrome P4503A is induced by 2-methyl-3-buten-2-ol, 3-methyl-1-penyn-3-ol (meparfynol), and tert-amyl alcohol). Xenobiotica. 1996;26(5):487-93.

26. Shipp E, Mehigh C, Helferich W. The effect of colupulone (a HOPS beta-acid) on hepatic cytochrome P-450enzymatic activity in the rat. Food and Chemical Toxicology. 1994;32(11):1007-14.

27. Yasukawa K, Yamaguchi A, Arita J, et al. Inhibitory effect of edible plant extracts on 12-O-tetradecanoylphorbol-13-acetate-induced ear oedema in mice. Phytotherapy Research. 1993;7:185-89.

28. Yasukawa K, Takeuchi M, Takido M. Humulon, a bitter in the hop, inhibits tumor promotion by 12-O-tetradecanoylphorbol-13-acetate in two stage carcinogenesis in mouse skin. Oncology. 1995;52(2):156-58.

29. Goetz P. Traitement des bouffees de chaleur par insuffisance ovarienne par l'extrait de houblon (Humuluslupulus). Rev. Phytother Prat. 1990;December(4):13-15.

30. O'Donovan W. Hops dermatitis. Lancet. 1924;2:597.

31. Newmark FM. Hops allergy and terepene sensitivity: An occupational disease. Annals of Allergy. 1978;41:311-12.

Horsechestnut

1. Barnes J, Anderson L, David Phillipson J. Herbal Medicines. 2nd ed. London: The Pharmaceutical Press; 2002.

2. Mills S, Bone K. Practice and Practice of Modern Phytotherapy. London: Churchill Livingstone; 2000:643.

3. Ernst E, ed. The Desktop Guide to Complementary and Alternative Medicine. London: Mosby; 2001:444.

4. Leung A, Foster S. Encyclopedia of Common Natural Ingredients Used in Food, Drugs and Cosmetics. 2nd ed. NY: John Wiley and Sons; 1996.

5. Ulbricht C, Tiffany N, Boon H, Smith M, Basch E. Horsechestnut: A multidisciplinary clinical review. Journal of Herbal Pharmacotherapy. 2002;2(1):71-85.

6. Brunner F, Hoffmann C, Schuller-Petrovic S. Responsiveness of human varicose saphenous veins to vasoactive agents. British Journal of Clinical Pharmacology. 2001;51(3):219-24.

7. Kreysel H. A possible role of lysosomal enzymes in the pathogenesis of varicosis and the reduction in their serum activity by Venostatin. Vasa. 1983;112:377-82.

8. Schulz V, Hansel R, Tyler V. Rational Phytotherapy: A Physicians Guide to Herbal Medicine. Berlin: Springer Verlag; 1998.

9. Diehm C, Trampisch H, Lange S, Schmidt C. Comparison of leg compression stocking and oral horse chestnut seed extract therapy in patients with chronic venous insufficiency. Lancet. 1996;347:593-96.

10. Pittler M, Ernst E. Horse-Chestnut seed extract for chronic venous insufficiency. A criteria based systematic review. Archives of Dermatology. 1998;134(11):1356-60.

11. Calabrese C, Preston P. Report of the results of a double-blind, randomised, single dose trial of a topical 2% escin gel versus placebo in the acute treatment of experimentally induced hematoma in volunteers. Planta Medica. 1993;59(5):394-97.

12. Williams M, Olsen J. Toxicity of seeds of three Aesculus spp. to chicks and hamsters. American Journal of Veterinary Research. 1984;45(3):539-42.

13. Greeske K, Pohlman B. Horse Chestnut seed extract — an effective therapy principle in general practice. Fortchr Med. 1996;114(15):196-200.

14. Comaish J, Kersey P. Contact dermatitis to extract of horse chestnut (esculin). Contact Dermatitis. 1980;6(2):150-51.

15. Rehn D, Unkauf M, Klein P, Jost V, Lucker P. Comparative clinical efficacy and tolerability of oxerutins and horsechestnut extract in patients with chronic venous insufficiency. Arzeimittelforschung. 1996;46(5):483-7.

16. DeSmet P, van den Eertwegh A, Lesterhuis W, Stricker B. Hepatotoxicty associated with herbal tablets. British Medical Journal. 1996;313:92.

17. Grazzo A, Corvaglia E. Two cases of suspected toxic tubulonephrosis due to escine. Gazz Med Ital. 1976;135:581-84.

18. Takegoshi K. A case of venoplant-induced hepatic injury. Gastroenterol Japonica. 1986;21:62-65.

Juniper

1. Hutchens A. Indian Herbology of North America. Boston, MA: Shambhala Press; 1991:382.

2. Newall C, Anderson L, Philipson JD. Herbal Medicines: A Guide for Health Care Professionals. London: The Pharmaceutical Press; 1996:296.

3. Leung A, Foster S. Encyclopedia of Common Natural Ingredients Used in Food, Drugs and Cosmetics. 2nd ed. New York, NY: John Wiley and Sons; 1996:649.

4. Evans W. Trease and Evan's Pharmacognosy. 13th ed. London: Bailliere Tindall; 1989:832.

5. Bergner P. Juniper berries. Medical Herbalism. 1994;6(2):13.

6. Tyler V. The Honest Herbal. 3rd ed. Binghamton, NY: Pharmaceutical Products Press; 1993:375.

7. Thomas AF, Ozainne M. 'Junionone' {1-(2,2-Dimethylcyclobutyl)but-1-2en-3-one], the first vegetable monocyclic cyclobutane monoterpenoid. J C S Chem Comm. 1973:746.

8. Chandler RF. An inconspicuous but insidious drug. Rev Pharm Can. 1986:563-6.

9. Friedrich H, Engelshowe R. Tannin producing monomeric substances in *Juniperus communis*. Planta Medica. 1978;33:251-57.

10. Wren R. Potter's New Encyclopaedia of Botanical Drugs and Preparations. Saffron Walden: C.W. Daniel Company; 1988:362.

11. Hoffmann D. Holistic Herbal. Rockport, CA: Element Books; 1996:256.

12. Weiss R. Herbal Medicine. 6th ed. Gothenburg, Sweden: AB Arcanum; 1988:362.

13. Mills S. The Essential Book of Herbal Medicine. 2nd ed. London: Penguin; 1991:677.

14. Chevallier A. The Encyclopedia of Medicinal Plants. London: Reader's Digest; 1996:336.

15. Sanchez de Medina F, Gamez M, Jimenez I, et al. Hypoglycemic activity of juniper "berries". Planta Medica. 1994;60(3):197-200.

16. Swanston-Flatt S, Day C, Bailey C, Flatt P. Traditional plant treatments for diabetes. Studies in normal and streptozotocin mice. Diabetologia. 1990;33(8):462-64.

17. Mascolo N, et al. Biological screening of Italian medicinal plants for anti-inflammatory activity. Phytotherapy Research. 1987;1:28-31.

18. Mathias CG, Maibach HI, Mitchell JC. Plant dermatitis-patch test results (1975-78). Note on Juniperus extract. Contact Dermatitis. 1979;5:336-37.

19. Tyler V. Herb's of Choice.The Therapeutic Use of Phytomedicinals. Binghampton, NY: Pharmaceutical Products Press; 1994:208.

20. Schilcher H, Heil BM. Nephrotoxicity of juniper berry preparations: A critical review of the literature from 1844 to 1993. Zeitschrift fur Phytother. 1994;15:203-13.

21. Bone K. Juniper berry is not a kidney irritant. Medical Herbalism. 1994;6(2):12.

22. Farnsworth N, Bingel A, Cordell G, et al. Potential value of plants as sources of new antifertility agents I. Journal of Pharmaceutical Sciences. 1975;64(4):535-98.

Kava

1. Leung AY, Foster S. Encyclopedia of Common Natural Ingredients Used in Food, Drugs, and Cosmetics. 2nd ed. Toronto, ON/New York, NY: John Wiley and Sons Inc; 1996.

2. Wren RC. Potter's New Encyclopaedia of Botanical Drugs and Preparations. Saffron Waldon, UK: C.W. Daniel Company; 1988.

3. Singh Y, Blumenthal M. Kava: an overview. Herbalgram. 1997;39:34-54.

4. Bone K. A safe herbal treatment for anxiety. British Journal of Phytotherapy. 1993/94;3(4):147-53.

5. Brown D. Herbal Prescriptions for Better Health. Rocklin, CA: Prima Publishing; 1995.

6. Hansel R. (translated by A. Clay and R. Reichert). Kava-kava in modern drug research: Portrait of a medicinal plant. Quarterly Review of Natural Medicine. 1996;4(4):259-274.

7. Farnsworth N. NAPRALERT natural product computer database. In: University of Illinois at Chicago program for Collaborative Research in the Pharmaceutical Sciences. Chicago; 1998.

8. Chevallier A. The Encyclopedia of Medicinal Plants. Westmount, QC: Readers Digest; 1996.

9. Pittler MH, Ernst E. Efficacy of kava extract for treating anxiety: Systematic review and meta-analysis. Journal of Clinical Psychopharmacology. 2000;20(1):84-89.

10. Blumenthal M, et al. The Complete German Commission E Monographs: Therapeutic Guide to Herbal Medicine. Austin, TX: American Botanical Council; 1998.

11. Mills S. Essential Book of Herbal Medicine. London: Penguin Books Limited; 1991.

12. Duke J. The Green Pharmacy. New York, NY: Rodale Press Inc.; 1997.

13. Jussofie A, Schmiz A, Hiemke C. Kavapyrone enriched extract from *Piper methysticum* as modulator of the GABA binding site in different regions of rat brain. Psychopharmacology (Berl). 1994;116(4):469-74.

14. Davies LP, Drew CA, Duffield P, Johnston GA, Jamieson DD. Kava pyrones and resin: studies on GABAA, GABAB and benzodiazepine binding sites in rodent brain. Pharmacology and Toxicology 1992;71(2):120-26.

15. Reichling J, Saller R. Quality control in the manufacturing of modern herbal remedies. Quarterly Review of Natural Medicine. 1998;6(1):21-28.

16. Schulz V, Hansel R, Tyler V. Rational Phytotherapy: A Physician's Guide to Herbal Medicine. Berlin: Springer-Verlag; 1998.

17. Backhauss C, Krieglstein J. Extract of kava (*Piper methysticum*) and its methysticin constituents protect brain tissue against ischemic damage in rodents. Eur J Pharmacol. 1992;215(2-3):265-69.

18. Gebner B, Cnota P. Extract of Kava-kava rhizome in comparison with diazepam and placebo. Zeitschrift fur Phytother. 1994;15:30-37.

19. Glietz J, Beile A, Peters T. Kawain inhibits vetradine-activated voltage-dependent Na+ channels in synaptosomes prepared from rat cerebral cortex. Neuropharmacology. 1995;24:1133-38.

20. Kretzschmar R, Meyer HJ. Comparative studies on the anticonvulsant activity of the pyrone compounds of *Piper methysticum* Forst [German]. Arch Int Pharmacodyn Ther. 1969;177(2):261-67.

21. Kretzschmar R, Meyer HJ, Teschendorf HJ, Zollner B. Antagonistic action of natural 5,6-hydrogenated Kava pyrones against strychnine poisoning and experimental local tetanus [German]. Arch Int Pharmacodyn Ther. 1969;182(2):251-68.

22. Meyer HJ, Kretzschmar R. Studies on the relations between molecular structure and pharmacological effect of C6-aryl-substituted 4-methoxy-alpha-pyrones of the kawa-pyrone type [German]. Arzneimittelforschung. 1969;19(4):617-23.

23. Duffield PH, Jamieson DD, Duffield AM. Effect of aqueous and lipid-soluble extracts of kava on the conditioned avoidance response in rats. Arch Int Pharmacodyn Ther. 1989;301:81-90.

24. Lehmann E, Kinzler E, Friedmann J. Efficacy of a special Kava extract (*Piper methysticum*) in patients with states of anxiety, tension and excitedness of non-mental origin: A double-blind placebo-controlled study of four weeks treatment. Phytomedicine. 1996;III(2):113-19.

25. Connor KM, Davidson JR. A placebo-controlled study of Kava kava in generalized anxiety disorder. Int Clin Psychopharmacol. 2002;17(4):185-88.

26. Schulz V, Hubner W, Ploch M. Clinical trials with phyto-psychopharmacological agents. Phytomedicine. 1997;4(4):379-87.

27. Wooltorton E. Herbal kava: Reports of liver toxicity. Canadian Medical Association Journal. 2002;166(6):777.

28. Health Canada. Advisory: Health Canada issues a stop-sale order for all products containing kava. In.: http://www.hc-sc.gc.ca/english/protection/warnings/2002/2002_56e.html; 2002.

29. Escher M, Desmeules J, Giostra E, Mentha G. Hepatitis associated with Kava, a herbal remedy for anxiety. British Medical Association Journal. 2001;322(7279):139.

30. Brauer RB, Stangl M, Stewart JR, Pfab R, Becker K. Acute liver failure after administration of herbal tranquilizer kava-kava (*Piper methysticum*). J Clin Psychiatry. 2003;64(2):216-18.

31. Ernst E. Cave kava? Focus on Alternative and Complementary Therapies. 2002;7(4):323-24.

32. Schmidt P, Boehncke WH. Delayed-type hypersensitivity reaction to kava-kava extract. Contact Dermatitis. 2000;42(6):363-64.

33. Munte TF, Heinze HJ, Matzke M, Steitz J. Effects of oxazepam and an extract of kava roots (*Piper methysticum*) on event-related potentials in a word recognition task. Neuropsychobiology. 1993;27(1):46-53.

34. Schelosky L, Raffauf C, Jendroska K, Poewe W. Kava and dopamine antagonism. J Neurol Neurosurg Psychiatry. 1995;58(5):639-40.

35. Brinker F. Herb Contraindications and Drug Interactions. 3rd ed. Sandy, OR: Eclectic Medical Publishers; 2001.

36. Herberg KW. Effect of Kava-Special Extract WS 1490 combined with ethyl alcohol on safety-relevant performance parameters [German]. Blutalkohol. 1993;30(2):96-105.

37. Almeida JC, Grimsley EW. Coma from the health food store: interaction between kava and alprazolam. Ann Intern Med. 1996;125(11):940-41.

Lemon Balm

1. Mills S. The Essential Book of Herbal Medicine. 2nd ed. London: Penguin Publ; 1991.

2. Leung AY, Foster S. Encyclopedia of Common Natural Ingredients Used in Food, Drugs, and Cosmetics. 2nd ed. Toronto/New York: John Wiley and Sons Inc; 1996.

3. Wren R. Potter's New Encyclopaedia of Botanical Drugs and Preparations. Saffron Walden: C.W Daniel Company; 1988.

4. Bove M. An Encylopedia of Natural Healing for Children and Infants. New Canaan, CT: Keats; 1996.

5. Mulkens A. Flavonoids of the leaves of *Melissa officianalis* L. Pharmaceutica Acta Helvetiae 1987;62(1):19-22.

6. Weiss R. Herbal Medicine. 6th ed. Gothenburg, Sweden: AB Arcanum; 1988.

7. Hoffmann D. Holistic Herbal. Rockport, CA: Element Books; 1996.

8. Chevalier A. The Encyclopedia of Medicinal Plants. London: Reader's Digest; 1996.

9. Koytchev R, Alken RG, Dundarov S. Balm mint extract (Lo-701) for topical treatment of recurring herpes labialis. Phytomedicine. 1999;6(4):225-30.

10. Soulimani R, et al. Neurotropic action of the hydroalcoholi extract of *Melissa officinalis* in the mouse. Planta Medica. 1991;57(2):105-9.

11. Dressing H, Riemann D, et al. Insomnia: Are valerian/balm combination of equal value to benzodiazepine? Therapiewoche. 1992;42:726-36.

12. Albrect M, Berger W, et al. Psychopharmaceuticals and safety in traffic. Zeits Allgemeinmed. 1995;71:1215-21.

13. Larrondo JV, Agut M, M C-T. Antimicrobial activity of essences from labiates. Microbios. 1995;82(332):171-72.

14. Kucera L, Cohen R, Herrmann E. Antiviral activites of extracts of the Lemon balm plant. Annals of the New York Academy of Sciences. 1965;130(1):474-82.

15. Kucera L, E H. Antiviral substances in plants of the mint family (labiatae). I. Tannin of *Melissa officianalis*. Proceedings of the Society for Experimental Biology and Medicine. 1967;124(3):865-69.

16. Wobling R, Leonhardt K. Local therapy of herpes simplex with dried extract from *Melissa officianalis*. Phytomedicine. 1994;1(1):25-31.

17. Dimitrova Z, al. e. Antiherpes effect of *Melissa officianalis* L. extracts. Acta Microbiologica Bulgarica. 1993;29:65-72.

18. Foster S. Clinical Assessment of *Melissa officianalis*(Lemon Balm) in Herpes Treatment. Quarterly Review of Natural Medicine. 1995;3(2):3-5.

19. Auf'mkolk M, et al. Antihormonal effects of plant extracts: Iodothyronine deiodinase of rat liver is inhibited by extracts and secondary metabolites of plants. Hormone and Metabolic Research. 1984;16(4):188-92.

20. Brinker F. Inhibition of endocrine function by botanical agents. Journal of Naturopathic Medicine. 1990;1(1):10-18.

21. Auf'mkolk M, et al. Inhibition by certain plant extracts of the binding and adenylate cyclase stimulatory effect of bovine thyrotropin in human thyroid membranes. Endocrinology. 1984;115(2):527-34.

22. Auf'mkolk M, Ingbar J, Kubota K, et al. Extracts and auto-oxidized constituents of certain plants inhibit the receptor-binding and the biological activity of Graves' immunoglobulin. Endocrinology. 1985;116(5):1687-93.

23. Lamaison J, et al. Medicinal Lamiaceae with antioxidant properties, a potential source of rosmarinic acid. Pharmaceutica Acta Helvetiae. 1991;66(7):185-88.

24. Englberger W, et al. Rosmarinic acid: A new inihibitor of complement C3-convertase with anti-inflammatory activity. International Journal of Immunopharmacology. 1988;10(6):729-37.

25. Peake P, et al. The inhibitory effect of rosmarinic acid on complement involves the C5 convertase. International Journal of Immunology. 1991;13(7):853-57.

26. Ramos Ruiz A, De la Toree R, Alonso N, A V, Betancourt J, Vizoso A. Screening of medicinal plants for induction of somatic segregation activity in *Aspergillus nidulans*. Journal of Ethnopharmacology.1996;52(3):123-27.

Licorice

1. Chandler RF. Licorice, more than just a flavour. Canadian Pharmaceutical Journal. 1985;September:421-24.

2. Tyler VE. Herbs of Choice. The Therapeutic Use of Phytomedicinals. Binghamton, NY: Pharmaceutical Products Press; 1994:209.

3. Chandler RF. *Glycyrrhiza glabra*. In: De Smet PAGM, Keller K, Hansel R, Chandler RF, eds. Adverse Effects of Herbal Drugs. Volume 3. New York, NY: Springer; 1997:67-87.

4. Snow JM. *Glycyrrhiza glabra* L. (Leguminaceae). The Protocol Journal of Botanical Medicine. 1996;1(3):9-14.

5. Murray MT. The Healing Power of Herbs. Rocklin, CA: Prima Publishing; 1992:246.

6. Leung A, Foster S. Encyclopedia of Common Natural Ingredients Used in Food, Drugs and Cosmetics. 2nd ed. New York, NY: John Wiley and Sons; 1996:649.

7. Foster S, Chongxi Y. Herbal Emissaries. Bringing Chinese Herbs to the West. Rochester, VT: Healing Arts Press; 1992:356.

8. Mizutani K, Kuramoto T, Tamura Y, et al. Sweetness of glycyrrhetic acid 3-O-beta-D-monoglucuronide and the related glycosides. Bioscience, Biotechnology and Biochemistry. 1994;58(3):554-55.

9. Spinks EA, Fenwick GR. The determination of glycyrrhizin in selected UK liquorice products. Food Additives and Contaminants. 1990;7:769-78.

10. Stormer FC, Reistad R, Alexander J. Glycyrrhizic acid in liquorice — evaluation of health hazard. Food and Chemical Toxicology. 1993;31:303-12.

11. Tyler V. The Honest Herbal. 3rd ed. Binghamton, N.Y.: Pharmaceutical Products Press; 1993:375.

12. Newall CA, Anderson LA, Phillipson JD. Herbal Medicines: A Guide for Health Care Professionals. London: The Pharmaceutical Press; 1996:296.

13. Kitagawa I, Chen WZ, Hori K, et al. Chemical studies of Chinese licorice-roots. I. Elucidation of five new flavonoid constituents from the roots of *Glycyrrhiza glabra* L. collected in Xinjiang. Chemical and Pharmaceutical Bulletin (Tokyo).1994;42(5):1056-62.

14. Walker BR, Edwards CR. Licorice-induced hypertension and syndromes of apparent mineralocorticoid excess. Endocrinology and Metabolism Clinics of North America. 1994;23(2):359-77.

15. Shimojo M, Stewart PM. Apparent mineralocorticoid excess syndromes. Journal of Endocrinological Investigation. 1995;18(7):518-32.

16. Schambelan M. Licorice ingestion and blood pressure regulating hormones. Steroids. 1994;59(2):127-30.

17. Biglieri EG. My engagement with steroids: A review. Steroids. 1995;60(1):52-58.

18. White PC, Mune T, Agarwal AK. 11 beta-Hydroxysteroid dehydrogenase and the syndrome of apparent mineralocorticoid excess. Endocrine Reveiws. 1997;18(1):135-56.

19. Stewart PM, Wallace AM, Valentino R, et al. Mineralcorticoid activity of liquoirce: 11-Beta-hydroxysteroid dehydrogenase deficiency comes of age. Lancet. 1987;II:821-24.

20. Armanini D, Lewicka S, Pratesi C, et al. Further studies on the mechanism of the mineralocorticoid action of licorice in humans. Journal of Endocrinological Investigation. 1996;19(9):624-29.

21. Armanini D, Karbowiak I, Funder J. Affinity of glycyrrhetinic acid and its derivatives for mineralocorticoid and glucocorticoid receptors. Clinical Endocrinology. 1983;19:609-12.

22. Epstein M, Espiner E, Donald R, Hughes H. Effect of eating liquorice on the renin-angiotensin

aldosterone axis in normal subjects. British Medical Journal. 1977;1:488-90.

23. Conn J, Rovner D, Cohen EL. Licorice-induced pseudoaldosteronism. Hypertension, hypokalaemia, aldosteroneopenia, and suppressed plasma renin activity. Journal of the American Medical Association. 1968;205:492-96.

24. Forslund T, Fyhrquist F, Froseth B, Tikkanen I. Effects of licorice on plasma atrial natriuretic peptide in healthy volunteers. Journal of Internal Medicine. 1989;225:95-99.

25. Krahenbuhl S, Hasler F, Frey BM, et al. Kinetics and dynamics of orally administered 18 beta-glycyrrhetinic acidin humans. Journal of Clinical Endocrinology and Metabolism. 1994;78(3):581-85.

26. Cantelli-Forti G, Maffei F, Hrelia P, et al. Interaction of licorice on glycyrrhizin pharmacokinetics. Environmental Health Perspectives. 1994;102(Suppl 9):65-68.

27. Raggi MA, Maffei F, Bugamelli F, Cantelli Forti G. Bioavailability of glycyrrhizin and licorice extract in rat and human plasma as detected by a HPLC method. Pharmazie. 1994;49(4):269-72.

28. Wang Z, Nishioka M, Kurosaki Y, et al. Gastrointestinal absorption characteristics of glycyrrhizin from glycyrrhiza extract. Biological and Pharmaceutical Bulletin. 1995;18(9):1238-41.

29. Nishioka Y, Kyotani S, Miyamura M, Kusunose M. Influence of time of administration of a Shosaiko-to extract granule on blood concentrations of its active constituents. Chemical and Pharmaceutical Bulletin. 1992;40:1335-37.

30. Ichikawa T, Ishida S, Sakiya Y, et al. Biliary excretion and enterohepatic cycling of glycyrrhizin in rats. Journal of Pharmaceutical Science. 1986;75:672-75.

31. Baker ME. Licorice and enzymes other than 11 beta-hydroxysteroid dehydrogenase: an evolutionary perspective. Steroids. 1994;59(2):136-41.

32. Morgan AG, McAdam WAF, Pacsoo C, Darnborough A. Comparison between cimetidine and Caved-S in the treatment of gastric ulceration, and subsequent maintenance therapy. Gut. 1982;23:545-51.

33. Glick L. Deglycyrrhizinated liquorice for peptic ulcer. Lancet. 1982;2:817.

34. Tewari SN, Wilson AK. Deglycyrrhizinated liquorice in duodenal ulcer. Practitioner. 1972;210:820-25.

35. Kassir ZA. Endoscopic controlled trial of four drug regimens in the treatment of chronic duodenal ulceration. Irish Medical Journal. 1985;78:153-56.

36. Pompei R, Pani A, Flore O, et al. Antiviral activity of glycyrrhizic acid. Experientia. 1980;36:304-05.

37. Utsunomiya T, Kobayashi M, Pollard RB, Suzuki F. Glycyrrhizin, an active component of licorice roots, reduces morbidity and mortality of mice infected with lethal doses of influenza virus. Antimicrobial Agents and Chemotherapy. 1997;41(3):551-56.

38. Hirabayashi K, Iwata S, Matsumoto H, et al. Antiviral activities of glycyrrhizin and its modified compounds against human immunodeficiency virus type 1 (HIV-1) and Herpes simplex virus type 1 (HSV-1) *in vitro*.

Chemical and Pharmaceutical Bulletin. 1991;39:112-15.

39. Dargan DJ, Subak-Sharpe JH. The effect of triterpenoid compounds on uninfected and herpes simplex virus-infected cells in culture. I. Effect on cell growth, virus particles and virus replication. Journal of General Virology. 1985;66:1771-84.

40. Baba M, Shigeta S. Antiviral activity of glycyrrhizin against *Varicella zoster virus in vitro*. Antiviral Research. 1987;7:999-107.

41. Crance JM, Biziagos E, Passagot J, et al. Inhibition of hepatitis A virus replication in vitro by antiviral compounds. Journal of Medical Virology. 1990;31:155-60.

42. Hattori T, Ikematsu S, Koito A, et al. Preliminary evidence for inhibitory effect of glycyrrhizin on HIV replication in patients with AIDS. Antiviral Research. 1989;11:255-62.

43. Ito M, Sato A, Hirabayashi K, et al. Mechanism of inhibitory effect of glycyrrhizin on replication of human immunodeficiency virus (HIV). Antiviral Research. 1988;10:289-98.

44. Abe N, Ebina T, Ishida N. Interferon induction by glycyrrhizin and glycyrrhetinic acid in mice. Microbiology and Immunology. 1982;26:535-59.

45. Partridge M, Poswillo D. Topical carbonoxolone sodium in the management of herpes simplex infection. British Journal of Oral Maxillofacial Surgery. 1984;22:138-45.

46. Csonka G, Tyrrell D. Treatment of herpes genitalis with carbonoxolone and cicloxolone creams: A double blind placebo controlled trial. British Journal of Venereal Disease. 1984;60:178-81.

47. Poswillo DE, Roberts GL. Topical carbonoxolone for orofacial herpes simplex infections. Lancet. 1981;2:142-44.

48. Mitscher L, Park Y, Clark D. Antimicrobial agents from higher plants. Antimicrobial isoflavonoids from *Glycyrrhiza glabra* L. var. typica. Journal of Natural Products. 1980;43:259-69.

49. Chen M, Theander TG, Christensen SB, et al. Licochalcone A, a new antimalarial agent, inhibits *in vitro* growth of the human malaria parasite *Plasmodium falciparum* and protects mice from *P. yoelii* infection. Antimicrobial Agents and Chemotherapy. 1994;38(7):1470-75.

50. Chen M, Christensen SB, Blom J, et al. Licochalcone A, a novel antiparasitic agent with potent activity against human pathogenic protozoan species of Leishmania. Antimicrobial Agents and Chemotherapy.1993;37(12):2550-56.

51. Christensen SB, Ming C, Andersen L, et al. An antileishmanial chalcone from Chinese licorice roots. Planta Medica. 1994;60(2):121-23.

52. Kroes BH, Beukelman CJ, van den Berg AJ, et al. Inhibition of human complement by beta-glycyrrhetinic acid. Immunology. 1997;90(1):115-20.

53. Mauricio I, Francischetti B, Monteiro RQ, Guimaraes JA. Identification of glycyrrhizin as a thrombin inhibitor. Biochemical and Biophysical Research Communications. 1997;225:259-63.

54. Hikino H, Kiso Y. Natural products for liver diseases. Economic and Medicinal Plant Research. 1988;2:39-72.

55. Sato H, Goto W, Yamamura J, et al. Therapeutic basis of glycyrrhizin on chronic hepatitis B. Antiviral Research. 1996;30 (2-3):171-77.

56. Yamashiki M, Nishimura A, Suzuki H, et al. Effects of the Japanese herbal medicine "Sho-saiko-to" (TJ-9) on in vitro interleukin-10 production by peripheral blood mononuclear cells of patients with chronic hepatitis C.Hepatology. 1997;25(6):1390-97.

57. Suzuki H, Ohta Y, Takino T, Fugisawa Kea. Effects of glycyrrhizin on biochemical tests in patients with chronic hepatitis — double blind trial. Asian Medical Journal. 1984;26:423-38.

58. Takahara T, Watanabe A, Shiraki K. Effects of glycyrrhizin on hepatitis B surface antigen: A biochemical and morphological study. Journal of Hepatology. 1994;21(4):601-09.

59. Kiso Y, Tohkin M, Hikino H, et al. Mechanism of antihepatotoxic activity of glycyrrhizin, I. effect on free radical generation and lipid peroxidation. Planta Medica. 1984;50:298-302.

60. Poswillo D, Partridge M. Management of recurrent aphthous ulcers. British Dentistry Journal. 1984;157:55-57.

61. Anderson DM, Smith WG. The antitussive activity of glycyrrhetinic acid and its derivatives. Journal of Pharmacy and Pharmacology. 1961;13:396-404.

62. Aida K, et al. Isoliquiritigenin: A new aldose reductase inhibitor from Glycyrrhizae radix. Planta Medica. 1990;56:254-58.

63. Yun-ping Z, Jia-qing Z. Oral baicalin and liquid extract of licorice reduce sorbital levels in red blood cells of diabetic rats. Chinese Medical Journal. 1989;102:203-06.

64. Kobayashi M, Schmitt DA, Utsunomiya T, et al. Inhibition of burn-associated suppressor cell generation by glycyrrhizin through the induction of contrasuppressor T cells. Immunology and Cell Biology. 1993;71(Pt 3):181-89.

65. Nakajima N, Utsunomiya T, Kobayashi M, et al. In vitro induction of anti-type 2 T cells by glycyrrhizin. Burns. 1996;22(8):612-17.

66. Zani F, Cuzzoni MT, Daglia M, et al. Inhibition of mutagenicity in Salmonella typhimurium by Glycyrrhiza glabra extract, glycyrrhizinic acid, 18 alpha- and 18 beta-glycyrrhetinic acids. Planta Medica. 1993;59(6):502-07.

67. Kitagawa K, Nishino H, Iwashima A. Inhibition of 12-0-tetradecanoylphorbol-13-acetate-stimulated 3-0-methyl-glucose transport in mouse Swiss 3T3 fibroblasts by glycyrrhetic acid. Cancer Letters. 1984;24:157-63.

68. Kato H, Kanaoka M, Yano S, Kobayashi M. 3-Monoglucuronyl-glycyrrhetinic acid is a major metabolite that causes licorice-induced pseudoaldosteronism. Journal of Clinical Endocrinology and Metabolism. 1995;80(6):1929-33.

69. Cibelli G, et al. Hypokalemic myopathy associated with liquorice ingestion [Italian]. Italian Journal of Neurological Science. 1984;5:463-66.

70. Shintani S, Murase H, Tsukagoshi H, Shiigai T. Glycyrrhizin (licorice) — induced hypokalemic myopathy. European Neurology. 1992;32:44-51.

71. Corrocher R, et al. Pseudoprimary hyperaldosteronism due to liquorice intoxication. European Review Med Pharmacol Sci. 1983;5:467-70.

72. Werner S, Brismar K, Olsson S. Hyperprolactinemia and liquorice. Lancet. 1979;1:319.

73. Nielsen I, Pedersen RS. Life-threatening hypokalemia caused by liquorice ingestion. Lancet. 1984;1:1305.

74. Megia A, Herranz L, Martin-Almendra MA, Martinez I. Angiotensin I-converting enzyme levels and renin-aldosterone axis recovery after cessation of chronic licorice ingestion. [Letter]. Nephron. 1993;65(2):329-30.

75. Chamberlain TJ. Licorice poisoning, pseudoaldosteronism, heart failure. Journal of the American Medical Association. 1970;213:1343.

76. Basso A, Dalla Paola L, Erle G, et al. Licorice ameliorates postural hypotension caused by diabetic autonomic neuropathy. Diabetes Care. 1994;17(11):1356.

77. Teelucksingh S, Mackie ADR, Burt D, et al. Potentiation of hydrocortisone activity in skin by glycyrrhetinic acid. Lancet. 1990;335:1060-63.

78. Schleimer RP. Potential regulation of inflammation in the lung by local metabolism of hydrocortisone. American Journal of Respiratory Cell and Molecular Biology. 1991;4:166-73.

79. Chen M-F, Shimada F, Kato H, et al. Effect of oral administration of glycyrrhizin on the pharmacokinetics of prednisone. Endocrinologica Japonica. 1991;38:167-74.

80. Blumenthal M, Brusse WR, Goldberg A, et al. The Complete German Commission E Monographs. Austin, TX: American Botanical Council; 1998:685.

Lobelia

1. Newall C, Anderson L, Phillipson J. Herbal Medicines: A Guide for Health Care Professionals. London: The Pharmaceutical Press; 1996:296.

2. Leung A, Foster S. Encyclopedia of Common Natural Ingredients Used in Food, Drugs and Cosmetics. 2nd ed. New York, NY: John Wiley and Sons; 1996:649.

3. Wren R. Potter's New Encyclopedia of Botanical Drugs and Preparations. Saffron Walden: CW Daniel Company; 1988:362.

4. Micheletti E, Winterberg A, Humbert G, et al. North American Folk Healing. Westmount, QC: Reader's Digest; 1998:408.

5. Chevallier A. The Encyclopedia of Medicinal Plants. London: Reader's Digest; 1996:336.

6. Reynolds J. Martindale: The Extra Pharmacopoeia. 13th ed. London: The Pharmaceutical Press; 1993:2363.

7. Saunders P. Personal Communication; 1998.

8. Subarnas A, Tadano T, Nakahata N, et al. A possible mechanism of antidepressant activity of beta-amyrin palmitate isolated from Lobelia inflata leaves in the forced swimming test. Life Sciences. 1993;52(3):289-96.

9. Krochmal A, Wilken L, Chien M. Lobeline content of four Appalachian lobelias. Lloydia. 1972;35(3):303-4.

10. Hoffman D. Holistic Herbal. Rockport, CA: Element Books; 1996:256.

11. Mills S. The Essential Book of Herbal Medicine. London: Penguin; 1991:677.

12. Health Canada. Drug Product Database, Ottawa: Health Canada; 1998.

13. Damaj MI, Patrick GS, Creasy KR, Martin BR. Pharmacology of lobeline, a nicotinic receptor ligand. Journal of Pharmacology & Experimental Therapeutics. 1997;282(1):409-10.

14. Rao TS, Correa LD, Lloyd GK. Effects of lobeline and dimethylphenylpiperazinium iodide (DMPP) on N-methyl-D-aspartate (NMDA)-evoked acetylcholine release *in vitro*: Evidence for a lack of involvement of classical neuronal nicotinic acetyl choline receptors. Neuropharmacology. 1997;36(1):39-50.

15. Cambar P, Shore S, Aviado D. Bronchopulmonary and gastrointestinal effects of lobeline. Archives Internationoves de Pharmacodynamie et de Therapie. 1969;177(1):1-27.

16. Murray M. The Healing Power of Herbs. 2nd ed. Rocklin, CA: Prima Publishing; 1995:410.

17. Korczyn AD, Bruderman I, Braun K. Cardiovascular effects of lobeline. Archives Internationales de Pharmacodynamie et de Therapie. 1969;182(2):370-75.

18. Becker L. Helping patients quit smoking. Journal of Family Practice. 1998;46(3):195-6.

19. Plakun A, Ambrus J, Bross I, Graham S, Levin M, Ross C. Clinical factors in smoking withdrawal: Preliminary report. American Journal of Public Health. 1966;56(3):434-41.

20. Ross C. Smoking withdrawal research clinics. American Journal of Public Health. 1967;57(4):677-81.

21. Ford S, Ederer F. Breaking the cigarette habit. Journal of the Amerian Medical Association. 1965;194(2):119-22.

22. Willard T. Wild Rose Scientific Herbal. Calgary, AB: Wild Rose College of Natural Healing; 1991:416.

23. Tyler V. Herbs of Choice. The Therapeutic Use of Phytomedicinals. Binghamton, NY: Pharmaceutical Products Press; 1994:209.

24. McLaren G. Sudden death in asthma. British Medical Journal. 1968;4(628):456.

Ma Huang

1. Leung AY, Foster S. Encyclopedia of Common Natural Ingredients Used in Food, Drugs, and Cosmetics. 2nd ed. Toronto, ON/New York, NY: John Wiley and Sons Inc; 1996.

2. Wren R. Potter's New Encyclopedia of Botanical Drugs and Preparations. Saffron Walden: C.W. Daniel Company; 1988.

3. Tyler VE. Herbs of Choice. The Therapeutic Use of Phytomedicinals. Binghamton, NY: Pharmaceutical Products Press; 1994.

4. Murray M. The Healing Power of Herbs. 2nd ed. Rocklin, CA: Prima Publishing; 1995.

5. Willard T. Wild Rose Scientific Herbal. Calgary, AB: Wild Rose College of Natural Healing; 1991.

6. Hoffmann D. Holistic Herbal. Rockport, CA: Element Books; 1996.

7. Chevallier A. The Encyclopedia of Medicinal Plants. London: Reader's Digest; 1996.

8. Mills S. The Essential Book of Herbal Medicine. 2nd ed. London: Penguin Publ; 1991.

9. Trease G, Evans W. Pharmacognosy. London: Bailliere and Tindall; 1989.

10. Olin B. The Review of Natural products; The Ephedras. St.Louis: Facts and Comparisons, a Wolters Kluwer Company; 1995.

11. Duke J. The Green Pharmacy. New York: Rodale Press Inc.; 1997.

12. Lee T, Stitzel R. Adrenomimetic drugs. In: Craig C, Stitzel R, eds. Modern Pharmacology. 4th ed. New York, NY: Little, Brown and Company; 1994:907.

13. Kasahara Y, Hikino H, Tsurufuji S, Watanabe M, Ohuchi K. Anti-inflammatory actions of ephedrines in acute inflammations. Planta Medica. 1985;51:325-31.

14. Bowman W, Rand M. Textbook of Pharmacology. London: Blackwell Scientific Publications; 1980.

15. Health Canada. Labelling Standard: Ephedra. In Ottawa: Health Canada Drugs Directorate; 1996.

16. Health Canada. Drug Product Database. In Health Canada; 1998.

17. King K. The treatment of asthma. Medical Journal of Australia. 1985;143:390-94.

18. Dulloo AG, Miller DS. The thermogenic properties of ephedrine/methylxanthine mixtures: animal studies. American Journal of Clinical Nutrition. 1986;43(3):388-94.

19. Tulp OL, Buck CL. Caffeine and ephedrine stimulated thermogenesis in LA-corpulent rats. Comparative Biochemistry & Physiology — C: Comparative Pharmacology & Toxicology. 1986;85(1):17-19.

20. Dulloo AG, Miller DS. Prevention of genetic fa/fa obesity with an ephedrine-methylxanthines thermogenic mixture. American Journal of Physiology. 1987;252(3 Pt 2):R507-13.

21. Breum L, Pedersen JK, Ahlstrom F, Frimodt-Moller J. Comparison of an ephedrine/caffeine combination and dexfenfluramine in the treatment of obesity. A double-blind multi-centre trial in general practice. International Journal of Obesity & Related Metabolic Disorders. 1994;18(2):99-103.

22. Daly PA, Krieger DR, Dulloo AG, Young JB, Landsberg L. Ephedrine, caffeine and aspirin: Safety and efficacy for treatment of human obesity. International Journal of Obesity & Related Metabolic Disorders. 1993;17(Suppl 1):S73-8.

23. Astrup A, Breum L, Toubro S, Hein P, Quaade F. The effect and safety of an ephedrine/caffeine compound compared to ephedrine, caffeine and placebo in obese subjects on an energy restricted diet. A double blind trial. International Journal of Obesity & Related Metabolic Disorders. 1992;16(4):269-77.

24. Norregaard J, Jorgensen S, Mikkelsen KL, Tonnesen P, Iversen E, Sorensen T, et al. The effect of ephedrine plus caffeine on smoking cessation and postcessation weight gain. Clinical Pharmacology & Therapeutics. 1996;60(6):679-86.

25. Dulloo AG, Miller DS. The thermogenic properties of ephedrine/methylxanthine mixtures: Human studies. International Journal of Obesity. 1986;10(6):467-81.

26. Astrup A, Lundsgaard C, Madsen J, Christensen NJ. Enhanced thermogenic responsiveness during chronic ephedrine treatment in man. American Journal of Clinical Nutrition. 1985;42(1):83-94.

27. Pasquali R, Cesari MP, Melchionda N, Stefanini C, Raitano A, Labo G. Does ephedrine promote weight loss in low-energy-adapted obese women? International Journal of Obesity. 1987;11(2):163-68.

28. Pasquali R, Baraldi G, Cesari MP, Melchionda N, Zamboni M, Stefanini C, et al. A controlled trial using ephedrine in the treatment of obesity. International Journal of Obesity. 1985;9(2):93-8.

29. Boozer CN, Nasser JA, Heymsfield SB, Wang V, Chen G, Solomon JL. An herbal supplement containing Ma Huang-Guarana for weight loss: A randomized, double-blind trial. Int J Obes Relat Metab Disord. 2001;25(3):316-24.

30. Boozer CN, Daly PA, Homel P, Solomon JL, Blanchard D, Nasser JA, et al. Herbal ephedra/caffeine for weight loss: A 6-month randomized safety and efficacy trial. Int J Obes Relat Metab Disord. 2002;26(5):593-604.

31. Dulloo AG, Miller DS. Aspirin as a promoter of ephedrine-induced thermogenesis: potential use in the treatment of obesity. American Journal of Clinical Nutrition. 1987;45(3):564-69.

32. Horton TJ, Geissler CA. Aspirin potentiates the effect of ephedrine on the thermogenic response to a meal in obese but not lean women. International Journal of Obesity. 1991;15(5):359-66.

33. Dulloo A. Ephedrine, xanthines and prostaglandin-inhibitors: Action and interactions in the stimulation of thermogenesis. International Journal of Obesity 1993;17((Suppl. 1)):S35-S40.

34. Astrup A. Thermogenesis in human brown adipose tissue and skeletal muscle induced by sympathomimetic stimulation. Acta Endocrinologica. Supplementum 1986;278:1-32.

35. Buemann B, Marckmann P, Christensen NJ, Astrup A. The effect of ephedrine plus caffeine on plasma lipids and lipoproteins during a 4.2 MJ/day diet. International Journal of Obesity & Related Metabolic Disorders 1994;18(5):329-32.

36. Clarkson PM, Thompson HS. Drugs and sport. Research findings and limitations. Sports Medicine 1997;24(6):366-84.

37. Nightingale SL. From the Food and Drug Administration. Journal of the American Medical Association. 1996;275(20):1534.

38. Chase SL. The FDA warns of the dangers of ephedrine. Rn. 1996;59(12):67.

39. Josefson D. Herbal stimulant causes US deaths [News]. British Medical Journal. 1996;312(7043):1378-79.

40. Maron B, Shirani J, Poliac L, Matherige R, Roberts W, Mueller F. Sudden death in young competitive athletes. Journal of the American Medical Association. 1996;276:199-204.

41. Theoharides TC. Sudden death of a healthy college student related to ephedrine toxicity from a ma huang-containing drink. Journal of Clinical Psychopharmacology. 1997;17(5):437-39.

42. Karch SB. Comments on "ma huang toxicity" letter by Dr. Theoharides. Journal of Clinical Psychopharmacology. 1999;19(2):196-99.

43. Samenuk D, Link MS, Homoud MK, Contreras R, Theohardes TC, Wang PJ, et al. Adverse cardiovascular events temporally associated with ma huang, an herbal source of ephedrine. Mayo Clin Proc. 2002;77(1):12-16.

44. Theoharides TC. Sudden death of a healthy college student related to ephedrine toxicity from a ma huang-containing drink [Letter]. Journal of Clinical Psychopharmacology. 1997;17(5):437-39.

45. Doyle H, Kargin M. Herbal stimulant containing ephedrine has also caused psychosis [Letter; Comment]. British Medical Journal. 1996;313(7059):756.

46. Capwell R. Ephedrine induced mania from a herbal diet supplement. Am J Psychiatry. 1995;152:647.

47. Nightingale SL. From the Food and Drug Administration. Journal of the American Medical Association. 1997;278(1):15.

48. Kikutani T. Countrary Views on Chinese Herbal drugs and Side Effects. International Journal of Oriental Medicine. 1990;15(4):184-88.

49. Canada H. Warning not to use products containing the herb ephedra, also known as ma huang. Health Canada News Release 1997;1997-38.

50. Nadir A, Agrawal S, King PD, Marshall JB. Acute hepatitis associated with the use of a Chinese herbal product, ma-huang [see Comments]. American Journal of Gastroenterology. 1996;91(7):1436-38.

51. Stockley I. Drug Interactions. A Sourcebook of Adverse Interactions, Their Mechanisms, Clinical Importance, and Management. 3rd ed. Cambridge, UK: Blackwell Scientific Press; 1994.

52. Blumenthal M, et al. The Complete German Commission E Monographs: Therapeutic Guide to Herbal Medicine. Austin, TX: American Botanical Council; 1998.

Meadowsweet

1. Newall C, Anderson L, Phillipson J. Herbal Medicines: A Guide for Health Care Professionals. London: The Pharmaceutical Press; 1996:296.

2. Wren R. Potter's New Encyclopedia of Botanical Drugs and Preparations. Saffron Walden: C.W. Daniel Company; 1988:362.

3. Stuart M. The Encylcopedia of Herbs and Herbalism. London: Orbis Publishing; 1979:304.

4. Krutch J. Herbal. London: Phaidon Press; 1976:255.

5. Scheer T, Wichtl M. On the occurence of Kampferol-4'-O-beta-D-glucopyranoside in *Filipendula ulmaria* and *Allium cepa* [German]. Planta Medica. 1987; 53:573-74.

6. Barnaulov OD, et al. Chemical composition and primary evaluation of the properties of preparations from *Filipendula ulmaria* (L.) Maxim flowers. Rastilil'nye Resursy. 1977; 13:661-69.

7. Valle MG, Nano GM, Tira S. Das atherische ol aus *Filipendula ulmaria*. Planta Medica. 1988; 54:181-82.

8. Thieme H. Isolierung eines neuen phenolischen glykosids aus den bluten von *Filipendula ulmaria* (L.) Maxim. Pharmazie. 1966; 21:123.

9. Hoffmann D. Holistic Herbal. Rockport, CA: Element Books; 1996:256.

10. Mills S. The Essential Book of Herbal Medicine. 2nd ed. London: Penguin Publ; 1991:677.

11. Weiss R. Herbal Medicine. Beaconsfield, UK: Beaconsfield Publishers Ltd; 1988: 362.

12. Barnaulov OD, Denisenko PP. Antiulcerogenic action of the decoction from flowers of *Filipendula ulmaria* (L.). Pharmakol-Toxicol (Moscow). 1980; 43:700-05.

13. Liapina L, Koval'chuk G. A comparative study of the action on the hemostatic system of extracts from the flowers and seeds of the meadowsweet (*Filipendula ulmaria* (L.) Maxim) [Russian]. Izv Akad Nauk Ser Biol. 993; July-Aug(4):625-28.

14. Peresun'ko A, Bespalov V, Limarenko A, Aleksandrov V. Clinico-experimental study using plant preparations from the flowers of *Filipendula ulmaria* (L.) Maxim for the treatment of precancerous changes and preparation of uterine cervical cancer. [Russian]. Voprosy Onkologii. 1993; 39(7-12):291-95.

15. Bradley P. British Herbal Compendium. Bournemouth, UK: BHMA; 1992.

Milk Thistle

1. Foster S. Milk Thistle. *Silybum marianum.* Houston, TX: American Botanical Council; 1991: Botanical Series No. 305.

2. Murray MT. The Healing Power of Herbs. Rocklin, CA: Prima Publishing; 1992.

3. Hikino H, Kiso Y. Natural products for liver diseases. Economic and Medicinal Plant Research. 1988;2:39-72.

4. Leung AY, Foster S. Encyclopedia of Common Natural Ingredients Used in Food, Drugs, and Cosmetics. 2nd ed. Toronto, ON /New York, NY: John Wiley and Sons Inc; 1996.

5. Brown D. Silymarin educational monograph. Townsend Newsletter for Doctors and Patients. 1994;136:1282-85.

6. Brown D. Silymarin Education Monograph. Herbal Research Update. 1993;Summer Quarter:23-36.

7. Leng-Peschlow E. Alcohol-related liver diseases — use of Legalon for therapy. Quarterly Review of Natural Medicine. 1996;summer:103-18.

8. Sonnenblicher J, Goldberg M, et al. Stimulating effects of silibinin on the DNA-synthesis in partially hepatectomized rat livers: Non-response in hepatoma and other malignant cell lines. Biochem Pharmacol. 1986;35:538-41.

9. Magliulo P, Carosi G, Minoli L, Gorini S. Studies on the regenerative capacity of the liver in rats subjected to partial hepatectomy and treated with silymarin. Arzneimittel Forschung (Drug Research). 1973;23:161-7.

10. Valenzuela A, Lagos C, Schmidt K, Videla LA. Silymarin protection against hepatic lipid peroxidation induced by acute ethanol intoxication in the rat. Biochem Pharmacol. 1985;34(12):2209-12.

11. Valenzuela A, Aspillaga M, Vial S, Guerra R. Selectivity of silymarin on the increase of the glutathione content in different tissues of the rat. Planta Medica. 1989;55:420-2.

12. Wagner H. Antihepatotoxic flavonoids. In: Cody V, Middleton E, Harbourne JB, editors. Plant Flavonoids in Biology and Medicine: Biochemical, Pharmacological, and Structure-Activity Relationships. New York, NY: Alan R Liss; 1986:545-48.

13. Adzet T. Polyphenolic compounds with biological and pharmacological activity. Herbs Spices Medicinal Plants. 1986;1:167-84.

14. Hikino H, Kiso Y, Wagner H, Fiebig. Antihepatotoxic actions of flavanolignans from *Silybum marianum* fruits. Planta Medica. 1984;50:248-50.

15. Campos R, Garrido A, Guerra R, Valenzuela A. Silybin dihemisuccinate protects against glutathione depletion and lipid peroxisation induced by acetaminophen in rat liver. Planta Medica. 1989;55:417-9.

16. Muzes G, Deak G, Land I, Nekam K, Gergely P, Feher J. Effect of the bioflavonoid silymarin on the *in vitro* activity and expression of superoxide dismutase (SOD) enzyme. Acta Physiologica Hungarica. 1991;78(1):3-9.

17. Fiebrich F, Koch H. Silymarin, an inhibitor of lipoxygenase. Experentia 1979;35:148-50.

18. Alarcon de la Lastra AC, Martin MJ, Motilva V, Jimenez M, La Casa C, Lopez A. Gastroprotection induced by silymarin, the hepatoprotective principle of *Silybum marianum* in ischemia-reperfusion mucosal injury: role of neutrophils. Planta Medica. 1995;61(2):116-19.

19. Dehmlow C, Erhard J, de Groot H. Inhibition of Kupffer cell functions as an explanation for the hepatoprotective properties of silibinin. Hepatology. 1996;23(4):749-54.

20. Tyler VE. Herbs of Choice. The Therapeutic Use of Phytomedicinals. Binghamton, NY: Pharmaceutical Products Press; 1994.

21. Blumenthal M, Brusse WR, Goldberg A, Gruenwald J, Hall T, Riggins CW, et al. The Complete German Commission E Monographs. Austin, TX: American Botanical Council; 1998.

22. Jacobs BP, Dennehy C, Ramirez G, Sapp J, Lawrence VA. Milk thistle for the treatment of liver disease: A systematic review and meta-analysis. American Journal of Medicine. 2002;113(6):506-15.

23. Weiss R. Herbal Medicine. 6th ed. Gothenburg, Sweden: AB Arcanum; 1988.

24. Hruby C. Silibinin in the treatment of deathcap fungus poisoning. Forum. 1984;6:23-26.

25. Faulstich H, Jahn W, Wieland T. Silybin inhibition of amatoxin uptake in the perfused rat liver. Arsneimittel Forschung. 1980;30(1):452-54.

26. Tuchweber B, Sieck R, Trost W. Prevention of silybin of phalloidin-induced acute hepatotoxicity. Toxicology and Applied Pharmacology. 1979;51:265-75.

27. Salami HA, Sarna S. Effect of silymarin on chemical, functional and morphological alterations of the liver. Scandinavian Journal of Gastroenterology. 1982;17:517-21.

28. Palasciano G, Portincasa P, Palmieri V, Ciani D, Vendemiale G, Altomare E. The effect of silymarin on plasma levels of malondialdehyde in patients receiving long-term treatment with psychotropic drugs. Current Therapeutic Research. 1994;55(5):537-45.

29. Buzzelli G, Moscarella S, et al. A pilot study on the liver protective effect of silybin-phosphatidylcholine complex (IdB1016) in chronic active hepatitis. Int J Clin Pharm Ther Toxicol. 1993;31(9):456-60.

30. Lirussi F, Okolicsanyi L. Cytoprotection in the nineties: Experience with ursodeoxycholic acid and silymarin in chronic liver disease. Acta Physiol Hungar. 1992;80(1-4):363-67.

31. Ferenci R, Gragosics B, et.al. Randomized controlled trial of silymarin treatment in patients with cirrhosis of the liver. Journal of Hepatology. 1989;9:105-13.

32. Pares A, Planas R, Torres M, Caballeria J, Viver JM, Acero D, et al. Effects of silymarin in alcoholic patients with cirrhosis of the liver: results of a controlled, double-blind, randomized and multicenter trial. Journal of Hepatology. 1998;28(4):615-21.

33. Weber G, Galle K. The liver, a therapeutic target in dermatoses. Medizinische Welt. 1983;34:108-11.

34. Anon. An adverse reaction to the herbal medication milk thistle (*Silybum marianum*). Adverse Drug Reactions Advisory Committee. Medical Journal of Australia. 1999;170(5):218-19.

35. Piscitelli SC, Formentini E, Burstein AH, Alfaro R, Jagannatha S, Falloon J. Effect of milk thistle on the pharmacokinetics of indinavir in healthy volunteers. Pharmacotherapy. 2002;22(5):551-56.

Nettle

1. Mills S. The Essential Book of Herbal Medicine. 2nd ed. London: Penguin Publ; 1991.

2. Newall CA, Anderson LA, Phillipson JD. Herbal Medicines. A Guide for Health Care Professionals. London: The Pharmaceutical Press; 1996.

3. Leung AY, Foster S. Encyclopedia of Common Natural Ingredients Used in Food, Drugs, and Cosmetics. 2nd ed. Toronto, ON/New York, NY: John Wiley and Sons Inc; 1996.

4. ESCOP. *Urticae Radix*/Nettle Root. In: Phytotherapy ESCo, ed. ESCOP Monographs (Fasicucle 2). Exeter: ESCOP; 1996:58.

5. ESCOP. *Urticae Folium*/Herba (Nettle Leaf). In: Phytotherapy) EESCo, ed. ESCOP Monographs /Fascicule 4. Exeter: ESCOP; 1997:58

6. Weiss R. Herbal Medicine. Beaconsfield, UK: Beaconsfield Publishers Ltd; 1988.

7. Chaurasia N, Wichtl M. Flavonolglykoside aus *Urtica dioica*. Planta Medica. 1987;53:432-24.

8. Andersen S, Wold JK. Water-soluble glycoprotein from *Urtica dioica* leaves. Phytochemistry. 1978;17:1875-77.

9. Barlow RB, Dixon ROD. Choline acetyltransferase in the nettle *Urtica dioica* L. Biochemistry Journal. 1973;132:15-18.

10. Chaurasia N, Wichtl M. Scopolectin, 3-B-sitosterin und 3-B-D-glucosid aus Brennesselwurzel (*Urtica radix*). Deutsch Apothek Zeitung. 1986;126:81-83.

11. Chaurasia N, Wichtl M. Sterols and steryl glycosides from *Urtica dioica*. Journal of Natural Products. 1987;50:881-85.

12. Hoffmann D. Holistic Herbal. Rockport, CA: Element Books; 1996.

13. Dreikorn K, Schonhofer P. Status of phytotherapeutic drugs in the treatment of benign prostatic hyperplasia [German]. Urologe A. 1995;34(2):119-29.

14. Buck A. Phytotherapy for the prostate. British Journal of Urology. 1996;78:325-36.

15. Schneider HJ, Honold E, Mashur T. Treatment of benign prostatic hyperplasia. Results of a surveilance study in the practices of urological specialists using a combined plant-based preparation. Forschr Med. 1995;113:37-40.

16. Hartmann R, Mark M, Soldati F. Inhibition of 5 alpha reductase and aromatase by PHL-00801 (Prostatonin), a combination of PY102 (*Pygeum africanum*) and UR102(*Urtica dioica*) extracts. Phytomedicine. 1996;3(2):121-28.

17. Hyrb D, Khan M, Romas N, Rosner W. The effect of estracts of the roots of the stinging nettle (*Urtica dioica*) on the interaction of SHBG with its receptor on human prostatic membranes. Planta Medica. 1995;61:31-32.

18. Sokeland J. Combined sabal and urtica extract compared with finasteride in men with benign prostatic hyperplasia: Analysis of prostate volume and therapeutic outcome. BJU Int. 2000;86(4):439-42.

19. Carraro JC, Raynaud JP, Koch G, et al. Comparison of phytotherapy (Permixon) with finasteride in the treatment of benign prostate hyperplasis: A randomized international study of 1,098 patients. Prostate. 1996;29:231-40.

20. McCaleb R. Synergistic action of pygeum and nettle root extracts in prostate disease. Herbalgram. 1996;40:18.

21. Obertreis B, Ruttkowski T, Teucher T, Behnke B, Schmitz H. *Ex-vivo in-vitro* inhibition of lipopolysaccharide stimulated tumor necrosis factor-alpha and interleukin-1 beta secretion in human whole blood by extractum *Urticae dioicae* foliorum [published erratum appears in Arzneimittelforschung 1996 Sep;46(9):936]. Arzneimittelforschung. 1996;46(4):389-94.

22. Chrubasik S, Enderlein W, Bauer R, Grabner W. Evidence for antirheumatic effectivenss of Herba *Urticae dioicae* in acute arthritis: A pilot study. Phytomedicine. 1997;4(2):105-08.

23. Rand J. Pilot study indicates that stewed herba urticae dioicae may potentiate the effects of diclofenac in acute arthritis. Focus on Alternative and Complementary Therapies. 1997;2(4):156-57.

24. Randall C, Randall H, Dobbs F, Hutton C, Sanders H. Randomized controlled trial of nettle sting for treatment of base-of-thumb pain. Journal of the Royal Societty of Medicine. 2000;93(6):305-09.

25. Mittman P. Randomized double-blind study of freeze-dried *Urtica diocia* in the treatment of allergic rhinitis. Planta Medica. 1990;56:44-47.

26. Bradley P. British Herbal Compendium. Bournemouth, UK: The British Herbal Medical Association; 1992.

Passionflower

1. Leung AY, Foster S. Encyclopedia of Common Natural Ingredients Used in Food, Drugs, and Cosmetics. 2nd ed. Toronto, ON/New York. NY: John Wiley and Sons Inc; 1996.

2. Newall CA, Anderson LA, Phillipson JD. Herbal Medicines. A Guide for Health Care Professionals. London: The Pharmaceutical Press; 1996.

3. Meier B. *Passiflora incarnata* L. — Passion flower. Portrait of a medicinal plant. Quarterly Review of Natural Medicine. 1995;Fall,3:191-202; Translated from the German Zeitschrift fur Phytotherapie. 1995;16:115-26.

4. Bergner P. Passionflower. Medical Herbalism. 1995;7(1-2):13-14,26.

5. Congora C, Proliac A, Raynaud J. Isolement et identification de deux glycosyl-luteolines mono-C-substituees et de la diglucosyl-6,8-luteoline di-C-substituee dans les tiges feuillees de *Passiflora incarnata* L. (Isolation and identification of two mono-C-glucosyl-luteolins and of the di-C-subsituted 6,8-diglucosyl-luteolin from the leafy stalks of *Passiflora incarnata* L.). Helv Chim Acta. 1986;69:251-53.

6. Quercia V, Turchetto L, Pierini N, Cuozzo V, Percaccio G. Identification and determination of vitexin and isovitexin in *Passiflora incarnata* extracts. Journal of Chromatography. 1978;161:396-402.

7. Pietta P, Manera E, Ceva P. Isocratic liquid chromatographic methiod for the simultaneous determination of *Passiflora incarnata* L. and *Crataegus monogyna* flavonoids in drugs. Journal of Chromatography. 1986;357:233-38.

8. Proliac A, Raynaud J. The presence of C-B-D-6-glucopyranosyl-C-a-L-arabinopyranosyl-8-apigenin in leafy stems of *Passiflora incarnata*. Pharmazie. 1986;41:673-74.

9. Geiger H, et al. The C-glycosylfavone pattern of *Passiflora incarnata* L. Zeitung Naturforsch. 1986;Sept/Oct:949-50.

10. Proliac A, Raynaud J. O-glucosyl-2"-C-glucosyl-6 apegenine de *Passiflora incarnata* L. (Passifloraceae). Pharm Acta Helv. 1988;63(6):174-75.

11. ESCOP. Passiflora Herba/Passiflora. In: Phytotherapy) EESCo, editor. ESCOP Monographs (Fascicule 4). Exeter: ESCOP; 1997:58.

12. Hoffmann D. Holistic Herbal. Rockport, CA: Element Books; 1996.

13. Weiss R. Herbal Medicine. Beaconsfield, UK: Beaconsfield Publishers Ltd; 1988.

14. Flynn J. The herbal management of stress. Australian Journal of Medical Herbalism. 1996;8(1):15-18.

15. Aoyagi N, Kimura R, Murata T. Studies on *Passiflora incarnata* dry extract. I. Isolation of maltol and pharmacological action of maltol and ethyl maltol. Chemical and Pharmaceutical Bulletin. 1974;22:1008-13.

16. Soulimani R, Younos C, Jarmouni S, Bousta D, Misslin R, Mortier F. Behavioural effects of *Passiflora incarnata* L. and its indole alkaloid and flavonoid derivatives and maltol in the mouse. Journal of Ethnopharmacology. 1997;57(1):11-20.

17. Della Loggia R, Tubaro A, Redaelli C. Valutazione dell'attivita sul S.N.C del topo di alcuni estratti vegetali e di una loro associazone [Italian]. Riv Neurol. 1981;51:297-310.

18. Speroni E, Minghetti A. Neuropharmacological activity of extracts from *Passiflora incarnata*. Planta Medica. 1988;54:488-491.

19. Wolfman C, Viola H, Paladini A, Dajas F, Medina JH. Possible anxiolytic effects of chrysin, a central benzodiazepine receptor ligand isolated from *Passiflora coerulea*. Pharmacol Biochem Behav. 1994;47(1):1-4.

20. Akhondzadeh S, Naghavi HR, Vazirian M, Shayeganpour A, Rashidi H, Khani M. Passionflower in the treatment of generalized anxiety: A pilot double-blind randomized controlled trial with oxazepam. Journal of Clinical Pharmacy. 2001;26(5):363-67.

21. Bourin M, Bougerol T, Guitton B, Broutin E. A combination of plant extracts in the treatment of outpatients with adjustment disorder with anxious mood: Controlled study versus placebo. Fundam Clin Pharmacol. 1997;11(2):127-32.

22. Akhondzadeh S, Kashani L, Mobaseri M, Hosseini SH, Nikzad S, Khani M. Passionflower in the treatment of opiates withdrawal: A double-blind randomized controlled trial. J Clin Pharm Ther 2001;26(5):369-73.

23. Hobbs C, Foster S. Hawthorn — a literature review. Herbalgram. 1990;22:19-33.

24. Tyler VE. Herbs of Choice. The Therapeutic Use of Phytomedicinals. Binghamton, NY: Pharmaceutical Products Press; 1994.

25. Smith GW, Chalmers TM, Nuki G. Vasculitis associated with herbal preparation containing Passiflora extract [Letter]. British Journal of Rheumatology. 1993;32(1):87-88.

26. Solbakken AM, Rorbakken G, Gundersen T. Nature medicine as intoxicant [Norwegian]. Tidsskr Nor Laegeforen. 1997;117(8):1140-41.

27. Fisher AA, Purcell P, Le Couteur DG. Toxicity of *Passiflora incarnata* L. J Toxicol Clin Toxicol. 2000;38(1):63-6.

28. Bradley P. British Herbal Compendium. Bournemouth, UK: The British Herbal Medical Association; 1992.

Peppermint

1. Wren R. Potter's New Encyclopedia of Botanical Drugs and Preparations. Saffron Walden: C.W. Daniel Company; 1988.

2. Murray MJ, Lincoln DE, Marble PM. Oil composition of *Mentha aquatica* x *M. sicata* F_1 hybrids in relation to the origin of *M. x piperita*. Canadian Journal of Genet Cytol. 1972;14:13-29.

3. Mills S. The Essential Book of Herbal Medicine. 2nd ed. London: Penguin Publ; 1991.

4. Foster S. Peppermint. *Mentha x piperita*. Austin, TX: American Botanical Council; 1991 February 19991. Report No.: Botanical Series No. 306.

5. Evans W. Trease and Evans' Pharmacognosy. 13th ed. London: Bailliere Tindall; 1989.

6. Tyler VE. Herbs of Choice. The Therapeutic Use of Phytomedicinals. Binghamton, NY: Pharmaceutical Products Press; 1994.

7. Sigmund CJ, McNally EF. The Action of a carminitive on the lower esophageal sphincter. Gastroenterology. 1969;56(1):13-18.

8. Murray M. The clinical uses of peppermint. The American Journal of Natural Medicine. 1995;2(2):10-13.

9. Leung AY, Foster S. Encyclopedia of Common Natural Ingredients Used in Food, Drugs, and Cosmetics. 2nd ed. Toronto, ON/New York, NY: John Wiley and Sons Inc; 1996.

10. Bauer K, Garbe D. Common Fragrance and Flavor Materials: Preparation, Properties and Uses. Deerfield Beach, FL: VCH Publishers; 1985.

11. Hoffmann D. Holistic Herbal. Rockport, CA: Element Books; 1996.

12. Weiss R. Herbal Medicine. 6th ed. Gothenburg, Sweden: AB Arcanum; 1988.

13. Blumenthal M. Herbalgram. 1990;49(23):32-33.

14. Blumenthal M, Brusse WR, Goldberg A, Gruenwald J, Hall T, Riggins CW, et al. The Complete German Commission E Monographs. Austin, TX: American Botanical Council; 1998.

15. Somerville KW, Richmond CR, Bell GD. Delayed release of peppermint oil capsules (Colpermin) for the spastic colon syndrome: A pharmacokinetic study. British Journal of Clinical Pharmacology 1984;18:638-40.

16. Rees WDW, Evans BK, Rhodes J. Treating irritable bowel syndrome with peppermint oil. British Medical Journal. 1979;October 6:835-36.

17. Dew MJ, Evans BK, Rhodes J. Peppermint oil for the irritable bowel syndrome: A multicentre trial. British Journal of Clinical Practice. 1984;38:394-98.

18. Kline RM, Kline JJ, Di Palma J, Barbero GJ. Enteric-coated, pH-dependent peppermint oil capsules for the treatment of irritable bowel syndrome in children. Journal of Pediatrics. 2001;138(1):125-28.

19. Hills JM, Aaronson PI. Mechanism of action of peppermint oil on GI smooth muscle. Gastroenterology. 1991;101:55-65.

20. Taylor BA, Luscombe DD, Duthie HL. Inhibitory effects of peppermint oil and menthol on isolated human coli. Gut. 1984;25:A1168-69.

21. Leicester RJ, Hunt RH. Peppermint oil to reduce colonic spasm during endoscopy. Lancet. 1982;30 October:989.

22. Jarvis LJ, Hogg JIC, Houghton CD. Topical peppermint oil for the relief of spasm at barium enema. Clincial Radiology. 1992;46:A435.

23. Sparks MJ, P OS, Herrington AA, Morcos SK. Does peppermint oil relieve spasm during barium enema? British Journal of Radiology. 1995;68(812):841-43.

24. Duthie HL. The effect of peppermint oil on colonic motility in man [Abstract only]. Surgical Research Society Abstracts:820.

25. May B, Kuntz HD, Kieser M, Kohler S. Efficacy of a fixed peppermint oil/caraway oil combination in non-ulcer dyspepsia. Arzneimittelforschung. 1996;46(12):1149-53.

26. Madisch A, Heydenreich CJ, Wieland V, Hufnagel R, Hotz J. Treatment of functional dyspepsia with a fixed peppermint oil and caraway oil combination preparation as compared to cisapride. A multicenter, reference-controlled double-blind equivalence study. Arzneimittelforschung. 1999;49(11):925-32.

27. Pattnaik S, Subramanyam VR, Kole C. Antibacterial and antifungal activity of ten essential oils *in vitro*. Microbios. 1996;86(349):237-46.

28. Pattnaik S, Rath C, Subramanyam VR. Characterization of resistance to essential oils in a strain of *Pseudomonas aeruginosa* (VR-6). Microbios. 1995;81(326):29-31.

29. Gobel H, Schmidt G, Soyka D. Effect of peppermint and eucalyptus oil preparations on neurophysiological and experimental algesimetric headache parameters. Cephalalgia. 1994;14(3):228-34; discussion 182.

30. Morton CA, Garioch J, Todd P, Lamey PJ, Forsyth A. Contact sensitivity to menthol and peppermint in patients with intra-oral symptoms. Contact Dermatitis. 1995;32(5):281-84.

31. Wilkinson SM, Beck MH. Allergic contact dermatitis from menthol in peppermint. Contact Dermatitis. 1994;30(1):42-43.

32. Sainio EL, Kanerva L. Contact allergens in toothpastes and a review of their hypersensitivity. Contact Dermatitis. 1995;33(2):100-05.

33. Tisserand R, Balacs T. Essential Oil Safety: A Guide for Health Care Professionals. London: Churchill Livingstone; 1995.

34. Sperl W, Stuppner H, Gassner I, Judmaier W, Dietze O, Vogel W. Reversible hepatic veno-occlusive disease in an infant after consumption of pyrrolizidine-containing herbal tea. European Journal of Pediatrics. 1995;154(2):112-16.

35. Thomas J. Peppermint fibrillation. Lancet. 1962;27 Jan:222.

36. Murray MT. The Healing Power of Herbs. Rocklin, CA: Prima Publishing; 1992.

Red Raspberry

1. Briggs C, Briggs K. Raspberry. Canadian Pharmacists Journal. 1997;April:41-43.

2. Chandler F, ed. Herbs: Everyday Reference for Health Professionals. 1st ed. Ottawa: Canadian Pharmacists' Association; 2000.

3. Blumenthal MT, Hall R, Rister B, eds. The German Commission E Monographs. Austin, TX: American Botanical Council; 1996.

4. Barnes J, Anderson L, David Phillipson J. Herbal Medicines. 2nd ed. London: Pharmaceutical Press; 2002.

5. Bradley P, ed. British Herbal Compendium. Bournemouth, UK: British Herbal Medical Association; 1992.

6. Zampieron E. Red Raspberry. Healthy and Natural Journal. 2000;7(4):7.

7. Yarnell E. Botanical medicine in pregnancy and lactation. Alternative and Complementary Therapies. 1997;April:93-101.

8. Ernst E, Schmidt K. Health risks over the internet: Advice offered by 'medical herbalists' to a pregnant woman. Wiener medizinische Wochenschrift. 2002;152(7-8):190-92.

9. Einarson A, Lawrimore T, Brand P, Gallo M, Rotatore C, Koren G. Attitudes and practices of physicians and naturopaths toward herbal products, including use during pregnancy and lactation. Canadian Journal of Clinical Pharmacology. 2000;7(1):45-49.

10. McFarlin B, Gibson M, O'Rear J, Harman P. A national survey of herbal preparation use by nurse-midwives for labor stimulation. Review of the literature and recommendations for practice. Journal of Nurse-Midwifery. 1999;44(3):205-16.

11. Wilkinson J. What do we know about herbal morning sickness treatments? A literature review. Midwifery. 2000;16(3):224-28.

12. Bamford D, Percival R, Tothill A. Raspberry leaf tea: A new aspect to an old problem. British Journal of Pharmacology. 1970;40:161-62.

13. McLean M. Journal Abstracts. Midwifery Today. 2001;59.

14. Schulz V, Hansel R, Tyler V. Rational Phytotherapy: A Physicians Guide to Herbal Medicine. Berlin: Springer Verlag; 1998.

Saw Palmetto

1. Newall CA, Anderson LA, Phillipson JD. Herbal Medicines. A Guide for Health Care Professionals. London: The Pharmaceutical Press; 1996.

2. Leung AY, Foster S. Encyclopedia of Common Natural Ingredients Used in Food, Drugs, and Cosmetics. 2nd ed. Toronto, ON/New York, NY: John Wiley and Sons Inc; 1996.

3. Awang DVC. Saw palmetto, African prune, and stinging nettle for benign prostatic hyperplasia (BPH). Canadian Pharmaceutical Journal. 1997;November:37-44,62.

4. Murray MT. The Healing Power of Herbs. Rocklin, CA: Prima Publishing; 1992.

5. Hutchens A. Indian Herbology of North America. Boston,MA: Shambhala; 1973.

6. Mills S. The Essential Book of Herbal Medicine. 2nd ed. London: Penguin Publ; 1991.

7. Brinker F. An overview of conventional, experimental and botanical treatments of non-malignant prostate conditions. British Journal of Phytotherapy. 1993/1994;3(4):154-76.

8. Snow JM. Serenoa repens Bartram (Palmae). The Protocol Journal of Botanical Medicine. 1996;1(3):15-16.

9. El-Sheikh MM, Dakkak MR, Saddique A. The effect of permixon on androgen receptors. Acta Obstetrica et Gynecologica Scandinavica. 1988;67:397-99.

10. Ravenna L, Di Silverio F, Russo MA, Salvatori L, Morgante E, Morrone S, et al. Effects of the lipidosterolic extract of Serenoa repens (Permixon) on human prostatic cell lines. Prostate. 1996;29(4):219-30.

11. Wilson JD. The pathogenesis of benign prostatic hyperplasia. American Journal of Medicine. 1980;68:745-55.

12. Carilla E, Briley M, Fauran Fea. Binding of Permixon, a new treatment for prostatic benign hyperplasia, to cytosolic androgen receptor in rat prostate. Journal of Steroid Biochem. 1984;20:521-23.

13. Sultan C, Terraza A, Devillier C, Carilla E, Briley M, Loire C, et al. Inhibition of androgen metabolism and binding by a liposterolic extract of Seronoa repens B in human foreskin fibroblasts. Journal of Steroid Biochemistry. 1984;20(1):515-19.

14. Briley M, Carilla E, et al. Inhibitory effect of Permixon on testosterone 5a-reductase activity of rat ventral prostate. British Journal of Pharmacology. 1984;83(supplement):401.

15. Delos S, Iehle C, Martin PM, Raynaud JP. Inhibition of the activity of 'basic' 5 alpha-reductase (type 1) detected in DU 145 cells and expressed in insect cells. Journal of Steroid Biochemistry and Molecular Biology. 1994;48(4):347-52.

16. Delos S, Carsol JL, Ghazarossian E, Raynaud JP, Martin PM. Testosterone metabolism in primary cultures of human prostate epithelial cells and fibroblasts. Journal of Steroid Biochemistry and Molecular Biology. 1995;55(3-4):375-83.

17. Iehle C, Delos S, Guirou O, Tate R, Raynaud JP, Martin PM. Human prostatic steroid 5 alpha-reductase isoforms—a comparative study of selective inhibitors. Journal of Steroid Biochemistry and Molecular Biology. 1995;54(5-6):273-79.

18. Rhodes L, Primka RL, Berman C, Vergult G, Gabriel M, Pierre-Malice M, et al. Comparison of Finasteride (Proscar), a 5a reductase inhibitor, and various commercial plant extracts in in vitro and in vivo 5a reductase inhibition. The Prostate. 1993;22:43-51.

19. Strauch G, Perles P, Vergult G, Gabriel M, Gibelin B, Cummings S, et al. Comparison of finasteride (Proscar) and Serenoa repens (Permixon) in the inhibition of 5-alpha reductase in healthy male volunteers. Eur Urol. 1994;26(3):247-52.

20. Breu W, Hagenlocher M, Redl K, Tittel G, Stadler F, Wagner H. Anti-inflammatory activity of Sabal fruit extracts prepared with supercritical carbon dioxide. In vitro antagonists of cyclooxygenase and 5-lipoxygenase metabolism. Arzeneim Forsch. 1992;42(4):547-51.

21. Elghamry MI, Hansel R. Activity and isolated phytoestrogen of shrub palmetto fruits (Serenoa repens Small), a new estrogenic plant. Experientia. 1969;25:828-29.

22. Di Silverio F, D'Eramo G, Lubrano C, et al. Evidence that Serenoa repens extract displays an antiestrogenic activity in prostatic tissue of benign prostatic hypertrophy patients. European Urology. 1992;21:309-14.

23. Casarosa C, Cosci di Coscio M, Fratta M. Lack of effects of a liposterolic extract of Serenoa repens on plasma levels of testosterone, FSH, and luteinizing hormone. Clinical Therapeutics. 1988;10:585-88.

24. Paubert-Braquet M, Richardson FO, Servent-Saez N, Gordon WC, Monge MC, Bazan NG, et al. Effect of Serenoa repens extract (Permixon) on estradiol/testosterone-induced experimental prostate enlargement in the rat. Pharmacology Research. 1996;34(3-4):171-79.

25. Cirillo-Marucco E, Pagliarulo A, Tritto G, et al. Extract of Serenoa repens (PermiconR) in the early treatment of prostatic hypertrophy. Urologia. 1983;5:1269-77.

26. Tripodi V, Giancaspro M, Pascarello M, et al. Treatment of prostatic hypertrophy with Serenoa repens extract. Medical Praxis. 1983;4:41-6.

27. Greca P, Volpi R. Experience with a new drug in the medical treatment of prostatic adenoma. Urologia. 1985;52:532-35.

28. Crimi A, Russo A. Serenoa repens for the treatment of the functional disturbances of prostate hypertrophy. Medical Praxis. 1983;4:47-51.

29. Braeckman J. The extract of Serenoa repens in the treatment of benign prostatic hyperplasia: a multicentre open study. Current Therap Research. 1994;55(7):776-85.

30. Romics I, Schmitz H, Frang D. Experience in treating benign prostatic hypertrophy with

Sabal serrulata for one year. International Urology and Nephrology. 1993;25(6):565-69.

31. Boccafoschi, Annoscia S. Comparison of *Serenoa repens* extract with placebo by controlled clinical trial in patients with prostatic adenomatosis. Urologia. 1983;50:1257-68.

32. Emili E, Lo Cigno M, Petrone U. Clinical trial of a new drug for treating hypertrophy of the prostate (Permixon). Urologia. 1983;50:1042-8.

33. Champault G, Bonnard AM, Cauquil J, Patel JC. Medical treatment of prostatic adenoma. Controlled trial: PA 109 vs placebo in 110 patients. Annals of Urology. 1984;18:407-10.

34. Tasca A, et al. Treatment of obstruction in prostatic adenoma using an extract of *Serenoa repens*. Double-blind clinical test v. placebo. Minnerva Urologica Nefrolologica. 1985;37:87-91.

35. Vahlensieck WJ, Volp A, Lubos W, Kuntze M. Benign prostatic hyperplasia — treatment with Sabal fruit extract. A treatment study of 1,334 patients. Fortschritte der Medizin. 1993;111:323-26.

36. Mohanty NK, Jha RJ, Dutt C. Randomized double-blind controlled clinical trial of *Serenoa repens* versus placebo in the management of patients with symptomatic grade I to grade II benign prostatic hyperplasia (BPH). Indian Journal of Urology. 1999;16(1).

37. Stepanov VN, Siniakova LA, Sarrazin B, Raynaud JP. Efficacy and tolerability of the lipidosterolic extract of *Serenoa repens* (Permixon) in benign prostatic hyperplasia: a double-blind comparison of two dosage regimens. Adv Ther. 1999;16(5):231-41.

38. Gerber GS, Kuznetsov D, Johnson BC, Burstein JD. Randomized, double-blind, placebo-controlled trial of saw palmetto in men with lower urinary tract symptoms. Urology. 2001;58(6):960-4; discussion 964-5.

39. Pannunzio E, et al. *Serenoa repens* in the treatment of human benign prostatic hypertrophy (BPH). Journal of Urology. 1987;137:226A.

40. Adriazola Semino M, et al. Symptomatic treatment of benign hypertrophy of the prostate. Arch Esp Urol. 1992;45:211-13.

41. Carraro JC, Raynaud JP, Koch G, et al. Comparison of phytotherapy (Permixon) with finasteride in the treatment of benign prostate hyperplasis: A randomized international study of 1,098 patients. Prostate. 1996;29:231-40.

42. Debruyne F, Koch G, Boyle P, Da Silva FC, Gillenwater JG, Hamdy FC, et al. Comparison of a phytotherapeutic agent (Permixon) with an alpha-blocker (Tamsulosin) in the treatment of benign prostatic hyperplasia: A 1-year randomized international study. European Urology. 2002;41(5):497-506; discussion 506-07.

43. Boyle P, Robertson C, Lowe F, Roehrborn C. Meta-analysis of clinical trials of permixon in the treatment of symptomatic benign prostatic hyperplasia. Urology 2000;55(4):533-9.

44. Wilt T, Ishani A, Stark G, MacDonald R, Mulrow C, Lau J. *Serenoa repens* for benign prostatic hyperplasia. Cochrane Database Syst Rev. 2000;2.

45. Wilt TJ, Ishani A, Stark G, MacDonald R, Lau J, Mulrow C. Saw palmetto extracts for treatment of benign prostatic hyperplasia. Journal of the American Medical Association. 1998;280(18):1604-1609.

46. Marks LS, Partin AW, Epstein JI, Tyler VE, Simon I, Macairan ML, et al. Effects of a saw palmetto herbal blend in men with symptomatic benign prostatic hyperplasia. Journal of Urology. 2000;163(5):1451-56.

47. Sokeland J. Combined sabal and urtica extract compared with finasteride in men with benign prostatic hyperplasia: Analysis of prostate volume and therapeutic outcome. BJU Int. 2000;86(4):439-42.

48. Prager N, Bickett K, French N, Marcovici G. A randomized, double-blind, placebo-controlled trial to determine the effectiveness of botanically derived inhibitors of 5-alpha-reductase in the treatment of androgenetic alopecia. Journal of Alternative and Complementary Medicine. 2002;8(2):143-52.

49. Blumenthal M, Brusse WR, Goldberg A, Gruenwald J, Hall T, Riggins CW, et al. The Complete German Commission E Monographs. Austin, TX: American Botanical Council; 1998.

Scullcap

1. Wren R. Potter's New Encyclopedia of Botanical Drugs and Preparations. Saffron Walden: C.W. Daniel Company; 1988:362.

2. Newall C, Anderson L, Phillipson J. Herbal Medicines: A Guide for Health Care Professionals. London: The Pharmaceutical Press; 1996:296.

3. Foster S, Chongxi Y. Herbal Emissaries. 1st ed. Rochester, VT.: Healing Arts Press; 1992:356.

4. Chevallier A. The Encyclopedia of Medicinal Plants. Westmount, QC: Reader's Digest, 1996.

5. Leung A, Foster S. Encyclopedia of Common Natural Ingredients Used in Food, Drugs and Cosmetics. New York, NY: John Wiley and Sons; 1996:649.

6. Kubo M, Matsuda H, Kimura Y, et al. *Scutellariae radix*. X. Inhibitory effects of various flavonoids on histamine release from rat peritoneal mast cells *in vitro*. Chemical and Pharmaceutical Bulletin. 1984;32(12):5051-54.

7. Tomimori T, Jin H, Miyaichi Y, et al. Studies on the constituents of Scutellaria species. VI. On the flavonoid constituents of the root *Scutellaria baicalensis* Georgi (5). Quantitative analysis of flavonoids in Scutellaria roots by high-performance liquid chromatography. Yakugaku Zasshi. 1985;105(2):148-55.

8. Hoffmann D. Holistic Herbal. Rockport, CA: Element Books; 1996:256.

9. Kimura Y, Okuda H, Tani T, Arichi S. Studies on *Scutellaria radix*. VI. Effects of flavanone compounds on lipid peroxidation in rat liver. Chemical and Pharmaceutical Bulletin. 1982;30(5):1792-95.

10. Kimura Y, Okuda H, Taira Z, et al. Studies on *Scutellaria radix*; IX. New component inhibiting lipid peroxidation in rat liver. Planta Medica. 1984;50:290-95.

11. Kubo M, Kimura Y, Odani T, et al. Studies on *Scutellaria radix*. Part II: The antibacterial substance. Planta Medica. 1981;43:194-201.

12. Kimura Y, Okuda H, Arichi S. Studies on *Scutellaria radix*; XIII. Effects of various flavonoids on arachidonate metabolism in leukocytes. Planta Medica. 1985;51:132-36.

13. Kimura Y, Kubo M, Kusaka K, et al. Studies on *Scutellaria radix*. V. Effects on ethanol-induced hyperlipemia and lipolysis in isolated fat cells. Chemical and Pharmaceutical Bulletin. 1982;30:219-22.

14. Kimura Y, Kubo M, Tani T, et al. Studies on *Scutellaria radix*. III. Effects on lipid metabolism in serum, liver and fat cells of rats. Chemical and Pharmaceutical Bulletin. 1981;29:2308-12.

15. Tyler VE. The Honest Herbal. 3rd ed. Philadelphia, PA: Pharmaceutical Products Press; 1993:375.

16. De Smet P. Scutellaria species. In: De Smet P, Keller K, Hansel R, Chandler R, eds. Adverse Effects of Herbal Drugs. Heidelberg: Springer-Verlag; 1993:289-96.

17. Perharic L, Shaw D, Colbridge M, et al. Toxicological problems resulting from exposure to traditional remedies and food supplements. Drug Safety. 1994;11:284-94.

18. De Smet P. Notes added in proof. In: De Smet P, Keller K, Hansel R, Chandler R, eds. Adverse Effects of Herbal Drugs. Heidelberg: Springer-Verlag; 1996:229-40.

19. Takeshita K, Saisho Y, Kitamura K, et al. Pneumonitis induced by ou-gon (skullcap). Internal Medicine. 40(8):764-68.

20. D'Arcy P. Adverse reactions and interactions with herbal medicines. Part 2 — Drug Interactions. Adverse Drug Reactions and Toxicological Reviews. 1993:1293: 147-162.

21. Bradley P. British Herbal Compendium. Bournemouth, UK: BHMA; 1992:239.

Slippery Elm

1. Hutchens A. Indian Herbology of North America. Boston, MA: Shambhala; 1973:382.

2. Newall C, Anderson L, Phillipson J. Herbal Medicines. A Guide for Health Care Professionals. London: The Pharmaceutical Press; 1996:296.

3. Wren R. Potter's New Encyclopedia of Botanical Drugs and Preparations. Saffron Walden: C.W. Daniel Company; 1988:362.

4. Evans W. Trease and Evans' Pharmacognosy. 13th ed. London: Bailliere Tindall; 1989:832.

5. Hoffmann D. Holistic Herbal. Rockport, CA: Element Books; 1996:256.

6. Tyler V. Herbs of Choice. The Therapeutic Use of Phytomedicinals. Binghampton: Pharmaceutical Products Press; 1994:209.

7. Mills S. The Essential Book of Herbal Medicine. 2nd ed. London: Penguin; 1991:677.

St John's Wort

1. Unknown. *Hypericum perforatum* (St John's Wort). The Canadian Journal of Herbalism. 1990;11(11):3-7.

2. Barnes J, Anderson L, Phillipson J. Herbal Medicines. 2nd ed. London: Pharmaceutical Press; 2002.

3. Upton R. St. John's Wort (*Hypericum perforatum*). In: Upton R, ed.. American Herbal Pharmacopoeia and Therapeutic Compendium: American Herbal Pharmacopoeia; 1997.

4. Tyler VE. Herbs of Choice. The Therapeutic Use of Phytomedicinals. Binghamton, NY: Pharmaceutical Products Press; 1994.

5. Marles RJ, Associate Professor, Department of Botany, Brandon University, Brandon, Manitoba. Review of Medicinal Plant Modules for CCNM; 1997.

6. Murray MT. The Healing Power of Herbs. Rocklin, CA: Prima Publishing; 1992.

7. Wagner H, Bladt S. Pharmaceutical quality of hypericum extracts. Journal Geriatric and Psychiatry Neurology. 1994;7(Suppl 1):S65-8.

8. Rath G, Potterat O, Mavi S, Hostettmann K. Xanthones from Hypericum roeperanum. Phytochemistry. 1996;43(2):513-20.

9. Rocha L, Marston A, Potterat O, Kaplan MA, Stoeckli-Evans H, Hostettmann K. Antibacterial phloroglucinols and flavonoids from Hypericum brasiliense. Phytochemistry. 1995;40(5):1447-52.

10. Kartnig T, Gobel I, Heydel B. Production of hypericin, pseudohypericin and flavonoids in cell cultures of various Hypericum species and their chemotypes. Planta Medica. 1996;62(1):51-53.

11. Staffeldt B, Kerb R, Brockmoller J, Ploch M, Roots I. Pharmacokinetics of hypericin and pseudohypericin after oral intake of the *Hypericum perforatum* extract LI 160 in healthy volunteers. Journal Geriatric and Psychiatry Neurology. 1994;7(Suppl 1):S47-53.

12. Kerb R, Brockmoller J, Staffeldt B, Ploch M, Roots I. Single-dose and steady-state pharmacokinetics of hypericin and pseudohypericin. Antimicrob Agents Chemother. 1996;40(9):2087-93.

13. Miskovsky P, Sureau F, Chinsky L, Turpin PY. Subcellular distribution of hypericin in human cancer cells. Photochem Photobiol. 1995;62(3):546-49.

14. Rocha L, Marston A, Kaplan MA, Stoeckli-Evans H, Thull U, Testa B, et al. An antifungal gamma-pyrone and xanthones with monoamine oxidase inhibitory activity from Hypericum brasiliense. Phytochemistry. 1994;36(6):1381-85.

15. Taylor RS, Manandhar NP, Hudson JB, Towers GH. Antiviral activities of Nepalese medicinal plants. Journal of Ethnopharmacology. 1996;52(3):157-63.

16. Hudson JB, Lopez-Bazzocchi I, Towers GH. Antiviral activities of hypericin. Antiviral Research. 1991;15(2):101-12.

17. Lopez-Bazzocchi I, Hudson JB, Towers GH. Antiviral activity of the photoactive plant pigment hypericin. Photochem Photobiol. 1991;54(1):95-8.

18. Takahashi I, Nakanishi S, Kobayashi E, Nakano H, Suzuki K, Tamaoki T. Hypericin and pseudohypericin specifically inhibit protein kinase C: Possible relation to their antiretroviral activity. Biochem Biophys Res Commun. 1989;165(3):1207-12.

19. Diwu Z. Novel therapeutic and diagnostic applications of hypocrellins and hypericins. Photochem Photobiol 1995;61(6):529-39.

20. Meruelo D, Lavie G, Lavie D. Therapeutic agents with dramatic antiretroviral activity and little toxicity at affective doses: Aromatic polycyclic diones hypericin and pseudohypericin. Proceedings of the National Academies of Science USA. 1988;85:5230-34.

21. Lavie G, Valentine F, et al. Studies of the mechanism of action of the antiretroviral agents hypericin and pseudohypericin. Proc Natl Acad Sci USA. 1989;86:5963-67.

22. Lenard J, Rabson A, Vanderoef R. Photodynamic inactivation of infectivity of human immunodeficiency virus and other enveloped viruses using hypericin and rose bengal: Inhibition of fusion and syncytia formation. Proceedings of the Natkional Academies of Science USA 1993;90(1):158-62.

23. De Smet PA, Nolen WA. St John's wort as an antidepressant [Editorial; Comment] [see Comments]. British Medical Journal. 1996;313(7052):241-42.

24. Linde K, Ramirez G, Mulrow CD, Pauls A, Weidenhammer W, Melchart D. St John's wort for depression — an overview and meta-analysis of randomised clinical trials [see Comments]. British Medical Journal. 1996;313(7052):253-58.

25. Jenike MA. Editorial. Journal of Geriatric Psychiatry and Neurology. 1994;7(suppl 1):S1.

26. Cott JM. In vitro receptor binding and enzyme inhibition by Hypericum perforatum extract. Pharmacopsychiatry. 1997;30 Suppl 2:108-12.

27. Perovic S, Muller WE. Pharmacological profile of hypericum extract. Effect on serotonin uptake by postsynaptic receptors. Arzneimittelforschung. 1995;45(11):1145-48.

28. Muller WE, Rolli M, Schafer C, Hafner U. Effects of hypericum extract (LI 160) in biochemical models of antidepressant activity. Pharmacopsychiatry. 1997;30 Suppl 2:102-7.

29. Muller WE, Rossol R. Effects of hypericum extract on the expression of serotonin receptors. Journal of Geriatric and Psychiatry Neurology. 1994;7(Suppl 1):S63-4.

30. Baureithel KH, Buter KB, Engesser A, Burkard W, Schaffner W. Inhibition of benzodiazepine binding in vitro by amentoflavone, a constituent of various species of Hypericum. Pharm Acta Helv. 1997;72(3):153-57.

31. Von SNO, Weischer ML. Experimental animal studies of the psychotropic activity of a Hypericum extract. Drug Research. 1987;37(1):10-13.

32. Von HM, Zoller M. Antidepressive effect of a Hypericum extract. Drug Research. 1984;34(2):918-920.

33. Thiele B, Brink I, Ploch M. Modulation of cytokine expression by hypericum extract. Journal of Geriatric and Psychiatry Neurology. 1994;7(Suppl 1):S60-62.

34. Suzuki H, Ohta Y, Takino T, Fugisawa Kea. Effects of glycyrrhizin on biochemical tests in patients with chronic hepatitis — double blind trial. Asian Medical Journal. 1984;26:423-38.

35. Bladt S, Wagner H. Inhibition of MAO by fractions and constituents of hypericum extract. Journal of Geriatric and Psychiatry Neurology. 1994;7(Suppl 1):S57-9.

36. Thiede HM, Walper A. Inhibition of MAO and COMT by hypericum extracts and hypericin. Journal of Geriatric and Psychiatry Neurology. 1994;7(Suppl 1):S54-6.

37. Ozturk Y. Testing the antidepressant effects of Hypericum species on animal models. Pharmacopsychiatry. 1997;30 Suppl 2:125-28.

38. Butterweck V, Wall A, Lieflander-Wulf U, Winterhoff H, Nahrstedt A. Effects of the total extract and fractions of Hypericum perforatum in animal assays for antidepressant activity. Pharmacopsychiatry. 1997;30 Suppl 2:117-24.

39. Payk TR. Treatment of depression. J Geriatr Psychiatry Neurol. 1994;7(Suppl 1):S3-5.

40. Harrer G, Schulz V. Clinical investigation of the antidepressant effectiveness of hypericum. Journal of Geriatric and Psychiatry Neurology. 1994;7(Suppl 1):S6-8.

41. Sommer H, Harrer G. Placebo-controlled double-blind study examining the effectiveness of an hypericum preparation in 105 mildly depressed patients. Journal of Geriatric and Psychiatry Neurology. 1994;7(Suppl 1):S9-11.

42. Hubner WD, Lande S, Podzuweit H. Hypericum treatment of mild depressions with somatic symptoms. Journal of Geriatric Psychiatry and Neurology. 1994;7(Suppl 1):S12-14.

43. Hansgen KD, Vesper J, Ploch M. Multicenter double-blind study examining the antidepressant effectiveness of the hypericum extract LI 160. Journal of Geriatric Psychiatry and Neurology. 1994;7(Suppl 1):S15-18.

44. Vorbach EU, Hubner WD, Arnoldt KH. Effectiveness and tolerance of the hypericum extract LI 160 in comparison with imipramine: Randomized double-blind study with 135 outpatients. Journal of Geriatric Psychiatry and Neurology. 1994;7(Suppl 1):S19-23.

45. Harrer G, Hubner WD, Podzuweit H. Effectiveness and tolerance of the hypericum extract LI 160 compared to maprotiline: A multicenter double-blind study. Journal of Geriatric Psychiatry and Neurology. 1994;7(Suppl 1):S24-28.

46. Martinez B, Kasper S, Ruhrmann S, Moller HJ. Hypericum in the treatment of seasonal affective disorders. Journal of Geriatric Psychiatry and Neurology. 1994;7(Suppl 1):S29-33.

47. Volz HP. Controlled clinical trials of hypericum extracts in depressed patients — an overview. Pharmacopsychiatry. 1997;30 Suppl 2:72-6.

48. Kim HL, Streltzer J, Goebert D. St. John's wort for depression: A meta-analysis of well-defined clinical trials. J Nerv Ment Dis. 1999;187(9):532-38.

49. Gaster B, Holroyd J. St John's wort for depression: A systematic review. Archives of Internal Medicine. 2000;160(2):152-56.

50. Stevinson C, Ernst E. Hypericum for depression. An update of the clinical evidence. Eur Neuropsychopharmacol. 1999;9(6):501-05.

51. Linde K, Mulrow CD. St John's wort for depression. Cochrane Database Syst Rev. 2000;2.

52. Kalb R, Trautmann-Sponsel RD, Kieser M. Efficacy and tolerability of hypericum extract WS 5572 versus placebo in mildly to moderately depressed patients. A randomized double-blind multicenter clinical trial. Pharmacopsychiatry. 2001;34(3):96-103.

53. Philipp M, Kohnen R, Hiller KO. Hypericum extract versus imipramine or placebo in patients with moderate depression: randomised multicentre study of treatment for eight weeks. British Medical Journal. 1999;319(7224):1534-38.

54. Lecrubier Y, Clerc G, Didi R, Kieser M. Efficacy of St. John's wort extract WS 5570 in major depression: A double-blind,

placebo-controlled trial. American Journal of Psychiatry. 2002;159(8):1361-66.

55. Laakmann G, Schule C, Baghai T, Kieser M. St. John's wort in mild to moderate depression: The relevance of hyperforin for the clinical efficacy. Pharmacopsychiatry. 1998;31(Suppl):54-59.

56. Laakmann G, Dienel A, Kieser M. Clinical significance of hyperforin for the efficacy of Hypericum extracts on depressive disorders of different severities. Phytomedicine. 1998;5(6):435-442.

57. Lenoir S, Degenring FH, Saller R. A double-blind randomised trial to investigate three different concentrations of a standardised fresh plant extract obtained from the shoot tips of *Hypericum perforatum* L. Phytomedicine. 1999;6(3):141-46.

58. Woelk H. Comparison of St John's wort and imipramine for treating depression: randomised controlled trial. British Medical Journal. 2000;321(7260):536-39.

59. Bergmann RJ, Nubner J, Demling J. Behandlung leichter bis mittelschwerer depressionen. Vergleich von *Hypericum perforatum* mit amitriptylin. TW Neurologie Psychiatrie. 1993;7:135-240.

60. Volz HP, Laux P. Potential treatment for subthreshold and mild depression: A comparison of St. John's wort extracts and fluoxetine. Compr Psychiatry. 2000;41(2 Suppl 1):133-37.

61. Friede M, Henneicke von Zepelin HH, Freudenstein J. Differential therapy of mild to moderate depressive episodes (ICD-10 F 32.0; F 32.1) with St. John's wort. Pharmacopsychiatry. 2001;34 Suppl 1:S38-41.

62. Schrader E. Equivalence of St John's wort extract (Ze 117) and fluoxetine: A randomized, controlled study in mild-moderate depression. International Clinical Psychopharmacology. 2000;15(2):61-68.

63. Harrer G, Schmidt U, Kuhn U, Biller A. Comparison of equivalence between the St. John's wort extract LoHyp-57 and fluoxetine. Arzneimittel-Forschung. 1999;49(4):289-96.

64. van Gurp G, Meterissian GB, Haiek LN, McCusker J, Bellavance F. St John's wort or sertraline? Randomized controlled trial in primary care. Canadian Family Physician. 2002;48:905-12.

65. Brenner R, Azbel V, Madhusoodanan S, Pawlowska M. Comparison of an extract of hypericum (LI 160) and sertraline in the treatment of depression: A double-blind, randomized pilot study. Clinical Therapeutics. 2000;22(4):411-19.

66. Shelton RC, Keller MB, Gelenberg A, Dunner DL, Hirschfeld R, Thase ME, et al. Effectiveness of St John's wort in major depression: A randomized controlled trial. Journal of the American Medical Association. 2001;285(15):1978-86.

67. Cott JM, Rosenthal N, Blumenthal M. St John's wort and major depression. Journal of the American Medical Association. 2001;286(1):42; author reply 44-45.

68. Fomous CM, Cardellina JH, 2nd. St John's wort and major depression. Journal of the American Medical Association. 2001;286(1):42; author reply 44-5.

69. Cohen HW, Marantz PR. St John's wort and major depression. Journal of the American Medical Association. 2001;286(1):42-3; author reply 44-5.

70. Brenner R, Madhusoodanan S, Pawlowska M, Czobor P. St John's wort and major depression. Journal of the American Medical Association. 2001;286(1):43; author reply 44-5.

71. Shelton RC, Crits-Cristoph P. St John's wort and major depression. Journal of the American Medical Association. 2001;286(1):42-45.

72. Hypericum Depression Trial Study Group. Effect of *Hypericum perforatum* (St John's wort) in major depressive disorder: a randomized controlled trial. Journal of the American Medical Association. 2002;287(14):1807-14.

73. Jonas W. St John's wort and depression. Journal of the American Medical Association. 2002;288(4):446; author reply 448-49.

74. Wheatley D. St. John's wort and depression. Journal of the American Medical Association. 2002;288(4):446-47.

75. Spielmans G. St. John's wort and depression. Journal of the American Medical Association. 2002;288(4):447.

76. Volp A. St. John's wort and depression. Journal of the American Medical Association. 2002;288(4):447.

77. Linde K, Melchart D, Mulrow C, Berner M. St. John's wort and depression. Journal of the American Medical Association. 2002;288(4):447-48.

78. Cott J. St. John's wort and depression. Journal of the American Medical Association. 2002;288(4):448.

79. Davidson J. St. John's wort and depression. Journal of the American Medical Association. 2002;288(4):448-49.

80. Kupfer D. St. John's wort and depression. Journal of the American Medical Association. 2002;288(4):449.

81. Vorbach EU, Arnoldt KH, Hubner WD. Efficacy and tolerability of St. John's wort extract LI 160 versus imipramine in patients with severe depressive episodes according to ICD- 10. Pharmacopsychiatry. 1997;30 Suppl 2:81-85.

82. Volz HP, Murck H, Kasper S, Moller HJ. St John's wort extract (LI 160) in somatoform disorders: Results of a placebo-controlled trial. Psychopharmacology (Berl). 2002;164(3):294-300.

83. Sindrup SH, Madsen C, Bach FW, Gram LF, Jensen TS. St. John's wort has no effect on pain in polyneuropathy. Pain. 2001;91(3):361-65.

84. Woelk H, Burkard G, Grunwald J. Benefits and risks of the hypericum extract LI 160: Drug monitoring study with 3250 patients. J Geriatr Psychiatry Neurol. 1994;7(Suppl 1):S34-38.

85. Ernst E, Rand JI, Barnes J, Stevinson C. Adverse effects profile of the herbal antidepressant St. John's wort (*Hypericum perforatum* L.). Eur J Clin Pharmacol. 1998;54(8):589-94.

86. Schempp CM, Muller K, Winghofer B, Schulte-Monting J, Simon JC. Single-dose and steady-state administration of *Hypericum perforatum* extract (St John's Wort) does not influence skin sensitivity to UV radiation, visible light, and solar-simulated radiation. Arch Dermatol. 2001;137(4):512-13.

87. Parker V, Wong AH, Boon HS, Seeman MV. Adverse reactions to St John's Wort. Canadian Journal of Psychiatry. 2001;46(1):77-79.

88. Ferko N, Levine MA. Evaluation of the association between St. John's wort and elevated thyroid-stimulating hormone. Pharmacotherapy. 2001;21(12):1574-78.

89. Bhopal JS. St John's wort-induced sexual dysfunction. Canadian Journal of Psychiatry. 2001;46(5):456-57.

90. Moses EL, Mallinger AG. St. John's wort: Three cases of possible mania induction. Journal of Clinical Psychopharmacology. 2000;20(1):115-17.

91. Schneck C. St. John's wort and hypomania. J Clin Psychiatry. 1998;59(12):689.

92. O'Breasail AM, Argouarch S. Hypomania and St John's wort. Canadian Journal of Psychiatry. 1998;43(7):746-7.

93. Nierenberg AA, Burt T, Matthews J, Weiss AP. Mania associated with St. John's wort. Biol Psychiatry. 1999;46(12):1707-08.

94. Barbenel DM, Yusufi B, O'Shea D, Bench CJ. Mania in a patient receiving testosterone replacement postorchidectomy taking St John's wort and sertraline. Journal of Psychopharmacology. 2000;14(1):84-86.

95. Patel S, Robinson R, Burk M. Hypertensive crisis associated with St. John's Wort. American Journal of Medicine. 2002;112(6):507-08.

96. Schulz H, Jobert M. Effects of hypericum extract on the sleep EEG in older volunteers. Journal of Geriatric Psychiatry and Neurology. 1994;7(Suppl 1):S39-43.

97. Johnson D, Ksciuk H, Woelk H, Sauerwein-Giese E, Frauendorf A. Effects of hypericum extract LI 160 compared with maprotiline on resting EEG and evoked potentials in 24 volunteers. Journal of Geriatric Psychiatry and Neurology. 1994;7(Suppl 1):S44-46.

98. Miller LG. Drug interactions known or potentially associated with St. John's wort. J Herb Pharmacotherapy. 2001;1(3):51-64.

99. Ernst E. The risk-benefit profile of commonly used herbal therapies: Ginkgo, St. John's wort, ginseng, echinacea, saw palmetto, and kava. Annals of Internal Medicine. 2002;136(1):42-53.

100. Ernst E. Possible interactions between synthetic and herbal medicinal products. Part 1: A systematic review of the indirect evidence. Perfusion. 2000;1:4-15.

101. Fugh-Berman A. Herb-drug interactions. Lancet. 2000;355(9198):134-38.

102. Bon S, Hartmann K, Kuhn M. Johanniskraut ein enzyminduktor? Schweitz Apoth. 1999;16:535-36.

103. Ernst E. Second thoughts about the safety of St. John's wort. Lancet. 1999;355:134-38.

104. Ruschitzka F, Meier PJ, Turina M, Luscher TF, Noll G. Acute heart transplant rejection due to Saint John's wort. Lancet. 2000;355(9203):548-49.

105. Moschella C, Jaber BL. Interaction between cyclosporine and *Hypericum perforatum* (St. John's wort) after organ transplantation. American Journal of Kidney Disease. 2001;38(5):1105-07.

106. Breidenbach T, Hoffmann MW, Becker T, Schlitt H, Klempnauer J. Drug interaction of St John's wort with cyclosporin. Lancet. 2000;355(9218):1912.

107. Karhova M, Treichel U, Malago M, Frilling A, Gerken G, Broelsch C. Interaction of *Hypericum perforatum* (St. John's wort) with cyclosporin A metabolism in a patient after liver transplantation. Journal of Hepatology. 2000;33:853-55.

108. Ahmed SM, Banner NR, Dubrey SW. Low cyclosporin-A level due to Saint-John's-wort in heart transplant patients. J Heart Lung Transplant. 2001;20(7):795.

109. Barone GW, Gurley BJ, Ketel BL, Lightfoot ML, Abul-Ezz SR. Drug interaction between St. John's wort and cyclosporine. Ann Pharmacother. 2000;34(9):1013-16.

110. Ernst E. St John's Wort supplements endanger the success of organ transplantation. Archives of Surgery. 2002;137(3):316-19.

111. Johne A, Brockmoller J, Bauer S, Maurer A, Langheinrich M, Roots I. Pharmacokinetic interaction of digoxin with an herbal extract from St John's wort (*Hypericum perforatum*). Clinical Pharmacology & Therapeutics. 1999;66(4):338-45.

112. Crowe S, McKeating K. Delayed emergence and St. John's wort. Anesthesiology. 2002;96(4):1025-27.

113. Piscitelli SC, Burstein AH, Chaitt D, Alfaro RM, Falloon J. Indinavir concentrations and St John's wort [Letter]. Lancet. 2000;355(9203):547-48.

114. Lantz MS, Buchalter E, Giambanco V. St. John's wort and antidepressant drug interactions in the elderly. Journal of Geriatric Psychiatry and Neurology. 1999;12(1):7-10.

115. Gordon JB. SSRIs and St.John's Wort: possible toxicity? [Letter]. American Family Physician. 1998;57(5):950,953.

116. Maurer A, Johne A, Bauer S, Brockmoller J, Donath F, Roots I, et al. Interaction of St. John's wort extract with phenprocoumon. Eur J Clin Chem Clin Pharmacol. 1999;55(3):A22.

117. Nebel A, Schneider BJ, Baker RK, Kroll DJ. Potential metabolic interaction between St. John's wort and theophylline [Letter]. Annals of Pharmacotherapy. 1999;33(4):502.

118. Demott K. St. John's wort tied to serotonin syndrome. Clin Psychiatry News. 1998;26:28.

119. Yue QY, Bergquist C, Gerden B. Safety of St John's wort (*Hypericum perforatum*) [Letter; Comment]. Lancet. 2000;355(9203):576-77.

120. Durr D, Steiger B, Kullak-Ublick GA, Rentsch KM, Steinert HC, Meier PJ, et al. St. John's wort induces intestinal P-glycoprotein/MDRI and intestinal and hepatic CYP3A4. Clinical Pharmacology and Therapeutics. 2000;68:598-604.

121. Moore LB, Goodwin B, Jones SA, Wisely GB, Serabjit-Singh CJ, Willson TM, et al. St. John's wort induces hepatic drug metabolism through activation of the pregnane X receptor. Proceedings of the National Academy of Sciences. 2000;97(13):7500-02.

122. Roby CA, Anderson GD, Kantor E, Dryer DA, Burstein AH. St. John's wort: Effect on CYP3A4 activity. Clinical Pharmacology and Therapeutics. 2000;67:451-57.

123. Brinker F. Herb Contraindications and Drug Interactions. 3rd ed. Sandy, OR: Eclectic Medical Publishers; 2001.

124. Chevalleir A. The Encyclopedia of Medicinal Plants. Westmount, QC: Reader's Digest, 1996.

Tea Tree Oil

1. Altman P. Australian tea tree oil. Aust. J Pharm. 1988;69:276-78.

2. Williams L, Home V. A comparative study of some essential oils for potential use in topical applications for the treatment of the yeast *Candida albicans*. Australian Journal of Medical Herbalism. 1995;7(3):57-62.

3. Leung AY, Foster S. Encyclopedia of Common Natural Ingredients Used in Food, Drugs, and Cosmetics. 2nd ed. Toronto, ON/New York,NY: John Wiley and Sons Inc; 1996.

4. Tyler VE. Herbs of Choice. The Therapeutic Use of Phytomedicinals. Binghamton, NY: Pharmaceutical Products Press; 1994.

5. Tyler V. The Honest Herbal. 3rd ed. Binghamton, NY: Pharmaceutical Products Press; 1993.

6. Buck D, Midorf D, Addino J. Comparison of two topical preparations for the treatment of onychomycosis: *Melaleuca alternifolia* (tea tree) oil and clotrimazole. Journal of Family Practice. 1994;38:601-05.

7. Caelli M, Porteous J, Carson CF, Heller R, Riley TV. Tea tree oil as an alternative topical decolonization agent for methicillin-resistant *Staphylococcus aureus*. J Hosp Infect. 2000;46(3):236-37.

8. Bassett I, et al. A comparative study of tea-tree oil versus benzoyl peroxide in the treatment of acne. Medical Journal of Australia. 1990;153:455-58.

9. Tong M, Altmann P, Barnetson R. Tea tree oil in the treatment of tinea pedis. Australian Journal of Dermatology. 1992;33:145-49.

10. Satchell AC, Saurajen A, Bell C, Barnetson RS. Treatment of interdigital tinea pedis with 25% and 50% tea tree oil solution: a randomized, placebo-controlled, blinded study. Australas J Dermatol. 2002;43(3):175-78.

11. Syed TA, Qureshi ZA, Ali SM, Ahmad S, Ahmad SA. Treatment of toenail onychomycosis with 2% butenafine and 5% *Melaleuca alternifolia* (tea tree) oil in cream. Trop Med Int Health. 1999;4(4):284-87.

12. Satchell AC, Saurajen A, Bell C, Barnetson RS. Treatment of dandruff with 5% tea tree oil shampoo. Journal of the American Academy of Dermatology. 2002;47(6):852-55.

13. Carson CF, Ashton L, Dry L, Smith DW, Riley TV. *Melaleuca alternifolia* (tea tree) oil gel (6%) for the treatment of recurrent herpes labialis. J Antimicrob Chemother. 2001;48(3):450-51.

14. Tisserand R, Balacs T. Essential Oil Safety: A Guide for Health Care Professionals. London: Churchill Livingstone; 1995.

15. Brown D. Topical tea tree oil for onychomycosis. Quarterly Review of Natural Medicine. 1995;Spring:11.

16. Brown D. Tea tree oil for athlete's foot. Quarterly Review of Natural Medicine. 1993;Winter:15.

Thyme

1. Newall C, Anderson L, Phillipson J. Herbal Medicines: A Guide for Health Care Professionals. London: The Pharmaceutical Press; 1996:296.

2. Leung A, Foster S. Encylopedia of Common Natural Ingredients Used in Food, Drugs and Cosmetics. New York, NY: John Wiley and Sons; 1996:649.

3. Tyler V. Herbs of Choice. The Therapeutic Use of Phytomedicinals. Binghampton, NY: Pharmaceutical Products Press; 1994:209.

4. Mills S. The Essential Book of Herbal Medicine. 2nd ed. London: Penguin 1991:677.

5. Tisserand R, Balacs T. Essential Oil Safety: A Guide for Health Care Professionals. London: Churchill Livingstone; 1995:279.

6. ESCOP. Thymi Herba/Thyme. In: ESCOP Monographs (Fascicule 1) Exeter: ESCOP; 1996:62.

7. Marles RJ, Associate Professor, Department of Botany, Brandon University, Brandon, Manitoba. Review of Medicinal Plant Modules for CCNM; 1998.

8. Hoffmann D. Holistic Herbal. Rockport, CA: Element Books; 1996:256.

9. Wren R. Potter's New Encyclopedia of Botanical Drugs and Preparations. Saffron Walden, UK: C.W. Daniel Company; 1988:362.

10. Van Den Broucke CO, Lernli JA. Pharmacological and chemical investigation of thyme liquid extracts. Planta Medica. 1981;41:129-35.

11. Van Den Broucke CO. The therapeutic value of Thymus species. Fitoterapia. 1983;4:171-74.

12. Agnihotri S, Vaidya AD. A novel approach to study antibacterial properties of volatile components of selected Indian medicinal herbs. Indian Journal of Experimental Biology. 1996;34(7):712-15.

13. Juven BJ, Kanner J, Schved F, Weisslowicz H. Factors that interact with the antibacterial action of thyme essential oil and its active constituents. Journal of Applied Bacteriology. 1994;76(6):626-31.

14. Tabak M, Armon R, Potasman I, Neeman I. *In vitro* inhibition of Helicobacter pylori by extracts of thyme. Journal of Applied Bacteriology. 1996;80(6):667-72.

15. Vukovic-Gacic B, Simic D. Identification of natural antimutagens with modulating effects on DNA repair. Basic Life Sciences. 1993;61:269-77.

16. Englberger W, Hadding U, Etschenberg E, et al. Rosmarinic acid: A new inhibitor of complement C3-convertase with anti-inflammatory activity. International Journal of Immunopharmacology. 1988;10:729-37.

17. Haraguchi H, Saito T, Ishikawa H, et al. Antiperoxidative components in *Thymus vulgaris*. Planta Medica. 1996;62(3):217-21.

18. Brinker F. The Toxicology of Botanical Medicines. 2nd ed. Portland, OR: National College of Naturopathic Medicine; 1983:141.

19. Lemiere C, Cartier A, Lehrer SB, Malo JL. Occupational asthma caused by aromatic herbs. Allergy. 1996;51(9):647-49.

20. Benito M, Jorro G, Morales C, et al. Labiatae allergy: Systemic reactions due to ingestion of oregano and thyme. Annals of Allergy Asthma and Immunology. 1996;76(5):416-18.

Turmeric

1. Tyler VE. Herbs of Choice. The Therapeutic Use of Phytomedicinals. Binghamton, NY: Pharmaceutical Products Press; 1994:209.

2. Leung A, Foster S. Encyclopedia of Common Natural Ingredients Used in Food, Drugs and Cosmetics 2nd Edition. New York: John Wiley and Sons; 1996:649.

3. Murray MT. The Healing Power of Herbs. Rocklin, CA: Prima Publishing; 1992:246.

4. Marles RJ, Associate Professor, Department of Botany, Brandon University, Brandon, Manitoba. Review of Medicinal Plant Modules for CCNM; 1998.

5. Srivastava R. Inhibition of neutrophil response by curcumin. Agents and Actions. 1989;28:298-303.

6. Ammon HP, Safayhi H, Mack T, Sabieraj J. Mechanism of antiinflammatory actions of curcumine and boswellic acids. Journal of Ethnopharmacology. 1993;38(2-3):113-19.

7. Chan MM. Inhibition of tumor necrosis factor by curcumin, a phytochemical. Biochemical Pharmacology. 1995;49(11):1551-56.

8. Srimal R, Dhawan B. Pharmacology of diferuloyl methane (curcumin), a non-steroidal anti-inflammatory agent. Journal of Pharmacy and Pharmacology. 1973;25:447-52.

9. Mukhopadhyay A, Basu N, Ghatak N, Gujral P. Anti-inflammatory and irritant activities of curcumin analogues in rats. Agents and Actions. 1982;12:508-15.

10. Srivastava R, Srimal RC. Modification of certain inflammation-induced biochemical changes by curcumin. Indian Journal of Medical Research. 1985;81:215-23.

11. Ramprasad C, Sirsi M. *Curcuma longa* and bile secretion: quantitative changes in the bile constituents induced by sodium curcuminate. J Sci Ind Res. 1957;16C:108-10.

12. Selvam R, Subramanian L, Gayathri R, Angayarkanni N. The anti-oxidant activity of turmeric (*Curcuma longa*). Journal of Ethnopharmacology. 1995;47(2):59-67.

13. Osawa T, Sugiyama Y, Inayoshi M, Kawakishi S. Antioxidative activity of tetrahydrocurcuminoids. Bioscience Biotechnology and Biochemistry. 1995;59(9):1609-12.

14. Chandra D, Gupta S. Anti-inflammatory and anti-arthritic activity of volatile oil of *Curcuma longa* (Haldi). Indian Journal of Medical Research. 1972;60:138-42.

15. Arora R, Basu N, Kapoor V, Jain A. Anti-inflammatory studies on *Curcuma longa* (tumeric). Indian Journal of Medical Research. 1971;60:138-42.

16. Ghatak N, Basu N. Sodium curcuminate as an effective anti-inflammatory agent. Indian Journal of Experimental Biology. 1972;10:235-6.

17. Deodhar SD, Sethi R, Srimal RC. Preliminary studies on antirheumatic activity of curcumin (di-feruloyl methane). Indian Journal of Medical Research. 1980;71:632-34.

18. Satoskar RR, Shah SJ, Shenony SG. Evaluation of anti-inflammatory property of curcumin (di-feruloyl methane) in patients with postoperative inflammation. International Journal of Clinical Pharmacology Therapy and Toxicology. 1986;24:651-54.

19. Rafatullah S, et al. Evaluation of turmeric (*Curcuma longa*) for gastric and duodenal antiulcer activity in rats. Journal of Ethnopharmacology. 1990;29(1):25-34.

20. Blumenthal M. Therapeutic Monographs on Medicinal Plants for Human Use of Special Expert Committee, Federal Health Agency, Germany. Austin, TX: American Botanical Council; 1998.

21. Duke J. The Green Pharmacy. New York: Rodale Press Inc.; 1997.

22. van Dau N, Ngoc Ham N, Huy Khac D, et al. The effects of a traditional drug, turmeric (*Curcuma longa*), and placebo on the healing of duodenal ulcer. Phytomedicine. 1998;5:29-34.

23. Kiso Y, Suzuki Y, Watanabe N, et al. Antihepatotoxic principles of *Curcuma longa* rhizomes. Planta Medica. 1983;49:185-87.

24. Lin SC, Lin CC, Lin YH, Supriyatna S, Teng CW. Protective and therapeutic effects of Curcuma xanthorrhiza on hepatotoxin-induced liver damage. American Journal of Chinese Medicine. 1995;23(3-4):243-54.

25. Huang MT, Lou YR, Ma W, Newmark HL, Reuhl KR, Conney AH. Inhibitory effects of dietary curcumin on forestomach, duodenal, and colon carcinogenesis in mice. Cancer Research. 1994;54(22):5841-47.

26. Azuine MA, Bhide SV. Adjuvant chemoprevention of experimental cancer: Catechin and dietary turmeric in forestomach and oral cancer models. Journal of Ethnopharmacology. 1994;44(3):211-17.

27. Ruby AJ, Kuttan G, Babu KD, Rajasekharan KN, Kuttan R. Anti-tumour and antioxidant activity of natural curcuminoids. Cancer Letters. 1995;94(1):79-83.

28. Limtrakul P, Lipigorngoson S, Namwong O, Apisariyakul A, Dunn FW. Inhibitory effect of dietary curcumin on skin carcinogenesis in mice. Cancer Letters. 1997;116(2):197-203.

29. Soni KB, Lahiri M, Chackradeo P, Bhide SV, Kuttan R. Protective effect of food additives on aflatoxin-induced mutagenicity and hepatocarcinogenicity. Cancer Letters. 1997;115(2):129-33.

30. Verma SP, Salamone E, Goldin B. Curcumin and genistein, plant natural products, show synergistic inhibitory effects on the growth of human breast cancer MCF-7 cells induced by estrogenic pesticides. Biochemical and Biophysical Research Communications. 1997;233(3):692-96.

31. Dahl TA, Bilski P, Reszka KJ, Chignell CF. Photocytotoxicity of curcumin. Photochemistry and Photobiology. 1994;59(3):290-94.

32. Mazumder A, Raghavan K, Weinstein J, Kohn KW, Pommier Y. Inhibition of human immunodeficiency virus type-1 integrase by curcumin. Biochemical Pharmacology. 1995;49(8):1165-70.

33. Sui Z, Salto R, Li J, Craik C, Ortiz de Montellano PR. Inhibition of the HIV-1 and HIV-2 proteases by curcumin and curcumin boron complexes. Bioorganic and Medicinal Chemistry. 1993;1(6):415-22.

34. Li CJ, Zhang LJ, Dezube BJ, Crumpacker CS, Pardee AB. Three inhibitors of type 1 human immunodeficiency virus long terminal repeat-directed gene expression and virus replication. Proceedings of the National Academy of Sciences of the USA. 1993;90:1839-42.

35. Kiuchi F, Goto Y, Sugimoto N, Akao N, Kondo K, Tsuda Y. Nematocidal activity of turmeric:

Synergistic action of curcuminoids. Chemical and Pharmaceutical Bulletin (Tokyo). 1993;41(9):1640-43.

36. Apisariyakul A, Vanittanakom N, Buddhasukh D. Antifungal activity of turmeric oil extracted from *Curcuma longa* (Zingiberaceae). Journal of Ethnopharmacology. 1995;49(3):163-69.

37. Shankar TNB, Muthy IAS. Effect of tumeric *Curcuma longa* fractions on the growth of some intestinal and pathogenic bacteria *in vitro*. Indian Journal of Experimental Biology. 1978;17:1363-66.

38. Tonnesen HH, de Vries H, Karlsen J, van Hengouwen GB. Studies on curcumin and curcuminoids IX: Investigation of the photobiological activity of curcumin using bacterial indicator systems. Journal of Pharmaceutical Sciences. 1987;76:371-73.

39. Dahl TA, McGowan WM, Shand MA, Srinivasan VS. Photokilling of bacteria by the natural dye curcumin. Archives of Microbiology. 1989;151:183-85.

40. Lal B, Kapoor AK, Asthana OP, et al. Efficacy of curcumin in the management of chronic anterior uveitis. Phytotherapy Research. 1999;13:318-22.

41. Roa SD, Chandrashekhera N, Satyanarayana N, Srinivasan M. Effect of curcumin on serum and liver cholesterol levels in the rat. Journal of Nutrition. 1970;100:1307-16.

42. Dixit VP, Jain P, Joshi SC. Hypolipidaemic effect of *Curcuma longa* L. and *Nardostachys jatamansi* DC in triton-induced hyperlipidaemic rats. Indian Journal of Physiol Pharmacol. 1988;32:299-304.

43. Shankar TNB, Shantha NV, Ramesh HP, et al. Toxicity studies on tumeric (*Curcuma longa*): Acute toxicity studies in rats, guinea pigs, and monkeys. Indian Journal of Experimental Biology. 1980;18:73-75.

44. Singh A, Singh SP, Bamezai R. Postnatal modulation of hepatic biotransformation system enzymes via translactational exposure of F1 mouse pups to turmeric and curcumin. Cancer Letters. 1995;96(1):87-93.

Uva-Ursi

1. Newall CA, Anderson LA, Phillipson JD. Herbal Medicines. A Guide for Health Care Professionals. London: The Pharmaceutical Press; 1996.

2. Leung AY, Foster S. Encyclopedia of Common Natural Ingredients Used in Food, Drugs, and Cosmetics. 2nd ed. Toronto, ON/New York, NY: John Wiley and Sons Inc; 1996.

3. Mills S. The Essential Book of Herbal Medicine. 2nd ed. London: Penguin Publ; 1991.

4. Tyler V. The Honest Herbal. 3rd ed. Binghamton, N.Y.: Pharmaceutical Products Press; 1993.

5. Evans W. Trease and Evans' Pharmacognosy. 13th Edition ed. London: Bailliere Tindall; 1989.

6. Jahodar L, Leifertova I. The evaluation of p-methoxyphenol in the leaves of *Arctostaphylos uva-ursi*. Pharmazie. 1979;34:188-89.

7. Karikas GA, et.al. Isolation of piceoside from *Arctostaphylos uva-ursi*. Planta Medica. 1987;53: 307-08.

8. Jahodar L, et al. Unedoside in *Arctostaphylos uva-ursi* roots. Pharmazie. 1981;36:294-96.

9. Jahodar L, et al. Investigation of iridoid substances in *Arctostaphylos uva-ursi*. Pharmazie. 1978;33:536-37.

10. ESCOP. Uvae Ursi Folium/Bearberry. In: Phytotherapy) EESCo, ed. ESCOP Monographs (Fascicule 5). Exeter: ESCOP; 1997:65.

11. Weiss R. Herbal Medicine. Beaconsfield, UK: Beaconsfield Publishers Ltd; 1988.

12. Tyler VE. Herbs of Choice. The Therapeutic Use of Phytomedicinals. Binghamton, NY: Pharmaceutical Products Press; 1994.

13. Hoffmann D. Holistic Herbal. Rockport, CA: Element Books; 1996.

14. Houghton P. Bearberry, dandelion and celery. The Pharmaceutical Journal. 1995;255:272-73.

15. Bradley P. British Herbal Compendium. Bournemouth, UK: The British Herbal Medical Association; 1992.

16. Frohne D. Untersuchungen zur Frage der Harndesinfizierenden Wirkungen von Barentraubenblatt-Extrakten. Planta Medica. 1970;18:23-25.

17. Grases F, Melero G, Costa-Bauza A, Prieto R, March J. Urolithiasis and Phytotherapy. International Urology and Nephrology. 1994;26(5):507-11.

18. Moskalenko SA. Preliminary screening of far-Eastern ethnomedicinal plants for antibacterial activity. Journal of Ethnopharmacology. 1986;15:231-59.

19. Schindler G, Patzak U, Brinkhaus B, von Niecieck A, Wittig J, Krahmer N, et al. Urinary excretion and metabolism of arbutin after oral administration of *Arctostaphylos uvae ursi* extract as film-coated tablets and aqueous solution in healthy humans. Journal of Clinical Pharmacology. 2002;42(8):920-27.

20. Merck. Merck Index. 10th ed. Rahway, NJ: Merck and Company; 1983.

Valerian

1. Newall CA, Anderson LA, Phillipson JD. Herbal Medicines. A Guide for Health Care Professionals. London: The Pharmaceutical Press; 1996.

2. Houghton PJ. The biological activity of valerian and related plants. Journal of Ethnopharmacology. 1988;22:121-42.

3. Hobbs C. Phu: Valerian and other anti-hysterics in European and American medicine (1733-1936). Pharm Hist. 1990;32(3):132-37.

4. Bos R, Woerdenbag HJ, De Smet PAGM, Scheffer JJC. Valerian Species. In: P.A.G.M DS, K K, Hansel R, Chandler RF, editors. Adverse effects of herbal drugs. Berlin, Heidelberg: Springer-Verlag; 1997:165-80.

5. Leathwood PD, Chauffard F, Heck E, Munoz-Box R. Aqueous extract of valerian root (*Valeriana officinalis*) improves sleep quality in man. Reduces sleep latency to fall asleep in man. Pharmacology Biochemistry and Behavior. 1982;17:65-71.

6. Tyler VE. Herbs of Choice. The Therapeutic Use of Phytomedicinals. Binghamton, NY: Pharmaceutical Products Press; 1994.

7. Murray MT. The Healing Power of Herbs. Rocklin, CA: Prima Publishing; 1992.

8. Fuchs R. Samtliche Werke (Collected Works). In Munich; 1895-1908.

9. European Scientific Cooperative on Phytotherapy. Monographs on the medicinal uses of plant drugs (Fasicule 4). Exeter: European Scientific Cooperative on Phytotherapy; 1997.

10. Hendriks H, et al. Eugenyl isovalerate and isoeugenyl isovalerate in the essential oil of Valerian root. Phytochemistry. 1977;16:1853-54.

11. Bos R, et al. Isolation of the sesquiterpene alcohol (-)-pacifigorgiol from Valeriana officinalis. Phytochemistry. 1986;25:1234-35.

12. Bos R, et al. Isolation and identification of valerenane sesquiterpenoids from Valeriana officinalis. Phytochemistry. 1986;25:133-35.

13. Holzl J, Godau P. Receptor binding studies with Valeriana officinalis on the benzodiazepine receptor. Planta Medica. 1989;55:642.

14. Mennini T, Bernasconi P, et al. In vitro study in the interaction of extracts and pure compounds from Valeriana officinalis roots with GABA, benzodiazepine and barbituate receptors. Fitoterapia. 1993;64:291-300.

15. Cavadas C, Araujo I, Cotrim MD, Amaral T, Cunha AP, Macedo T, et al. In vitro study on the interaction of Valeriana officinalis L. extracts and their amino acids on GABAA receptor in rat brain. Arzneimittelforschung. 1995;45(7):753-55.

16. Bodesheim U, Holzl J. Isolation and receptor binding properties of alkaloids and lignans from Valeriana officinalis L. Pharmazie. 1997;52(5):386-91.

17. Santos MS, Ferreira F, Cunha AP, Carvalho AP, Macedo T. An aqueous extract of valerian influences the transport of GABA in synaptosomes [Letter]. Planta Medica. 1994;60(3):278-79.

18. Santos MS, Ferreira F, Faro C, Pires E, Carvalho AP, Cunha AP, et al. The amount of GABA present in aqueous extracts of valerian is sufficient to account for [3H]GABA release in synaptosomes [Letter]. Planta Medica. 1994;60(5):475-76.

19. Riedel E, et al. Inhibition of gamma-aminobutyric acid catabolism by valerenic acid derivatives. Planta Medica. 1982;48:219-20.

20. Holzl J. Baldrian - Ein mittel gegen Schlafstorungen und Nervositat. Dtsch Apoth Ztg. 1996;136:751-59.

21. Balduini W, Cattabeni F. Displacement of [3H]-N6-cyclohexladenosine binding to rat cortical membranes by an hydroalcoholic extract of Valeriana officinalis. Medical Science and Research. 1989;17:639-40.

22. Hazelhoff B, et.al. Antispasmodic effects of Valeriana compunds: an in-vivo and in-vitro study on the guinea-pig ileum. Archives Int Pharmacodyn. 1982;257:274-87.

23. Shrivastava SC, Sisodia CS. Analgetic studies on Vitex Negundo and Valeriana wallichii. Indian Veterinary Journal. 1970;47:170-75.

24. Girgune JB, Jain NK, Grag BD. Antimicrobial activity of the essential oil from Valeriana wallichii D.C. (Valerianaceae). Indian Journal of Microbiology. 1980;20:142-43.

25. Chen S, Xie X, Du B, et al. Infantile rotavirus enteritis treated with herbal Valeriana jatamansi (VJ). Journal of Traditional Chinese Medicine. 1984;4:297-300.

26. Hansel R, Keller K, Rimpler H, Schneider G. Hagers Handbuch der Parmzeutischen Praxis. 5th ed. Berlin: Springer-Verlag; 1994.

27. Torrent MT, Iglesias J, Adzet T. Valoracion experimental de la actividad sedante de la tinctura de Valeriana officinalis L. Circular Farmaceutica. 1972;30:107-12.

28. Sakamoto T, Mitani Y, Nakajima K. Psychotropic effects of Japanese valerian root extract. Chemical and Pharmaceutical Bulletin (Tokyo) 1992;40(3):758-61.

29. Hikino H, Hikino Y, Kobinata H, Aizawa A. Sedative properties of valerian roots. Shoyakugako Zasshi 1980;34:19-24.

30. Takamura K, Kawaguchi M, Nabata H. The preparation and pharmacological screening of kessoglycol derivative. Yakugaku Zasshi. 1975;95:1198-1204.

31. Takamura K, Nabata H, Kawaguchi M. The pharmacological action on the kessoglycol-8-monoacetate. Yakugaku Zasshi. 1975;95:1205-09.

32. Hendriks H, et al. Central nervous system depressant activity of valerenic acid in the mouse. Planta Medica. 1985;51:28-31.

33. Hendriks R, Bos, Allersma DP, Malingre TM, Koster S. Pharmacological screening of valerenal and some other components of essential oil of Valeriana officinalis. Planta Medica. 1981;42:62-68.

34. Veith J, et al. The influence of some degradation products of valepotriates on the motor activity of light-dark synchronized mice. Planta Medica. 1986;52:179-83.

35. Wagner H, et al. Comparative studies on the sedative action of Valeriana extracts, valepotriates and their degradation products. Planta Medica. 1980;39:358-65.

36. Leuschner J, Muller J, Rudmann M. Characterisation of the central nervous depressant activity of a commercially available valerian root extract. Arzneimittelforschung. 1993;43(6):638-41.

37. Hiller K-O, Zetler G. Neuropharmacological studies on ethanol extracts of Valeriana officinalis L. behavioural and anticonvulsant properties. Phytotherapy Research. 1996;10:145-51.

38. Oshima Y, Matsuoka S, Ohizumi Y. Antidepressant principles of Valeriana fauriei roots. Chemical and Pharmaceutical Bulletin. (Tokyo) 1995;43(1):169-70.

39. Brattstrom A. Evidence of efficacy for herbal remedies exemplified for a fixed combination of hops and valerian. Forsch Komplementarmed. 1996;3(4):188-95.

40. Holm E, Kowollik H, Reinecke A, von Henning GE, F. B, Scherer H-D. Vergichende neurophysiologische Untersuchungen mit Valtratum/Isovaltratum und Extractum Valerianae an Katzen. Medizinische Welt. 1980;31:982-90.

41. Krieglstein J, Grusla D. Zentral dampfende Inhaltsstoffe im Baldrian. Valpotriate, Valerensaure, Valeranon and atherisches Ol sind jedoch unwirksam. Deutsch Apotheker Zeituug. 1988;128:2041-46.

42. Grusla D, Holzl J. J.K. Baldrianwirkungen im Gehirn der Ratte. Deutsch Apotheker Zeituug. 1986;126:2249-53.

43. Houghton P. Valerian. Pharmaceutical Journal. 1994;253:95-96.

44. Lindahl O, Lindwall L. Double blind study of a valerian preparation. Pharmacology Biochemistry and Behavior. 1989;32:1065-66.

45. Leathwood PD, Chauffard F. Quantifying the effects of mild sedatives. Journal of Psychiatric Research. 1983;17:115-22.

46. Leathwood PD, et al. Effect of St. John's wort *Valeriana officinalis* L. on subjective and objective sleep parameters. In: Sleep 1982, 6th European Congress on Sleep Research; 1983; Zurich: Karger; 1983:402-05.

47. Chauffard F, et al. Detection of mild sedative effects: Valerian and sleep in man. Experimentia. 1982;37:622.

48. Balderer G, Boebely AA. Effect of valerian on human sleep. Psychopharmacology. 1985;87:406-9.

49. Leathwood PD, Chauffard F. Aqueous extract of valerian reduces latency to fall asleep in man. Plana Medica. 1985;51:144-48.

50. Donath F, Quispe S, Diefenbach K, Maurer A, Fietze I, Roots I. Critical evaluation of the effect of valerian extract on sleep structure and sleep quality. Pharmacopsychiatry. 2000;33(2):47-53.

51. Poyares DR, Guilleminault C, Ohayon MM, Tufik S. Can valerian improve the sleep of insomniacs after benzodiazepine withdrawal? Prog Neuropsychopharmacol Biol Psychiatry. 2002;26(3):539-45.

52. Schulz H, Stolz C, Muller J. The effect of valerian extract on sleep polygraphy in poor sleepers: a pilot study. Pharmacopsychiatry. 1994;27(4):147-51.

53. Herrera-Arellano A, Luna-Villegas G, Cuevas-Uriostegui ML, Alvarez L, Vargas-Pineda G, Zamilpa-Alvarez A, et al. Polysomnographic evaluation of the hypnotic effect of *Valeriana edulis* standardized extract in patients suffering from insomnia. Planta Medica. 2001;67(8):695-99.

54. Andreatini R, Sartori V, Seabra M, Leite J. Effect of valepotriates (valerian extract) in generalized anxiety disorder: A randomized placebo-controlled pilot study. Phytotherapy Research. 2002;16:650-54.

55. Francis AJ, Dempster RJ. Effect of valerian, *Valeriana edulis*, on sleep difficulties in children with intellectual deficits: Randomised trial. Phytomedicine. 2002;9(4):273-79.

56. Kuhlmann J, Berger W, Podzuweit H, Schmidt U. The influence of valerian treatment on "reaction time, alertness and concentration" in volunteers. Pharmacopsychiatry. 1999;32(6):235-41.

57. Braun R, et al. Influence of valtrate/isovaltrate on the hematopoiesis and metabolic liver activity in mice *in vivo*. Planta Medica. 1984;50:1-4.

58. Keochanthala-Bounthanh C, Haag-Berrurier M, Beck JP, Anton R. Effects of thiol compounds versus the cytotoxicity of valepotriates on cultured hepatoma cells. Planta Med. 1990;56(2):190-92.

59. Keochanthala-Bounthanh C, Beck JP, Haag-Berrurier M, Anton R. Effects of two monoterpene esters, valtrate and didrovaltrate, isolated from *Valerian wallichii*, on the ultrastructure of hepatoma cells in culture. Phytotherapy Research. 1993;7:124-27.

60. MacGregor FB, Abernethy VE, Dahabra S, Cobden I, Hayes PC. Hepatotoxicity of herbal remedies. British Medical Jounral. 1989;299(6708):1156-57.

61. Shepherd C. Sleep disorders. Liver damage warning with insomnia remedy. British Medical Journal. 1993;306(6890):1477.

62. Bounthanh C, et al. The action of valepotriates on the synthesis of DNA and proteins of cultured hepatoma cells. Planta Medica. 1983;49:138-42.

63. Tufik S, Fuhita K, Seabra MdL, Lobo LL. Effect of a prolonged administrationof valepotriates in rats on the mothers and their offspring. Journal of Ethnopharmacology. 1996;41(1-2):39-44.

64. Berglund F, Flodh H, Lundborg P, Prame B, Sannerstedt R. Drug use during pregnancy and breast-feeding. A classification system for drug information. Acta Obstet Gynecol Scand Suppl. 1984;126:1-55.

65. ADE C. Medicines in pregnancy. An Australian categorization of risk. Canberra: Australian Government Publishing Service; 1989.

66. Takamura K, Kakimoto M, Kawaguchi M, Iwasaki T. Pharmacological studies on the constituents of crude drugs and plants. Yakugaku Zasshi - Journal of the Pharmaceutical Society of Japan. 1973;93:599-606.

Wild Yam

1. Wren R. Potter's New Encyclopedia of Botanical Drugs and Preparations. Saffron Walden, UK: C.W. Daniel Company; 988:362.

2. Chevalier A. The Encyclopedia of Medicinal Plants. London: Reader's Digest; 1996:336.

3. Evans W. Trease and Evans' Pharmacognosy. 13th ed. London: Bailliere Tindall; 1989:832.

4. Grieve M. A Modern Herbal. London: Penguin; 1984:912.

5. Hudson T. Wild Yam, Natural Progesterone, Unraveling the Confusion. Townsend Letter for Doctors and Patients. 1996; July:125-27.

6. Hoffmann D. Holistic Herbal. Rockport, CA: Element Books; 1996:256.

7. Araghiniknam M, Chung S, Nelson-White T, Eskelson C, Watson RR. Antioxidant activity of dioscorea and dehydroepian drosterone (DHEA) in older humans. Life Sciences. 1996;59(11):147-57.

8. Dollbaum C. Lab analyses of salivary DHEA and progesterone following ingestion of yam-containing products. Townsend Letter for Doctors and Patients. 1996;159:104.

9. Craddick J. Potential hazards of Mexican Yam. Townsend Letter for Doctors and Patients. 1996;August/September:101.

10. Park HS, Kim MJ, Moon HB. Occupational asthma caused by two herb materials, *Dioscorea batatas* and *Pinellia ternata*. Clinical and Experimental Allergy. 1994;24(6):575-81.

Willow

1. Newall CA, Anderson LA, Phillipson JD. Herbal Medicines. A Guide for Health Care Professionals. London: The Pharmaceutical Press; 1996.

2. Marles RJ, Associate Professor, Department of Botany, Brandon University, Brandon, Manitoba. Review of Medicinal Plant Modules for CCNM; 1998.

3. Hutchens A. Indian Herbology of North America. Boston,MA: Shambhala; 1973.

4. Tyler VE. Herbs of Choice. The Therapeutic Use of Phytomedicinals. Binghamton, NY: Pharmaceutical Products Press; 1994.

5. Meier B, et al. Pharmaceutical aspects of the use of willows in herbal remedies. Planta Medica. 1988;54:559-60.

6. Karl C, et al. Flavonoide aus *Salix alba*, die Struktur des terniflorins und eines Weiteren Acylflavonoides. Phytochemistry. 1976;15:1084-85.

7. ESCOP. *Salicis Cortex*/Willow Bark. In: Phytotherapy EESCO, ed. ESCOP Monograph/Fascicule 4. Exeter: ESCOP; 1997:58.

8. Meier B, et al. Identifikation und Bestimmung von je acht Phenolglykosiden in *Salix purpurea* und *Salix daphnoides* mit moderner HPLC. Pharm Acta Helvetica. 1985;60:269-74.

9. Hoffmann D. Holistic Herbal. Rockport, CA: Element Books; 1996.

10. Chrubasik S, Eisenberg E, Balan E, Weinberger T, Luzzati R, Conradt C. Treatment of low back pain exacerbations with willow bark extract: A randomized double-blind study. American Journal of Medicine. 2000;109(1):9-14.

11. Schmid B, Ludtke R, Selbmann HK, Kotter I, Tschirdewahn B, Schaffner W, et al. Efficacy and tolerability of a standardized willow bark extract in patients with osteoarthritis: Randomized placebo-controlled, double blind clinical trial. Phytotherapy Research. 2001;15(4):344-50.

12. Baker S, Thomas PS. Herbal medicine precipitating massive haemolysis. Lancet. 1987(i):1039-40.

13. Krivoy N, Pavlotzky E, Chrubasik S, Eisenberg E, Brook G. Effect of *Salicis cortex* extract on human platelet aggregation. Planta Medica. 2001;67(3):209-12.

14. Bradley P. British Herbal Compendium. Bournemouth, UK: The British Herbal Medical Association; 1992.

Index